A Complete MRCP(UK) Parts 1 and 2 Written Examination Revision Guide

A systems-based competencies approach

SHIBLEY RAHMAN

*Queen's Scholar, BA (1st Class Honours), MA,
MB, BChir, PhD (all Cambridge), MRCP(UK),
LLB(Hons), LLM(Commendation), FRSA, MSB
YWS Consultancy Ltd. (non-acute medical sections)*

with

AVINASH SHARMA

*MB, BS, MRCP(UK)
Consultant Physician
Luton and Dunstable NHS Foundation Trust (acute medical sections)*

Foreword by

NEIL BLACK

*MB, BCh (with Honours), MD, MRCP(UK)
Consultant Physician
Endocrinology and Diabetes and Acute Medicine
Western Health and Social Care Trust
Lead Clinician, Insulin Pump Service
Chair, Insulin Safety Group, WHCST*

Radcliffe Publishing
London • New York

Radcliffe Publishing Ltd
33–41 Dallington Street
London
EC1V 0BB
United Kingdom

www.radcliffepublishing.com

British Library Cataloguing in Publication Data

A catalogue record for this book is available from the British Library.

ISBN-13: 978 184619 481 8

The paper used for the text pages of this book is FSC® certified. FSC (The Forest Stewardship Council®) is an international network to promote responsible management of the world's forests.

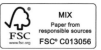

Typeset by Darkriver Design, Auckland, New Zealand
Printed and bound by TJ International Ltd, Padstow, Cornwall, UK

Contents

Foreword

This is a practical manual of clinical medicine, arranged systematically and concisely as a wide-ranging systems-based survey of the main points of clinical practice. As such, it is perfectly geared towards study for the MRCP(UK) Part 1 and Part 2 written examinations.

It is only really clear what form a study aid should take after that stage of professional study is itself complete. This book is certainly the fruit of such experience. It has few parallels in clinical medicine that survey clinical systems and specialties as succinctly. The content is clinically orientated and so complements the excellent basic science study aids that are available for MRCP(UK) Part 1. Due to these features it also lends itself readily to act as a rapid clinical review to help in preparation for early post-graduate medical training itself and for medical finals.

The book comes as the first such comprehensive clinical review available at this level after the issue of the MRCP(UK) specialty training curricula for General Internal Medicine in 2009.

Dr Neil Black MB, BCh (with Honours), MD, MRCP(UK)
Consultant Physician, Endocrinology and Diabetes and Acute Medicine
Western Health and Social Care Trust
Lead Clinician, Insulin Pump Service
Chair, Insulin Safety Group, WHCST
October 2011

Preface

The first thing to note is that you should consult the official MRCP(UK) website for the most current information about this examination.

Passing all parts of the MRCP(UK) is still a pivotal part of the completion of a junior physician's medical training, although the Deaneries will ensure that all aspects of the 'Core Medical Training' will be satisfied.

To help candidates, a syllabus was compiled and edited for the MRCP(UK) Part 1 examination over a decade ago in 1999. This has been a very helpful sign-post as to what the Royal Colleges have felt would be appropriate to examine in their examination. Many have therefore appreciated what the MRCP(UK) Central Office have, in fact, been doing to help candidates, as much as they can, in preparation for this difficult assessment.

Exactly a decade later, the Specialty Advisory Committee for General Internal Medicine under the direction of the Joint Royal Colleges of Physicians Training Board (JRCPTB) produced the *MRCP(UK) specialty training curriculum for General Internal Medicine*, a landmark document which was published in 2009. This document describes the competencies required to practise General Internal Medicine in a patient-centred manner.

The syllabus is based in system competencies, surgical presentations, system-specific competencies and procedural competencies. This book provides comprehensive coverage of these system-specific competencies, and it is anticipated that listing the specific conditions aims to advise the trainee on the conditions that require detailed comprehension. Information in this book should not be relied upon to make actual clinical decisions; it is for the purpose of your exam revision.

You are advised to download a copy of this syllabus, as well as the complete description of details of the Foundation Programme, to guide your personal learning.

What exactly does this exam test and how?

The MRCP(UK) Part 1 Examination is designed to assess a candidate's knowledge and understanding of the clinical sciences relevant to medical practice and of common or important disorders to a level appropriate for entry to specialist training.

Candidates will be tested on a wide range of common and important disorders in General Medicine. There is reassuringly much convergence between what has been examined in the MRCP(UK) examination previously in the last decade, and the framework for the knowledge to be acquired by the learner. For each condition, this ideally includes a working definition, pathophysiology, epidemiology, features of the history, typical examination findings, investigations indicated, and detailed initial management and principles of ongoing management.

However, the book does not apologise for its coverage of the common general medical emergencies which should be understood well by the medical physician of any specialty.

Dr Avinash Sharma has comprehensively reviewed the current medical practice for these acute medical topics. Dr Neil Black has thoroughly reviewed the substantive points of the endocrinology and diabetes chapter (Chapter 3) in keeping with contemporaneous best practice guidelines. However, the authors should like to emphasise that the reader should consult the latest guidelines and protocols for everything, and not rely on any information in this book for actual clinical practice.

The MRCP(UK) Part 1 Examination has – presently – a two-paper format. Each paper is three hours in duration and contains 100 multiple choice questions in one from five ('best of five') format, where a candidate chooses the best answer from five possible answers.

Currently, the balance in the MRCP(UK) question bank is very large. For each question, their system keeps track of which diets it has appeared in, its statistical performance in every exam, and all revisions that have been made to the question's content. This new book has been written based on what we know about the contents of this question bank from the feedback of candidates, and the new GIM curriculum (2009).

When to take this exam

This new curriculum, which specifies what candidates are expected to know for the MRCP(UK) examination, has been put together with the Core Medical Training (CMT) in CMT occupies the Specialty Training years 1 and 2 (ST 1–2), and aims to take trainees who have completed the Foundation Programme (or have equivalent experience and qualifications) and train them in acute medicine and the medical specialties as outlined in the CMT curriculum.

All trainees who have entered CMT after August 2009 should have passed

MRCP(UK) PACES by the end of the CMT2 year to complete their core training. Any current Foundation Trainee who is contemplating applying to CMT, is strongly advised to try and pass MRCP(UK) Part 1 before completing the F2 year.

You should not wait unduly before sitting MRCP(UK) Part 1, and you will find it useful reading about it in your Foundation Years, even if you intend to do something totally different such as general surgery, a general surgical specialty, or general practice. However, you should set yourself a reasonable target for when to take this examination (by careful selection of the correct diet off the MRCP(UK) website), and prepare diligently for it.

How to use this book

The Foundation Programme and MRCP(UK) Part 1 syllabus (from the JRCPMTB) specify what is required in terms of competencies, skills and knowledge from junior physicians in core medical training. You are advised to carefully consult this syllabus, which emphasises the importance of basic medical sciences as well as a competent level of applied clinical practice.

There are no electronic citations given in the text, as the authors were concerned that pages might rapidly become outdated.

You will hopefully find this book useful as well for later parts of the examination (the MRCP(UK) Part 2 written and PACES). In PACES, you will be assumed to know your general medicine well, especially for the history taking, communication skills and ethics and focused clinical problem stations.

Finally, you should ideally not use this book in isolation. It has really been written as an '*aide memoire*' to what is currently important. You should use it as a way of referring to things which you find interesting in the syllabuses or in your favourite textbooks; also you should always refer to up-to-date official guidance, which may be more up-to-date than this book. This is particularly important for the BNF and NICE guidelines. Such information is normally subject to continual revision.

And finally . . .

. . . best of luck!

Dr Shibley Rahman
with **Dr Avinash Sharma**
October 2011

This book is dedicated to Dr Muhammad Khalilur Rahman, the father of Dr Shibley Rahman, who died on the same day as the birth of Keiran Sharma, the son of Dr Avinash Sharma. The authors devote this book to these two, without whom the book would not have been possible.

Acknowledgements

The authors would like to acknowledge the contribution of expert subject-reviewers for these chapters: Dr Sandeep Kalra (cardiology) (King's College Hospital NHS Foundation Trust); Dr Ritwick Banerjee (endocrinology) (Luton and Dunstable Hospital NHS Foundation Trust); Dr Ameet Dhar (gastroenterology and hepatology) (Imperial School of Medicine); Dr Daniel Patterson (clinical haematology, clinical immunology and oncology) (Royal Hampshire County Hospital); Dr Siva Kumar (infectious diseases, tropical medicine and sexually transmitted diseases) (Colchester Hospital NHS Foundation Trust); Dr M Suresh (nephrology) (East and North Hertfordshire NHS Trust, Stevenage); Dr Yohan Samarsinghe (clinical pharmacology, toxicology and therapeutics) (Frimley Park Hospital); and Dr Gary Davies (respiratory medicine) (Chelsea and Westminster Hospitals NHS Foundation Trust).

List of figures

Chapter 1

Cardiovascular medicine

The Foundation Programme and MRCP(UK) Part 1 syllabus (from the JRCPMTB) specify what is required in terms of competencies, skills and knowledge from junior physicians in core medical training in cardiovascular medicine. You are advised to carefully consult this syllabus, which emphasises the importance of basic medical sciences as well as a competent level of applied clinical practice.

A. Common cardiology syndromes

1. Constrictive pericarditis

Causes

- recurrent acute pericarditis (e.g. viral infections – coxsackie virus)
- post purulent pericarditis
- TB
- uraemia (causes a 'fibrinous' pericarditis)
- trauma
- post MI, Dressler's syndrome
- connective tissue disease
- hypothyroidism
- drugs (e.g. hydralazine)
- radiotherapy
- pericardial malignancy

ECG changes

- electric alternans (swinging QRS axis)
- low voltage QRS

Clinical signs

- low BP
- raised JVP
- impalpable apex
- CCF

Investigations

- echocardiogram (thickened pericardium, pericardial effusion, constrictive physiology)
- CT (can reveal a calcified pericardium)
- right + left heart catheterisation (ventricular inter-dependence)

BOX 1.1   A note on calcification in constrictive pericarditis

The most probable cause for this is prior tuberculous (TB) infection, which may have occurred many years previously. Acute TB would usually cause a constrictive pericarditis secondary to a pericardial effusion, but this is not normally associated with calcification.

(Uraemia can cause a constrictive pericarditis, as can a pericardial malignancy and coxsackie virus (secondary to a pericarditis), but calcification would be unusual.)

Management

- VERY difficult to manage
- medical therapy for CCF
- *'pericardial stripping'*

2. Pericardial effusion

Causes

+ acute pericarditis
+ all causes of constrictive pericarditis
+ aortic dissection
+ iatrogenic due to pacing or cardiac catheterisation (rare)
+ ischaemic heart disease with ventricular rupture (rare)
+ anticoagulation associated with acute pericarditis

ECG changes

+ electrical alternans – *'swinging QRS axis'*
+ small voltages
+ widespread 'saddle-shaped' ST elevation (acute pericarditis)
+ PR depression (acute pericarditis)

Echocardiogram

One of the applications that first brought echocardiography to the general attention of clinicians was its unique ability to detect pericardial effusion. It remains the most sensitive technique for the detection of this disorder.

Around the heart there exists a potential cavity between the visceral and parietal layers of the serous pericardium, into which the heart is invaginated during its development. There is normally a little fluid in this cavity that acts as a lubricant for heart movement, but the two layers of the serous pericardium essentially remain in contact. However, if the amount of fluid increases as a result of exudate from the pericardium, haemorrhage or the inadvertent infusion of fluid, the two layers become more widely separated.

3. Cardiac tamponade

Features

+ raised JVP, with an absent Y descent – this is due to the limited right ventricular filling (B)
+ tachycardia
+ absent apex beat (B)
+ hypotension (B)
+ muffled heart sounds

- pulsus paradoxus
- *Kussmaul's sign* (a rise in jugular venous pressure on inspiration – the opposite to normal which is seen in both constrictive pericarditis and pericardial tamponade, but it is in fact more likely to be present in the former)
- ECG: electrical alternans
  (B) = Beck's triad

BOX 1.2   A note on pulsus paradoxus

The right heart responds directly to changes in intrathoracic pressure, while the filling of the left heart depends on the pulmonary vascular volume. At high respiratory rates, with severe airflow limitation (for example, acute asthma) there is an increased and sudden negative intrathoracic pressure on inspiration and this will enhance the normal fall in blood pressure.

The **key differences** between constrictive pericarditis and cardiac tamponade are summarised in Table 1.1 below. These are worth knowing for the exam.

TABLE 1.1 Comparison between cardiac tamponade and constrictive pericarditis

	Cardiac tamponade	Constrictive pericarditis
JVP	Absent Y descent	X + Y present
Pulsus paradoxus	Present	Absent
Kussmaul's sign	Rare	Present
Characteristic features		Pericardial calcification on CXR

A commonly used mnemonic to remember the absent Y descent in cardiac tamponade is TAMponade = TAMpaX.

4. Infective endocarditis

The **strongest risk factor** for developing infective endocarditis is a previous episode of endocarditis.

Other factors include:

* previously normal valves (50%, typically acute presentation)
* rheumatic valve disease (30%)
* prosthetic valves
* congenital heart defects
* intravenous drug users (IVDUs, e.g. typically causing right-sided valve lesion)
* immunocompromise (chemotherapy, AIDS, malignancy, age)
* instrumentation

Causes

* *Streptococcus viridans* (most common cause – 40%–50%)
* *Staphylococcus epidermidis* (especially prosthetic valves)
* *Staphylococcus aureus* (especially acute presentation, IVDUs)
* *Streptococcus bovis* is associated with colorectal cancer
* Non-infective: systemic lupus erythematosus (Libman-Sacks), malignancy: marantic endocarditis. (Marantic endocarditis has platelet-fibrin thrombi that are prone to embolising. This form of non-infective endocarditis tends to be seen in persons who are very debilitated or who have a hypercoagulable state.)

Culture negative causes

* prior antibiotic therapy
* *Coxiella burnetii*
* *Bartonella*
* *Brucella*
* 'HACEK': *Haemophilus, Actinobacillus, Cardiobacterium, Eikenella, Kingella* – slow growing
* non-infective (see above)

Symptoms

◆ constitutional (fever, malaise, night sweats, anorexia, weight loss, myalgia, CCF, embolic phenomenon – see below)

Clinical features

◆ fever

◆ new cardiac murmur (regurgitant)

◆ hepatosplenomegaly

◆ embolic stigmata (e.g. Roth spots, retinopathy, Janeway lesions, splinter haemorrhages, nail fold infarcts, Osler's nodes)

Antibiotics following prosthetic valve surgery

Following prosthetic valve surgery, *Staphylococcus epidermidis* is the most common organism in the first two months and is usually the result of perioperative contamination.

Late endocarditis observed after two years post-surgery is found in 0.5%–1% of cases and is typically due to *Streptococci*, and typically group A haemolytic *Streptococci*, otherwise known as *Strep. viridans*.

NICE guidelines on infective endocarditis prophylaxis

The 2008 NICE guidelines have fundamentally changed the approach to infective endocarditis prophylaxis. What is not yet clear is if there are any circumstances in which NICE would recommend using antibiotic prophylaxis.

NICE recommends the following procedures do not require prophylaxis:

• dental procedures

• upper and lower gastrointestinal tract procedures

• genitourinary tract (this includes urological, gynaecological and obstetric procedures and childbirth)

• upper and lower respiratory tract; this includes ear, nose and throat procedures and bronchoscopy.

The guidelines do, however, suggest that:

• any episodes of infection in people at risk of infective endocarditis should be investigated and treated promptly to reduce the risk of endocarditis developing

• if a person at risk of infective endocarditis is receiving antimicrobial therapy because they are undergoing a gastrointestinal or genitourinary procedure at a site where there is a suspected infection, they should be given an antibiotic that covers organisms that cause infective endocarditis.

Modified Duke criteria

Infective endocarditis is diagnosed if:

◈ pathological criteria is positive, or

◈ there are 2 major criteria, or

◈ there are 1 major and 3 minor criteria, or

◈ there are 5 minor criteria

Pathological criteria

Positive histology or microbiology of pathological material obtained at autopsy or cardiac surgery (valve tissue, vegetations, embolic fragments or intracardiac abscess content).

Major criteria

Positive blood cultures

◈ two positive blood cultures showing typical organisms consistent with infective endocarditis, such as *Streptococcus viridans* and the HACEK group, or

◈ persistent bacteraemia from two blood cultures taken >12 hours apart or three or more positive blood cultures where the pathogen is less specific such as *Staphyloccus aureus* and *Staphyloccus epidermidis*, or

◈ positive serology for *Coxiella burnetii, Bartonella* species or *Chlamydia psittaci*, or

◈ positive molecular assays for specific gene targets

Evidence of endocardial involvement

◈ positive echocardiogram (mobile masses, abscess formation, new valvular regurgitation or dehiscence of prosthetic valves)

Minor criteria

◈ predisposing heart condition or intravenous drug use

◈ microbiological evidence does not meet major criteria

* positive echo not meeting major criteria
* fever >38°C
* vascular phenomena: major emboli, splenomegaly, clubbing, splinter haemorrhages, petechiae or purpura
* immunological phenomena: glomerulonephritis, Osler's nodes, Roth spots, Janeway lesions
* elevated ESR or CRP

Clinical features *see above*

As well as cardiac murmurs detected at auscultation, there are several other characteristic features of infective endocarditis:

* systemic signs of fever and retinopathy
* signs in hands and feet (e.g. splinter haemorrhages, Osler's nodes, clubbing, needle tracks, Janeway lesions)
* retinopathy
* hepatosplenomegaly
* signs of arterial embolism

Prognosis and management
Poor prognostic factors

* *Staphylococcus aureus* infection
* prosthetic valve (especially 'early', acquired during surgery)
* culture negative endocarditis
* low complement levels

Mortality according to organism

* *staphylococci* – 30%
* bowel organisms – 15%
* *streptococci* – 5%

Current antibiotic guidelines

Please check the current edition of the BNF for correct guidance.

- initial blind therapy – flucloxacillin + gentamicin (benzylpenicillin + gentamicin if symptoms less severe)
- initial blind therapy if prosthetic valve is present or patient is penicillin allergic – vancomycin + rifampicin + gentamicin
- endocarditis caused by staphylococci – flucloxacillin (vancomycin + rifampicin if penicillin allergic or MRSA)
- endocarditis caused by streptococci – benzylpenicillin + gentamicin (vancomycin + gentamicin if penicillin allergic)

(Source: British National Formulary)

Indications for surgery

- severe valvular incompetence
- aortic abscess (often indicated by a lengthening PR interval)
- infections resistant to antibiotics/fungal infections
- cardiac failure refractory to standard medical treatment
- recurrent emboli after antibiotic therapy

5. Restrictive cardiomyopathy

In **restrictive cardiomyopathy**, the heart is of normal size or only slightly enlarged. However, it cannot relax normally during diastole in early stages. The most common causes of restrictive cardiomyopathy are amyloidosis and scarring of the heart from an unknown cause (idiopathic myocardial fibrosis). It frequently occurs after a heart transplant.

Other causes of restrictive cardiomyopathy include:

- carcinoid
- rare diseases of the heart lining (endocardium), such as endomyocardial fibrosis and Loeffler's syndrome (rare)
- haemochromatosis
- radiation fibrosis
- sarcoidosis
- scleroderma
- neoplasms of the heart

Symptoms

Symptoms of heart failure are most common. Usually, these symptoms develop slowly over time. However, sometimes symptoms start very suddenly and are severe.

B. Valvular heart disease

You are advised to consider a good cardiology textbook for a detailed description of this topic. For sake of brevity, a possible approach to the **aortic valve disorders** is given only.

1. Aortic stenosis

Features of aortic stenosis

- narrow pulse pressure (S)
- slow rising pulse (S)
- ESM radiating to carotid arteries
- soft/absent S2 (S)
- LV heave
- CCF (pulmonary oedema, raised JVP, S3, peripheral oedema) (S)
- pulmonary hypertension (raised JVP, RV heave, S3, TR, peripheral oedema, ascites)

[S = severe]

Causes of aortic stenosis

- degenerative calcification (most common cause in elderly patients)
- bicuspid aortic valve (most common cause in younger patients)
- rheumatic valve disease
- William's syndrome (supravalvular aortic stenosis)
- subvalvular: HOCM

Echocardiography

- valve area (mild $>1.5\,cm^2$, moderate $1-1.5\,cm^2$, severe $<1\,cm^2$)
- transvalvular gradient (severe $>50\,mmHg$)
- LVH
- LV dysfunction and pulmonary hypertension in advanced disease

Management

◆ asymptomatic: observe

◆ medical: treat symptoms of CCF

◆ surgery: Symptoms (chest pain, SOB, syncope, CCF)
And/Or
Prognostic (severe AS on echo, LV dysfunction on echo, pulmonary hypertension on echo)

◆ balloon valvuloplasty or percutaneous valve replacement (TAVI) is limited to patients with critical aortic stenosis who are not fit for conventional valve replacement

2. Aortic incompetence

Causes and risk factors

Acute: infective endocarditis, trauma

Chronic:

◆ primary valvular (rheumatic fever, bicuspid aortic valve, Marfan's syndrome, Ehlers-Danlos syndrome, ankylosing spondylitis, systemic lupus erythematosus)

◆ diseases of the aortic root (syphilitic aortitis, osteogenesis imperfecta, aortic dissection, Behçet's disease, reactive arthritis, systemic hypertension)

Symptoms

◆ heart failure symptoms (such as dyspnoea on exertion, orthopnoea and paroxysmal nocturnal dyspnoea)

◆ palpitations

◆ angina pectoris

Signs

◆ increased pulse pressure

◆ diastolic de-crescendo murmur best heard at the left sternal border

◆ *'water hammer pulse'*

◆ Austin Flint murmur

◆ displaced apex

◆ possible third heart sound

Management

If stable and symptomatic, use conservative treatment such as a low sodium diet, diuretics, vasodilators (such as hydralazine or prazosin), digoxin, ACE inhibitors/AT2 receptor antagonists, calcium channel blockers and avoiding strenuous activity.

Aortic valve replacement in symptomatic patients, or progressive left ventricular dilatation or systolic ventricular diameter >55 mm on echocardiography; or immediately if acute. [See also above for antibiotic prophylaxis for endocarditis.]

C. General medicine and valvular disease

1. Turner's syndrome

Turner's syndrome is a chromosomal disorder affecting around 1 in 2500 females. It is caused by either the presence of only one sex chromosome (X) or a deletion of the short arm of one of the X chromosomes. Turner's syndrome is denoted as 45,XO or 45,X.

Features

- short stature
- shield chest, widely spaced nipples
- webbed neck
- bicuspid aortic valve (15%), coarctation of the aorta (5%–10%)
- primary amenorrhoea
- high-arched palate
- short fourth metacarpal
- multiple pigmented naevi
- lymphoedema in neonates (especially feet)

There is also an increased incidence of autoimmune disease (especially autoimmune thyroiditis) and Crohn's disease.

In Turner's syndrome, essential hypertension is still the most likely cause of hypertension. In a small proportion, causes can include coarctation of the aorta and renal dysfunction due to horseshoe kidney.

D. Acute coronary syndromes

1. Pathophysiology of the acute coronary syndromes

The **acute coronary syndromes** constitute a spectrum of diseases caused by sudden onset myocardial ischaemia where the common underlying pathology is rupture or erosion of a coronary artery plaque, leading to intracoronary thrombosis. The resulting clinical syndrome depends on whether it is only partially/transiently occluded (producing a non-ST elevation/non-Q-wave MI or unstable angina) or totally occluded (producing an ST elevation or Q-wave MI).

The distinction between unstable angina and non-ST elevation MI is often made retrospectively (after cardiac enzymes/troponin measured). Both unstable angina and non-ST elevation MI can have normal or ischaemic ECGs (ST depression or T wave inversion).

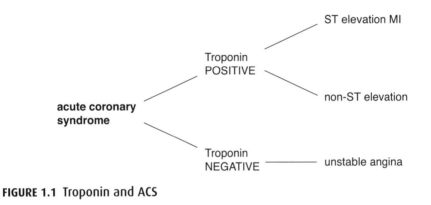

FIGURE 1.1 Troponin and ACS

Prognostic factors

There are several risk stratification models to predict outcome post-ACS, of which GRACE and TIMI score are the most used.

The **Global Registry of Acute Coronary Events** (GRACE) study has been used to derive regression models to predict death in hospital and death after discharge in patients with acute coronary syndrome. The **Thrombolysis in Myocardial Infarction** (TIMI) score, similarly, was developed to provide a simple risk score that has broad applicability, is easily calculated at patient presentation, does not require a computer, and identifies patients with different responses to treatments for unstable angina or NSTEMI.

Poor prognostic factors

◆ age

◆ development (or history) of heart failure

◆ peripheral vascular disease

◆ reduced systolic blood pressure

◆ Killip class (system used to stratify risk post myocardial infarction)

◆ initial serum creatinine concentration

◆ elevated initial cardiac markers

◆ cardiac arrest on admission

◆ ST segment deviation

It is felt that, across the entire spectrum of ACS and in general clinical practice, this model provides excellent ability to assess the risk for death and can be used as a simple nomogram to estimate risk in individual patients.

Management
An ECG diagnosis of myocardial infarction can be made on ECG.

2. STEMI (ST elevation MI)

Medical management
NICE produced guidelines on the management of patients following a myocardial infarction (MI) in 2007. Some key points are listed below:

All patients should be offered the following drugs:

◆ ACE inhibitor

◆ β-blocker

◆ aspirin

◆ statin

Clopidogrel

◆ After an ST segment elevation MI, patients treated with a combination of aspirin and clopidogrel during the first 24 hours after the MI should continue this treatment for at least 4 weeks.

◆ After a non-ST segment elevation MI clopidogrel should be given for the first 12 months.

Aldosterone antagonists

Patients who have had an acute MI and who have symptoms and/or signs of heart failure and left ventricular systolic dysfunction, treatment with an aldosterone antagonist licensed for post-MI treatment should be initiated within 3–14 days of the MI, preferably after ACE inhibitor therapy.

3. Cardiac enzymes

In fact, the evolution of Q waves is the most suggestive of an infarct. **Cardiac enzymes** may be elevated in pulmonary embolism (PE), renal failure and raised ST segments associated with pericarditis. Interpretation of the various cardiac enzymes has now largely been superseded by the introduction of troponin T and I. Questions still however commonly appear in the MRCP(UK).

Please note the following key points for the exam:

◆ Myoglobin is the first cardiac enzyme to rise.

◆ CK-MB is useful to look for reinfarction as it returns to normal after 2–3 days (troponin T remains elevated for up to 10 days).

However, you may be interested for the CK-MB fraction/level in addition to the troponin T level for your everyday clinical activity. A picture of the changes in these enzymes is given below.

Troponin is not related to infarct size, but CK is directly proportional.

The exact changes in cardiac enzymes are as follows.

TABLE 1.2 Timecourse of changes in cardiac enzymes

	Begins to rise	Peak value	Returns to normal
Myoglobin	1–2 hours	6–8 hours	1–2 days
CK-MB	2–6 hours	16–20 hours	2–3 days
CK	4–8 hours	16–24 hours	3–4 days
Trop T	4–6 hours	12–24 hours	7–10 days
AST	12–24 hours	36–48 hours	3–4 days
LDH	24–48 hours	72 hours	8–10 days

Causes of ST elevation

◆ STEMI

◆ acute pericarditis

◆ high take off/early repolarisation

◆ coronary artery spasm

◆ oesophageal spasm

◆ cardiac contusion

◆ ventricular aneurysm

◆ acute cerebral injury

Complications of STEMI: (Sudden Death on PRAED Street)

◆ cardiac arrest (or sudden death)

◆ pump failure + pericarditis (P)

◆ rupture of ventricle, septum, papillary muscle (R)

◆ aneurysm + arrythmia (A)

◆ embolism from LV aneurysm (E)

◆ Dressler's syndromes (D)

◆ heart failure

E. Heart failure

1. Medical management and interventional therapy

A number of drugs have been shown to improve mortality in patients with chronic heart failure:
- ACE inhibitors (CONSENSUS)
- spironolactone (RALES)
- beta-blockers (CIBIS II, MERIT HF, COPERNICUS)
- hydralazine with nitrates (VHEFT-1)

BOX 1.3 Historical development of the pharmacological rationale

The historical development of this is actually very interesting. In 1987 the results of the CONSENSUS study were published, and showed that enalapril, an angiotensin converting enzyme inhibitor (ACEI), was able to modify the clinical course of the heart failure syndrome thereby reducing mortality. Other ACEIs later demonstrated the same effect on the different degrees of symptomatic heart failure, left ventricular dysfunction, myocardial infarction and more recently in diabetic patients.

In 1996, studies on the beta-blockers carvedilol, bisoprolol and metoprolol showed their efficacy in reducing deaths due to progressive heart impairment and sudden death in chronic heart failure. The RALES study showed that small doses of spironolactone also improved the prognosis on this disease. Digitalis improves the quality of life but not the survival rate. Only amiodarone (among the anti-arrhythmics) reduces sudden death. Other drugs and groups of drugs cannot be considered for chronic outpatient treatment of heart failure.

Multi-centre trials make it possible to obtain scientific evidence for establishing rational treatments. Many groups of patients such as women, elderly people and the more severe cases of the disease are often not included in these trials.

Whilst spironolactone has been shown to improve prognosis in patients with chronic heart failure, no long-term reduction in mortality has been demonstrated for loop diuretics such as furosemide.

NICE produced guidelines on management in 2003, key points include:
- All patients should be given an ACE inhibitor unless contraindications exist.
- Once an ACE inhibitor has been introduced, a beta-blocker should be started regardless of whether the patient is still symptomatic.
- Offer annual influenza vaccine.
- Offer pneumococcal vaccine.

ACE inhibitors remain one of the cornerstones of the treatment of heart failure. There is clear evidence that higher doses exert greater benefit. They are usually very well tolerated, especially in milder cases.

Digoxin has also not been proven to reduce mortality in patients with heart failure. It may however improve symptoms due to its ionotropic properties. Digoxin is strongly indicated if there is coexistent atrial fibrillation.

In poorly controlled heart failure despite the above medical therapy, biventricular pacing should be considered (in the context of a broad QRS complex at rest and cardiac dyssynchrony).

F. Resuscitation

1. Cardiac arrest

ALS algorithm

You should go to the Resuscitation Council (UK)'s website for the most up-to-date algorithm.

For immediate post-cardiac arrest treatment:

◆ use ABCDE approach

◆ controlled oxygenation and ventilation

◆ 12-lead ECG

◆ treat precipitating cause

◆ temperature control/therapeutic hypothermia

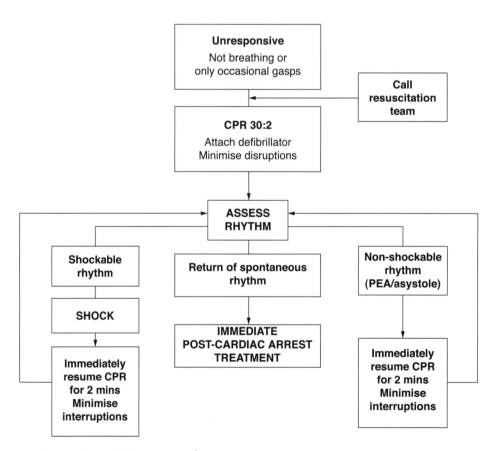

FIGURE 1.2 Resuscitation protocol

During CPR

◆ ensure high-quality CPR

◆ plan actions before interrupting CPR

◆ give oxygen

◆ consider airway and advanced capnography

◆ continuous chest compressions when advanced airway in place

◆ vascular access

◆ give adrenaline every 3–5 minutes

◆ correct reversible causes

Reversible causes (4 Hs and 4 Ts)

◆ Hypoxia

◆ Hypovolaemia

◆ Hypo-/Hyper-kalaemia/Metabolic

◆ Hypothermia

◆ Thrombosis

◆ Tamponade

◆ Toxins

◆ Tension pneumothorax

G. Arrhythmias and the ECG

1. Atrial fibrillation (AF)

Classification

An attempt was made in the Joint American Heart Association (AHA), American College of Cardiology (ACC), and European Society of Cardiology (ESC) 2002 guidelines to simplify and clarify the classification of atrial fibrillation (AF).

It is recommended that atrial fibrillation should be classified into three patterns:

- First-detected episode (irrespective of whether it is symptomatic or self-terminating).
- Recurrent episodes, when a patient has two or more episodes of AF. If episodes of AF terminate spontaneously then the term paroxysmal AF is used. Such episodes last less than 7 days (typically <24 hours). If the arrhythmia is not self-terminating then the term 'persistent AF' is used. Such episodes usually last greater than 7 days.
- In permanent AF there is continuous atrial fibrillation which cannot be cardioverted or if attempts to do so are deemed inappropriate. Treatment goals are therefore rate control and anticoagulation if appropriate.

Cardioversion

Onset <48 hours

If atrial fibrillation (AF) is of less than 48 hours onset patients should be heparinised and a transthoracic echocardiogram performed to exclude a thrombus. Following this patients may be cardioverted, either:

- electrical – 'DC cardioversion'

- pharmacology – amiodarone if structural heart disease, flecainide in those without structural heart disease. Following electrical cardioversion, if AF is confirmed as being less than 48 hours in duration, further anticoagulation is arguably unnecessary.

Onset >48 hours

If AF is of greater than 48 hours then patients should have therapeutic anticoagulation for at least 4 weeks. If there is a high risk of cardioversion failure (e.g. previous failure or AF recurrence) then it is recommended to have at least 4 weeks of amiodarone or sotalol prior to electrical cardioversion. Following electrical cardioversion, patients should be anticoagulated for at least 4 weeks.

After this time decisions about anticoagulation should be taken on an individual basis depending on the risk of recurrence.

Pharmacological cardioversion

> The Royal College of Physicians and NICE published guidelines on the management of atrial fibrillation (AF) in 2006. The following is also based on the joint American Heart Association (AHA), American College of Cardiology (ACC) and European Society of Cardiology (ESC) 2002 guidelines.

Agents with proven efficacy in the pharmacological cardioversion of atrial fibrillation

✦ amiodarone

✦ flecainide (if no structural heart disease)

✦ others (less commonly used in UK): quinidine, dofetilide, ibutilide, propafenone, dronedarone

Less effective agents

✦ beta-blockers (including sotalol)

✦ calcium channel blocks

✦ digoxin

✦ disopyramide

✦ procainamide

Rate control and maintenance of sinus rhythm

Table 1.3 indicates some of the factors which may be considered when choosing either a rate control or rhythm control strategy.

TABLE 1.3 Rate versus rhythm control in atrial fibrillation

Factors favouring rate control	Factors favouring rhythm control
• Older than 65 years	• Younger than 65 years
• History of ischaemic heart disease	• Symptomatic
	• First presentation
	• Lone AF or AF secondary to a corrected precipitant (e.g. alcohol)
	• Congestive heart failure

Amiodarone has been shown to be superior in maintaining sinus rhythm following DC cardioversion of atrial fibrillation; however, it is associated with more toxic side effects than the other agents mentioned.

Anticoagulation

The guidelines suggest a stroke risk stratification approach when determining how to anticoagulate a patient, as detailed below:

TABLE 1.4 Relative annual risk of stroke

Low risk – annual risk of stroke = 1%	Moderate risk – annual risk of stroke = 4%	High risk – annual risk of stroke = 8%–12%
Age <65 years with no moderate or high risk factors	Age >65 years with no high-risk factors, or	Age >75 years with diabetes, hypertension or cardiovascular disease
Use aspirin	Age <75 years with diabetes, hypertension or cardiovascular disease	Previous TIA, ischaemic stroke or thromboembolic event
	Use aspirin or warfarin depending on individual circumstances	Valve disease, heart failure or impaired left ventricular function
		Use warfarin

An alternative approach is the CHADS2 score for atrial fibrillation stroke risk.

The CHADS2 score is probably the best validated clinical prediction rule for determining the risk of stroke and who should be anticoagulated. It assigns points (0–6) depending on the presence or absence of co-morbidities. To compensate for the increased risk of stroke, anticoagulation may be necessary. However, with warfarin, if a patient has a yearly risk of stroke that is less than 2%, then the risks associated with taking warfarin outweigh the risk of getting a stroke from atrial fibrillation.

TABLE 1.5 The CHADS2 score

	Condition	Points
C	Congestive heart failure	1
H	Hypertension (or treated hypertension)	1
A	Age >75 years	1
D	Diabetes	1
S2	Prior Stroke or TIA	2

Table 1.6 shows a suggested anticoagulation strategy based on the score.

TABLE 1.6 Anticoagulation strategy based on the CHADS2 score

Score	Anticoagulation
0	Aspirin
1	Aspirin or warfarin, depending on patient preference and individual factors
2	Warfarin if not contraindicated

2. ECG: hypothermia

The following ECG changes may be seen in hypothermia:

◆ bradycardia

◆ 'J' wave – small hump at the end of the QRS complex

◆ first degree heart block

◆ long QT interval

◆ atrial and ventricular arrhythmias

Features

◆ syncope

◆ heart failure

◆ regular bradycardia (30–50 bpm)

◆ wide pulse pressure

◆ JVP: cannon waves in neck

◆ variable intensity of S1

3. Bradycardia
Causes of bradycardia
There are many potential causes of bradycardia. Some are directly cardiac-related, while others have a consequential effect on the cardiac muscle or conduction. These include:

◆ ischaemic heart disease

◆ drug induced: digoxin, β-blocker

◆ hypoxia

◆ metabolic disturbances

◆ myocardial infarction

◆ cardiomyopathy

◆ hypothermia

Recommended pacemaker codes for indications of pacing

This is a frequent exam topic.

This is shown in Table 1.7.

TABLE 1.7 Recommended pacemaker codes for common pacemaker indications

Diagnosis	Incidence	Appropriate pacemaker mode
Sinus node disease	25	AAIR
AV block	42	VDDR
Sinus node disease and AV block	10	DDDT
Chronic atrial fibrillation with AV block	13	VVIR
Carotid sinus syndrome	10	DD+hysteresis

4. The PR interval
Causes of a prolonged PR interval
◆ idiopathic

◆ ischaemic heart disease

◆ digoxin toxicity

◆ hypokalaemia

◆ rheumatic fever

◆ aortic root pathology, e.g. abscess secondary to endocarditis

◆ Lyme disease

◆ sarcoidosis

◆ myotonic dystrophy

A prolonged PR interval may also be seen in athletes.

5. Causes of a shortened PR interval
Pre-excitation

◆ Wolff-Parkinson-White (WPW) syndrome

◆ Low-Ganong-Levine syndrome

Other

◆ ventricular extrasystole after P wave (i.e. artefactual short PR)

◆ AV junctional rhythm

◆ low atrial rhythm

◆ coronary sinus escape rhythm

6. Peri-arrest rhythms: tachycardia

> The joint European Resuscitation Council and Resuscitation Council (UK) (2005) guidelines have simplified the advice given for the management of peri-arrest tachycardias.

Separate algorithms for the management of broad complex tachycardia, narrow complex tachycardia and atrial fibrillation have been replaced by one unified treatment algorithm.

Following basic ABC assessment, patients are classified as being stable or unstable according to the presence of any adverse signs:

◆ systolic BP <90 mmHg

◆ reduced conscious level

◆ chest pain

◆ heart failure

If any of the above adverse signs are present then synchronised DC shocks should be given.

Treatment following this is given according to whether the QRS complex is narrow or broad and whether the rhythm is regular or irregular. The full treatment algorithm can be found at the Resuscitation Council website.

7. Supraventricular tachycardia

Whilst strictly speaking the term **supraventricular tachycardia** (SVT) refers to any tachycardia that is not ventricular in origin, the term is generally used in the context of paroxysmal SVT. Episodes are characterised by the sudden onset of a narrow complex tachycardia, typically an atrioventricular nodal re-entry tachycardia (AVNRT). Paroxysmal SVT would start and stop suddenly, not gradually. Other causes include atrioventricular re-entry tachycardias (AVRT) and junctional tachycardias.

Acute management
+ vagal manoeuvres: e.g. Valsalva manoeuvre
+ adenosine
+ electrical cardioversion

Prevention of episodes
+ beta-blockers
+ radio-frequency ablation

Tachyarrhythmias may increase during pregnancy although the causes are not entirely clear. Regarding the termination of acute SVT, adenosine appears to be safe in pregnancy. In the case of the prevention of recurrent SVT, verapamil or beta-blockers have data supporting their use. Current AHA/EHA criteria for the treatment of SVTs in pregnancy do suggest using metoprolol (level of evidence 1B) rather than verapamil (C), although they recommend avoiding the former in the first trimester.

Wolff-Parkinson-White
Wolff-Parkinson-White (WPW) syndrome is caused by a congenital accessory conducting pathway between the atria and ventricles leading to an atrioventricular re-entry tachycardia (AVRT). As the accessory pathway does not slow conduction, AF can degenerate rapidly to VF.

Possible ECG features include:

- short PR interval
- wide QRS complexes with a slurred upstroke – 'delta wave'
- left axis deviation if right-sided accessory pathway
- right axis deviation if left-sided accessory pathway

Differentiating between type A and type B

- type A (left-sided pathway): dominant R wave in V1
- type B (right-sided pathway): no dominant R wave in V1

Associations of Wolff-Parkinson-White

- HOCM
- mitral valve prolapse
- Ebstein's anomaly
- thyrotoxicosis
- secundum ASD

Management

- definitive treatment: radiofrequency ablation of the accessory pathway
- medical therapy: sotalol, amiodarone, flecainide

8. Broad-complex tachycardia

Regular

- assume ventricular tachycardia (unless previously confirmed SVT with bundle branch block)
- loading dose of amiodarone followed by 24-hour infusion

Irregular

- 1. AF with bundle branch block – treat as for narrow complex tachycardia.
- 2. Polymorphic VT (e.g. torsade de pointes) – IV magnesium if true torsade, will degenerate into VF very rapidly, so usually DCC is treatment of choice before VF occurs.

Management of ventricular tachycardia

Whilst a broad complex tachycardia may result from a supraventricular rhythm with aberrant conduction, the **European Resuscitation Council** advise that in a peri-arrest situation it is assumed to be ventricular in origin.

If the patient has adverse signs (systolic BP <90 mmHg, chest pain, heart failure or rate >150 beats/min) then immediate cardioversion is indicated. In the absence of such signs antiarrhythmics may be used. If these fail, then electrical cardioversion may be needed with synchronised DC shocks.

Drug therapy

+ amiodarone: ideally administered through a central line
+ lidocaine: use with caution in severe left ventricular impairment
+ procainamide

Verapamil should **NOT** be used in VT. Verapamil may cause fatal hypotension in VT (due to negative inotropic and peripheral vasodilatory effects).

If drug therapy fails:

+ electrophysiological study (EPS)
+ implant able cardioverter-defibrillator (ICD) – this is particularly indicated in patients with significantly impaired LV function

Features of a broad complex tachycardia consistent with VT

+ RBBB + LAD
+ very wide QRS
+ chest lead concordance
+ P wave dissociation
+ capture beats
+ fusion beats

The most common cause of VT is ischaemic heart disease; acute myocardial ischaemia can present with VT although scar-related VT from a previous infarct is more common.

Other causes include:

+ metabolic derangement
+ drug induced

✦ cardiomyopathy

✦ long QT syndrome + other inherited channelopathies

Catecholaminergic polymorphic ventricular tachycardia (CPVT)

CPVT is a form of inherited cardiac disease which is also associated with sudden cardiac death. It is inherited in an autosomal dominant fashion and has a prevalence of around 1:10000.

9. ECG: coronary territories

Table 1.8 shows the correlation between ECG changes and coronary territories

TABLE 1.8 ECG changes and coronary territories

	ECG changes	Coronary artery
Anteroseptal	V1–V4	Left anterior descending
Inferior	II, III, aVF	Right coronary
Anterolateral	V4–6, I, aVL	Left anterior descending or left circumflex
Lateral	I, aVL +/– V5–6	Left circumflex
Posterior	Tall R waves V1–2	Usually left circumflex, also right coronary

10. Long QT syndrome

Long QT syndrome is associated with delayed repolarisation of the ventricles. It is important to recognise as it may lead to ventricular tachycardia and can therefore cause collapse/sudden death. The most common variants of LQTS (LQT1 & LQT2) are caused by defects in the alpha subunit of the slow delayed rectifier potassium channel. A normal corrected QT is less than 440 ms in males and 450 ms in females.

Causes

Congenital

Jervell-Lange-Nielsen syndrome includes deafness as well, and is due to mutations in the KCNE1 and KCNQ1 genes. The KCNE1 and KCNQ1 genes provide instructions for making proteins that work together to form a channel across cell membranes. These channels transport positively charged potassium atoms (ions) out of cells. The movement of potassium ions through these channels is critical for maintaining the normal functions of inner ear structures and cardiac muscle.

Romano-Ward syndrome is purely a cardiac electrophysiological disorder, characterised by QT prolongation and T-wave abnormalities on the ECG. It is in fact the most common form of inherited long QT syndrome, affecting an esti-mated 1 in 7000 people worldwide. Mutations in the KCNE1, KCNE2, KCNH2, KCNQ1, and SCN5A genes cause Romano-Ward syndrome.

Brugada syndrome is a form of inherited cardiovascular disease which again may present with sudden cardiac death. It is inherited in an autosomal dominant fashion and has an estimated prevalence of 1:5000–10000. Brugada syndrome is more common in Asians. It has a genetic basis that thus far has been linked only to mutations in SCN5A, the gene that encodes the β-subunit of the sodium channel.

Drugs – THIS LIST IS VERY IMPORTANT

- amiodarone
- sotalol
- class 1a antiarrhythmic drugs
- tricyclic antidepressants
- chloroquine
- terfenadine
- erythromycin

Other causes

- electrolyte: hypocalcaemia, hypokalaemia, hypomagnesaemia
- acute MI
- myocarditis
- hypothermia
- subarachnoid haemorrhage

Management

Beta-blockers are the mainstay of treatment in long QT syndrome. The most commonly used drugs are propranolol and nadolol, but metoprolol and atenolol are also used. Implantable cardioverter-defibrillators are the most effective treat-ment in high-risk cases.

H. Cardiomyopathy

1. HOCM

Hypertrophic obstructive cardiomyopathy (HOCM) is an autosomal dominant disorder of muscle tissue caused by defects in the genes encoding contractile proteins. The estimated prevalence is 1 in 500.

Features

The history of sudden arrhythmia in a young, previously well, individual is suggestive of hypertrophic cardiomyopathy; relatives should be screened for the condition.

These are the commonly recognised features:

- often asymptomatic
- dyspnoea, angina, syncope
- sudden death (most commonly due to ventricular arrhythmias), arrhythmias, heart failure
- jerky pulse, large 'a' waves, double apex beat
- ejection systolic murmur: increases with Valsalva manoeuvre and decreases on squatting.

Associations of HOCM

- Friedreich's ataxia
- Wolff-Parkinson-White syndrome

Investigations in HOCM
Echocardiography

- systolic anterior motion (SAM) of the anterior mitral valve leaflet
- left ventricular hypertrophy, with asymmetric septal hypertrophy (ASH)
- mitral regurgitation
- elevated gradient across the left ventricular outflow tract

ECG

- left ventricular hypertrophy
- progressive T wave inversion
- deep Q waves
- atrial fibrillation may occasionally be seen

Holter monitoring

✦ non-sustained VT

Prognostic factors

Hypertrophic obstructive cardiomyopathy (HOCM) is an autosomal dominant disorder of muscle tissue caused by defects in the genes encoding contractile proteins. Mutations to various proteins including beta-myosin, alpha-tropomyosin and troponin T have been identified. Septal hypertrophy causes left ventricular outflow obstruction. It is an important cause of sudden death in apparently healthy individuals.

Poor prognostic factors

✦ syncope

✦ family history of sudden death

✦ young age at presentation

✦ non-sustained ventricular tachycardia on 24- or 48-hour Holter monitoring

✦ abnormal blood pressure changes on exercise

✦ increased septal wall thickness

Management

✦ medical therapy to decrease the left ventricular outflow gradient: Bblocker +/−

✦ disopyramide

✦ medical therapy for any CCF symptoms

✦ high-risk individuals should have an ICD implanted

✦ RV pacing, surgical myomectomy and alcohol septal ablation are also used, but less commonly

I. General cardiology management issues

1. Percutaneous coronary intervention

Percutaneous coronary intervention (PCI) is a technique used to restore myocardial perfusion in patients with ischaemic heart disease, both in patients with stable angina and acute coronary syndromes. Stents are implanted in around 95% of patients – it is now rare for just balloon angioplasty to be performed.

Following stent insertion, migration and proliferation of smooth muscle cells and fibroblasts occur to the treated segment. The stent struts eventually become covered by endothelium. Until this happens there is an increased risk of platelet aggregation leading to thrombosis.

Two main complications may occur:

- **Stent thrombosis**: due to platelet aggregation as above. Occurs in 1%–2% of patients, most commonly in the first month. Usually presents with acute myocardial infarction.

- **Re-stenosis**: due to excessive tissue proliferation around stent. Occurs in around 5%–20% of patients, most commonly in the first 3–6 months. Usually presents with the recurrence of angina symptoms. Risk factors include diabetes, renal impairment and stents in venous bypass grafts.

Types of stent

- bare-metal stent (BMS)
- drug-eluting stents (DES): stent coated with paclitaxel or rapamycin which inhibit local tissue growth. Whilst this reduces restenosis rates the stent thrombosis rates are increased as the process of stent endothelisation is slowed.

Following insertion the most important factor in preventing stent thrombosis is antiplatelet therapy. Aspirin should be continued indefinitely. The length of clopidogrel treatment depends on the type of stent, reason for insertion and consultant preference.

2. Driving Vehicle Licensing Authority (DVLA)

The guidelines below relate to car/motorcycle use unless specifically stated. For obvious reasons, the rules relating to drivers of heavy goods vehicles tend to be much stricter.

Specific rules

◆ angioplasty (elective) – 1 week off driving

◆ CABG – 4 weeks off driving

◆ acute coronary syndrome – 4 weeks off driving, 1 week if successfully treated by angioplasty

◆ angina – driving must cease if symptoms occur at rest/at the wheel

◆ pacemaker insertion – 1 week off driving

◆ implantable cardioverter-defibrillator: if implanted for sustained ventricular arrhythmia: cease driving for 6 months. If implanted prophylactically then cease driving for 1 month

◆ successful catheter ablation – 2 days off driving

◆ aortic aneurysm >6 cm – notify DVLA. Licensing will be permitted subject to annual review. An aortic diameter of 6.5 cm or more disqualifies patients from driving.

3. Implantable cardiac defibrillators
Indications based on NICE guidance
Primary prevention
For patients with a previous myocardial infarction, who have:

◆ LV ejection fraction <35%, non-sustained VT on Holter AND inducible VT on EP testing

Or

◆ LV ejection fraction <30% AND broad QRS on resting ECG

Secondary prevention
For patients who have survived a cardiac arrest secondary to ventricular arrhythmia, sustained VT with haemodynamic compromise OR sustained VT with poor LV function. In the absence of any identifiable cause of VF/VT.

Other
Familial conditions with high risk of sudden cardiac death

◆ long QT syndrome

◆ hypertrophic obstructive cardiomyopathy

◆ Brugada syndrome

◆ ARVD

Evidence-based medicine

The **Antiarrhythmics Versus Implantable Defibrillators** (AVID) trial (1999) consisted of 1016 patients, and deaths in those treated with AAD were more frequent (n = 122) compared with deaths in the ICD groups (n = 80, p <0.001).

In 2002 **the MADITII trial** showed benefit of ICD treatment in patients after myocardial infarction with reduced left ventricular function (EF <30).

4. Vasovagal syncope

The gradual onset of the attack is typical. It is common for patients with syncope to have jerking of their limbs while they are unconscious.

Vasovagal syncope is common during dental procedures, mainly induced by pain (as the dentist started drilling). It is common to have jerking of limbs due to brain hypoxia.

Warning symptoms of darkening/blurring of vision, dizziness, and feeling hot, are characteristic in syncope. Patients usually recover very quickly after the event.

A **tilt table test** is a useful test to support the diagnosis of vasovagal syncope. An ECG is always normal.

5. Congenital heart disease

Types
Acyanotic – most common causes

◆ ventricular septal defects (VSD) – most common, accounts for 30%

◆ atrial septal defect (ASD)

◆ patent ductus arteriosus (PDA)

◆ coarctation of the aorta

◆ aortic valve stenosis

VSDs are more common than ASDs. However, in adult patients ASDs are the more common new diagnosis as they generally present later.

Cyanotic – most common causes

◆ tetralogy of Fallot

◆ transposition of the great arteries (TGA)

◆ tricuspid atresia

◆ pulmonary valve stenosis

Fallot's tetraology is much more common than TGA. However, at birth TGA is the more common lesion as patients with Fallot's generally present at around 1–2 months.

6. Primary pulmonary arterial hypertension
Features and management
Primary pulmonary arterial hypertension (PAH) may be defined as a sustained elevation in mean pulmonary arterial pressure of greater than 25 mmHg at rest or 30 mmHg after exercise, without any discernible underlying cause. The pathophysiology is thought to involve an imbalance between vasoconstrictors and vasodilators.

Secondary pulmonary hypertension occurs secondary to cardiac (e.g. valvular, ischaemic, hypertension), respiratory (e.g. COPD) or haematological (e.g. sickle cell) diseases.

Features are:

◆ exertional dyspnoea is the most frequent symptom

◆ chest pain and syncope may also occur

◆ loud P2

◆ left parasternal heave (due to right ventricular hypertrophy)

◆ raised JVP

◆ tricuspid regurgitation

◆ hepatomegaly

◆ peripheral oedema

Management should first involve treating any underlying conditions, for example with anticoagulants or oxygen. Following this, it has now been shown that acute vasodilator testing is central to deciding on the appropriate management strategy. Acute vasodilator testing aims to decide which patients show a significant fall in pulmonary arterial pressure following the administration of vasodilators such as intravenous epoprostenol or inhaled nitric oxide.

If there is a positive response to acute vasodilator testing:

◆ oral calcium channel blockers

If there is a negative response to acute vasodilator testing:

◆ prostacyclin analogues: treprostinil, iloprost

◆ endothelin receptor antagonists: bosentan

◆ phosphodiesterase inhibitors: sildenafil

Secondary PAH should be managed in the first instance by treating the underlying cause.

7. Hypertension – including investigation and management
Management

NICE published updated guidelines for the management of hypertension in June 2006

Initial drug choice
- patients <55 years old: ACE inhibitor
- patients >55 years old or of Afro-Caribbean origin: calcium channel blocker or thiazide diuretic

The target blood pressure is 140/90 mmHg.
   If this fails to control the blood pressure then use a combination of an ACE inhibitor plus either a calcium channel blocker or thiazide diuretic.
   If this still fails then a combination of an ACE inhibitor + calcium channel blocker + thiazide diuretic should be used.

Isolated systolic hypertension
Isolated systolic hypertension (ISH) is common in the elderly, affecting around 50% of people older than 70 years old. It is defined as a systolic BP >160 and diastolic BP <90 mmHg, which is the typical hypertension in the elderly population and is associated with a greater risk than combined systolic/diastolic hypertension.

BOX 1.4   A note on evidence-based guidelines for the management of ISH

Based upon studies such as SHEP and Syst-Eur, guidelines suggest treatment with either calcium antagonists or diuretics.

   The **Systolic Hypertension in the Elderly Program** (SHEP) back in 1991 established that treating ISH reduced both strokes and ischaemic heart disease. Drugs such as thiazides were recommended as first line agents.

   This approach is not contraindicated by the 2006 NICE guidelines which recommend treating ISH in the same stepwise fashion as standard hypertension.

Centrally acting anti-hypertensives

Examples of **centrally acting anti-hypertensives** include:

- methyldopa: used in the management of hypertension during pregnancy
- moxonidine: used in the management of essential hypertension when conventional anti-hypertensives have failed to control blood pressure
- clonidine: the anti-hypertensive effect is mediated through stimulating alpha-2 adrenoceptors in the vasomotor centre

Secondary hypertension

Ninety per cent of hypertension is idiopathic. In young patients or resistant hypertension, secondary causes should be considered:

- endocrine: Cushing's syndrome, Conn's syndrome, Liddle's syndrome, Acromegaly, phaeochromocytoma
- renal: any cause of CRF, renal artery stenosis
- other: pregnancy, coarcation of the aorta, drug induced (steroids, oral contraceptive pill, illicit)

Malignant hypertension

Malignant hypertension is a sudden and rapid development of extremely high blood pressure. The lower (diastolic) blood pressure reading, which is normally around 80 mmHg, is often above 130 mmHg; the upper (systolic) blood pressure is often above 200 mmHg. Patients often have left systolic dysfunction. Complications include papilloedema, convulsions and pulmonary oedema (thus excluding the use of a beta-blocker in the acute setting). This constitutes a medical emergency, with nitroprusside being the treatment of choice.

BOX 1.5   A note on new medications for hypertension

Aliskiren is a direct renin inhibitor and represents the first new class of drug available in over a decade for the treatment of hypertension.

Renin has long been recognised as a possible site for blockade of the renin-angiotensin-aldosterone system (RAS) because it prevents conversion of angiotensinogen to angiotensin I and is a rate-limiting step in the RAS cascade.

Aliskiren binds to the active site of the renin molecule, blocking angiotensinogen cleavage, thus preventing the formation of angiotensin I.

Clinical studies have demonstrated at least equivalent blood pressure-lowering efficacy compared with existing drugs with a favourable side-effect profile.

---

8. Patent ductus arteriosus
Overview
+ acyanotic congenital heart defect
+ connection between the pulmonary trunk and descending aorta
+ more common in premature babies, born at high altitude or maternal rubella infection in the first trimester

Features
+ left subclavicular thrill
+ continuous 'machinery' murmur
+ absent S2
+ large volume, collapsing pulse
+ wide pulse pressure
+ heaving apex beat

Management
+ indomethacin closes the connection in the majority of cases
+ if associated with another congenital heart defect amenable to surgery then prostaglandin E1 is useful to keep the duct open until after surgical repair
+ percutaneous occluder or surgical ligation

9. Aortic dissection
Classification
+ type A – ascending aorta (⅔ of cases)
+ type B – descending aorta, distal to left subclavian origin (⅓ of cases)

Type A
+ surgical management, but blood pressure should be controlled to a target systolic of 100–120 mmHg whilst awaiting intervention

Type B
+ conservative management
+ bed rest
+ reduce blood pressure, for example by IV labetalol to prevent progression

10. Paradoxical embolisation

An example in the MRCP(UK) Part 1 examination might be a young lady presenting with a history of sudden onset right-sided weakness and dysphasia lasting eight hours. She has possibly returned to the UK after a long international plane trip.

This is termed the **paradoxical embolus**, so-called because a thrombus arising from the venous circulation can end up in the systemic circulation. For a right-sided thrombus (e.g. DVT) to cause a left-sided embolism (e.g. stroke) it must pass from the right-to-left side of the heart.

The following cardiac lesions may cause such events:

+ patent foramen ovale – present in around 20% of the population
+ atrial septal defect – a much less common cause

Transoesophageal echocardiography is the investigation of choice to investigate for a patent foramen ovale, although transthoracic echocardiography with contrast may be an alternative.

11. Orthostatic hypotension

When a person stands up from sitting or lying down, the body must work to adjust to that change in position. It is especially important for the body to push blood upward and supply the brain with oxygen. If the body fails to do this adequately, blood pressure falls, and a person may feel lightheaded or even pass out. **Orthostatic hypotension** is the term used to describe the fall in blood pressure when a person stands.

Causes
+ haemorrhage
+ anaemia
+ dehydration
+ medications (including sildenafil, isosorbide mononitrate, tricyclic antidepressants such as amitriptyline)

Possible investigations
+ Blood tests (FBC, U&Es)
+ ECG

◈ Lying-standing BPs

◈ Tilt-table test

Management

The treatment for orthostatic hypotension depends upon the underlying diagnosis.

If the cause is dehydration, then fluid replacement will resolve the symptoms. If it is due to medication, then an adjustment of the dose or change in the type of medicine taken may be required.

Compression stockings may be considered to help prevent fluid from pooling in the legs when a person is sitting or lying down. This allows for more blood flow to be available to the brain when changes in position occur.

Medications may be of use, again depending upon the underlying cause of the orthostatic hypotension. For those who are otherwise healthy and have no specific illness that must be treated, increased salt and fluid intake may be recommended.

Some patients may be a candidate for fludrocortisone to increase the volume of fluid in the blood vessels. This medication does have significant side effects, however.

Reference

Granger CB, Goldberg RJ, Dabbous O, *et al.* Predictors of hospital mortality in the global registry of acute coronary events. *Arch Intern Med.* 2003 Oct 27; **163**(19): 2345–53.

Chapter 2

Dermatology

The Foundation Programme and MRCP(UK) Part 1 syllabus (from the JRCPMTB) specify what is required in terms of competencies, skills and knowledge from junior physicians in core medical training in dermatology. You are advised to consult carefully this syllabus, which emphasises the importance of basic medical sciences as well as a competent level of applied clinical practice.

A. Common clinical presentations

In particular, you should know the differential diagnosis and plan of investigation of patients who present with the following cutaneous signs or symptoms which may indicate internal disease.

1. Itch

Endocrine

- hypothyroidism
- hyperthyroidism
- diabetes mellitus
- diabetes insipidus

Haematology

- iron-deficiency anaemia
- polycythaemia rubra vera
- lymphoma
- leukaemia
- myeloma

Drugs

- opiates
- gold
- alcohol
- hepatotoxic drugs
- oral contraceptive pill

Other causes

- intestinal parasites
- scabies
- chronic renal failure
- obstructive biliary disease
- pregnancy
- psychogenic
- senile pruritus

2. Urticaria

Aetiology of urticaria

- idiopathic
- immunological
- autoimmune (autoantibodies against FccRI or IgE)
- allergic (IgE-mediated type I hypersensitivity reaction)
- immune complex (urticarial vasculitis)
- complement-dependent (C1 esterase inhibitor deficiency)
- non-immunological
- direct mast-cell releasing agents (e.g. opiates)
- drugs (see section above)

Drug causes of urticaria

The following drugs commonly cause urticaria:

- aspirin
- penicillins

◆ NSAIDs

◆ opiates

Management of urticaria

Grattan *et al.* (2007) published an influential paper on the analysis and management of urticaria in adults and children.

Advice on general measures and information can be helpful for most patients with urticaria, especially if an avoidable physical or dietary trigger can be identified.

◆ Over 40% of hospitalised patients with urticaria show a good response to antihistamines, which continue to be the first-line or 'mainstay' of therapy. It has become common practice to increase the dose of second-generation H_1 antihistamines above the manufacturer's licensed recommendation for patients when the potential benefits are considered to outweigh any risks. Combinations of non-sedating H_1 antihistamines with other agents, such as H_2 antihistamines, sedating antihistamines at night or the addition of antileukotrienes, can be useful for resistant cases.

◆ Oral corticosteroids should be restricted to short courses for more severe cases, i.e. severe acute urticaria or angio-oedema affecting the mouth, although more prolonged treatment may be necessary for delayed pressure urticaria or urticarial vasculitis.

◆ Immunomodulating therapies for chronic autoimmune urticaria should be restricted to patients with disabling disease who have not responded to optimal conventional treatments.

3. Hyperpigmentation
Endocrine

◆ Addison's disease

◆ Cushing's syndrome

◆ acromegaly

◆ Nelson's syndrome

◆ pregnancy

Metabolic

- porphyria
- renal failure
- cirrhosis
- haemochromatosis

Nutritional

- vitamin B$_{12}$ deficiency
- pellagra

Other causes

- amyloid
- acanthosis nigricans
- lymphoma
- Peutz-Jehgers syndrome

Drugs

- amiodarone
- oral contraceptive pill
- minocycline

4. Hirsutism

Hirsutism is often used to describe androgen-dependent hair growth in women, with hypertrichosis being used for androgen-independent hair growth.

Causes of hirsutism

- polycystic ovarian syndrome
- Cushing's syndrome
- congenital adrenal hyperplasia
- androgen therapy
- adrenal tumour
- androgen-secreting ovarian tumour
- drugs: phenytoin

5. Causes of hypertrichosis

◆ drugs: minoxidil, cyclosporin, diazoxide

◆ congenital hypertrichosis lanuginosa, congenital hypertrichosis terminalis

◆ porphyria cutanea tarda

◆ anorexia nervosa

6. Loss of hair

Alopecia may be divided into scarring (destruction of hair follicle) and non-scarring (preservation of hair follicle).

Scarring alopecia

◆ trauma, burns

◆ radiotherapy

◆ lichen planus

◆ discoid lupus

◆ *tinea capitis*

Non-scarring alopecia

◆ male-pattern baldness

◆ drugs: cytotoxic drugs, carbimazole, heparin, oral contraceptive pill, colchicine

◆ nutritional: iron and zinc deficiency

◆ autoimmune: alopecia areata

◆ *telogen effluvium* (In a normal healthy person's scalp about 85% of the hair follicles are actively growing hair and 15% are resting. If there is some shock to the system, as many as 70% of the scalp hairs can be precipitated into a resting state, thus reversing the usual ratio.)

BOX 2.1 A note on *telogen effluvium*

Typical precipitants include illnesses, operations, accidents and childbirth. The resting scalp hairs, now in the form of club hairs, remain firmly attached to the hair follicles at first. It is only about two months after the shock that the new hairs coming up through the scalp push out the 'dead' club hairs and increased hair fall is noticed. Thus, paradoxically, with this type of hair loss, hair fall is a sign of hair regrowth. As the new hair first comes up through the scalp and pushes out the dead hair a fine fringe of new hair is often evident along the forehead hairline. At first, the fall of club hairs is profuse and a general thinning of the scalp hair may become evident but after several months a peak is reached and hair fall begins to lessen, gradually tapering back to normal over six to nine months. As the hair fall tapers off, the scalp thickens back up to normal, but recovery may be incomplete in some cases.

Alopecia areata

Alopecia areata is a presumed autoimmune condition causing localised, well-demarcated patches of hair loss. At the edge of the hair loss, there may be small, broken 'exclamation mark' hairs.

Note that the combination of vitiligo and alopecia areata can co-exist and have similar autoimmune aetiology. Discrete areas of hair loss and normal texture on the scalp are highly suggestive of alopecia areata. Hair will re-grow in 50% of patients by 1 year, and in 80–90% eventually.

The Guidelines for the management of alopecia areata published in the *British Journal of Dermatology* (2003) recommend various therapies, on an evidence-basis.

The Group emphasises that alopecia areata is difficult to treat and few treatments have been assessed in randomised controlled trials. The tendency to spontaneous remission and the lack of adverse effects on general health are important considerations in management, and not treating is the best option in many cases. On the other hand, alopecia areata may cause considerable psychological and social disability and in some cases, particularly those seen in secondary care, it may be a chronic and persistent disease causing extensive or universal hair loss.

In those cases where treatment is appropriate, there is reasonable evidence to support the following:

Limited patchy hair loss: intralesional corticosteroid
Intralesional corticosteroids stimulate hair regrowth at the site of injection. The effect is temporary, lasting a few months, and it is unknown whether the long-term outcome is influenced.

Extensive patchy hair loss: contact immunotherapy

7. Clubbing

Primary

Familial

Hypertrophic osteoarthropathy

Cardiac

Cyanotic heart disease

Infective endocarditis

Lung disease

Lung cancers

Tuberculosis

Interstitial lung disease

Empyema

Mesothelioma

Cryptogenic fibrosing alveolitis

Gastrointestinal disease

Ulcerative colitis

Crohn's disease

Liver cirrhosis

Primary biliary cirrhosis

FIGURE 2.1 Causes of clubbing

8. Onycholysis
Onycholysis describes the separation of the nail plate from the nail bed.

Causes
- idiopathic
- trauma, e.g. excessive manicuring
- infection: especially fungal
- skin disease: psoriasis, dermatitis
- impaired peripheral circulation, e.g. Raynaud's
- systemic disease: hyper- and hypothyroidism

B. Specific skin conditions/diseases
1. Erythema nodosum
- inflammation of subcutaneous fat
- typically causes tender, erythematous, nodular lesions
- usually occurs over shins, may also occur elsewhere (e.g. forearms, thighs)
- usually resolves within six weeks
- lesions heal without scarring

Key signs
Flat, red, tender, nodular large lesions on the shins, associated with fever and arthralgia.

Signs of a cause, e.g. sore throat or systemic manifestations of sarcoidosis. Investigations: history, may be due to sarcoid, check ACE and CXR, ?TB.

Causes
Include:
- *Streptococcus*, salmonella or campylobacter gastroenteritis
- sarcoidosis
- tuberculosis
- ulcerative colitis, Crohn's disease
- lymphoma/malignancy
- viral/chlamydial infection

◆ pregnancy

◆ oral contraceptive pill, sulphonamides, tetracyclines, penicillin

Management
Often self-resolving, treat sarcoid if required, or remove cause. Other skin manifestations of sarcoidosis: nodules and plaques (red/brown seen particularly around the face, nose, ears and neck). Demonstrates Koebner's phenomenon and lupus pernio (bluish/brown plaque with central small papules commonly affecting the nose).

2. Erythema multiforme
◆ target lesions (typically worse on peripheries, e.g. palms and soles)

◆ severe = Stevens-Johnson syndrome (blistering and mucosal involvement)

Causes
◆ viruses: herpes simplex, orf

◆ idiopathic

◆ bacteria: *Mycoplasma, Streptococcus*

◆ drugs: penicillin, sulphonamides, carbamazepine, allopurinol, NSAIDs, oral contraceptive pill, nevirapine

◆ connective tissue disease, e.g. systemic lupus erythematosus

◆ sarcoidosis

◆ malignancy

3. Purpura
Purpura fall largely into two groups: vessel disorders and platelet disorders.

The distribution of the lesions is worth examining, e.g. senile purpura/steroids often affect backs of hands and forearms. Henoch-Schönlein purpura classically appears over lower limbs and buttocks. Scurvy over lower limbs/backs of thighs with perifollicular haemorrhages plus corkscrew hairs; look for woollen gums.

One should examine palate for petechial haemorrhages, gums for ulceration and haemorrhage (suggests neutropaenia and thrombocytopaenia), conjunctivae and fundi for haemorrhages (fundal haemorrhages only in severe thrombocytopaenia); also look for evidence of cause ?Cushingoid (steroid), ?rheumatoid disease, SLE, infective endocarditis, ?chronic liver disease, ?Ehlers-Danlos syndrome.

4. Ulceration

Ulceration due to herpes simplex virus

There are two strains of the herpes simplex virus (HSV) in humans: HSV-1 and HSV-2. Whilst it was previously thought HSV-1 accounted for oral lesions (cold sores) and HSV-2 for genital herpes it is now known there is considerable overlap.

Features

◈ primary infection: may present with a severe gingivostomatitis

◈ cold sores

◈ painful genital ulceration

Venous ulceration

Venous ulceration is typically seen above the medial malleolus.

Investigations

◈ Ankle-brachial pressure index (ABPI) is important in non-healing ulcers to assess for poor arterial flow which could impair healing.

◈ A 'normal' ABPI may be regarded as between 0.9 and 1.2. Values below 0.9 indicate arterial disease. Interestingly, values above 1.3 may also indicate arterial disease, in the form of false-negative results secondary to arterial calcification (e.g. in diabetics).

Management

◈ compression bandaging, usually four layer (only treatment shown to be of real benefit)

◈ oral pentoxifylline, a peripheral vasodilator, improves healing rate

◈ small evidence base supporting use of flavinoids

◈ little evidence to suggest benefit from hydrocolloid dressings, topical growth factors, ultrasound

5. Psoriasis

A genetically determined, inflammatory and proliferative disorder of the skin, occurring in 1%–2% of the UK population.

Aetiology unknown. Association with HLA Cw6, B13 and B17 in skin disease and B27 in psoriatic arthropathy.

More common in 2nd and 6th decades, with females generally developing psoriasis at a younger age than males.

Numerous symmetrical well-demarcated/sharply defined salmon pink/red plaques of varying sizes with silvery white scaling surfaces.

The plaques are most prominent on extensor surfaces (elbows, knees)/scalp and hairline/behind the ears/at the umbilicus. Extent of severity of plaque psoriasis, presence of variant psoriasis, presence of arthropathy.

Note the character of the lesions (scales, thickness, erythema, pustulation), the extent of cover, the degree of itching, and complications such as joint involvement. Skin staining from treatment.

BOX 2.2 A note on signs associated with psoriasis

Koebner's phenomenon: localised lesions at the site of trauma (other causes include lichen planus, vitiligo, viral warts, *molluscum contagiosum*).

Auspitz's sign: punctuate bleeding spots on scraping the scales (other associations are lichen planus, viral warts, vitiligo and sarcoid).

Types of psoriasis

- palmoplantar pustular variant: yellow/brown sterile pustules and erythema, affects palms and soles
- erythodermic psoriasis: severe systemic upset with fever, raised WBC, inflammatory markers and dehydration; confluent areas affecting most of the skin surface
- flexural psoriasis: affects axillae, submammary areas and natal cleft; often smooth, red and glazed looking
- guttate: an acute eruption of multiple 'drop-like' lesions on trunk and limbs following a streptococcal infection
- nail psoriasis
- chronic plaque

Associations

- gout and arthropathy
- malabsorption (Crohn's disease and ulcerative colitis)

Factors which exacerbate psoriasis

- trauma (Kobner's phenomenon)
- infection (including HIV)

◆ endocrine (psoriasis generally tends to improve during pregnancy and deteriorate during the post-partum period)

◆ drugs (beta-blockers, lithium, antimalarials and the withdrawal of oral steroids can exacerbate psoriasis)

◆ alcohol

◆ stress (severe physical or psychological)

Investigations

Most patients do not require any investigations.

Skin biopsy can be used to detect psoriasiform papillomatosis, acanthosis, hyperkeratosis and parakeratosis, with intra-dermal collections of neutrophils.

Management

A careful explanation of the disease process and the likely necessity for long-term treatment should always be given.

The type of psoriasis and severity influences the choice of treatment. It is usual to use topical agents as the first-line treatment.

Treatments include:

◆ topical (emollients such as oil/soap emollients and moisturisers control scale)

◆ calcipotriol ointment (vitamin D_3 analogues)

◆ coal tar (smell, stains brown)

◆ dithranol (stains purple and burns normal skin, usually effective)

◆ topical retinoids such as tazarotene, hydrocortisone

For widespread or severe disease, further treatment options include:
Systemic:

Cytotoxics

◆ methotrexate and cyclosporin (methotrexate is used in widespread plaque, acute generalised pustular and erythrodermic psoriasis, and psoriatic arthropathy as short-term or maintenance treatment)

◆ retinoids are effective particularly in acral or generalised pustular psoriasis), retinoids (acitretin, safe and teratogenic)

Phototherapy

UVB narrowband (311–313 nm) is now replacing broadband UVB (290–320 nm) (for chronic plaque and guttate psoriasis), psoralen + UVA (PUVA).

Other biological agents (promising new treatments but as yet not licensed for psoriasis include etanercept and efalizumab, presently under review):

◆ efalizumab humanised monoclonal antibody – blocks T cell activation/ migration

◆ alefacept – recombinant fusion protein which interferes with activation/ proliferation of T cells

◆ etanercept – human fusion protein of the TNF receptor which acts as a TNF inhibitor

◆ infliximab – monoclonal antibody which binds TNFα

Complications

◆ psoriatic arthropathy 10% (five forms: DIP involvement, large joint mono/ oligoarthritis, seronegative, sacroilitis, *arthritis mutilans*), erythroderma

◆ guttate psoriasis: associated with streptococcal throat infection, resolves in 3 months

6. Eczema
Diagnosis

> ### UK Working Party diagnostic criteria for atopic eczema
>
> Hanifin and Rajka originally laid the groundwork for the compilation of useful diagnostic criteria for this important condition in 1980. Subsequently Williams and colleagues (1999) published the UK Working Party guidance with this helpful definition:
>
> *'This is an itchy skin condition in the last 12 months.'*
> Plus **three or more** of:
> - onset below age 2 years
> - history of flexural involvement
> - history of generally dry skin
> - personal history of other atopic disease
> - visible flexural dermatitis

Treatment: topical steroids

The general principle is that you should preferably use weakest steroid cream which controls the patient's symptoms. Table 2.1 shows topical steroids by potency.

TABLE 2.1 Steroids by potency

Mild	Moderate	Potent	Very potent
Hydrocortisone 0.5%–2.5%	Betamethasone valerate 0.025% (Betnovate RD)	Betamethasone dipropionate 0.025% (Propaderm)	Clobetasol propionate 0.05% (Dermovate)
	Clobetasone butyrate 0.05% (Eumovate)	Betamethasone valerate 0.1% (Betnovate)	

Fingertip rule

1 fingertip unit (FTU) = 0.5 g, sufficient to treat a skin area about twice that of the flat of an adult hand.

Topical steroid doses for eczema in adults are given in Table 2.2.

TABLE 2.2 Fingertip units per areas of body

Area of skin	Fingertip units per dose
Hand and fingers (front and back)	1.0
A foot (all over)	2.0
Front of chest and abdomen	7.0
Back and buttocks	7.0
Face and neck	2.5
An entire arm and hand	4.0
An entire leg and foot	8.0

7. Superficial fungal infections

Dermatophytosis

Dermatophytosis (*tinea*) infections are fungal infections caused by dermato-phytes – a group of fungi that invade and grow in dead keratin.

They tend to grow outwards on skin producing a ring-like pattern, hence the term 'ringworm'.

They are very common and affect different parts of the body.

They can usually be successfully treated but success depends on the site of infection and on compliance with treatment.

The infection can be transmitted to humans by anthropophilic (between people), geophilic (from soil) and zoophilic (from animals) spread.

The most common organisms are:

- *Trichophytons rubrum, Trichophytons tonsurans, Trichophytons interdigitale* and *Trichophytons mentagrophytes*
- *Microsporum canis*
- *Epidermophyton floccosum*

Clinical classification is according to site:

- Scalp – *Tinea capitis*
- Feet – *Tinea pedis*
- Hands – *Tinea manuum*
- Nail – *Tinea unguum*
- Beard area – *Tinea barbae*
- Groin – *Tinea cruris*

Management

- For most skin infections it is sufficient to apply an imidazole cream twice daily.
- Clotrimazole or miconazole is recommended topically for pregnant or breastfeeding women.
- Agents containing a corticosteroid are not usually necessary.
- Offer advice on hygiene measures.
- Continue school and sports activities.
- Cover feet in communal changing areas.

◆ Systemic agents are appropriate for tinea capitis and onychomycosis (although topical nail preparations can be used in limited distal nail disease).
◆ Referral may be needed if diagnosis is in doubt.

BOX 2.3   A note on Tinea capitis

Tinea capitis is a dermatophyte infection of the scalp most often caused by *Trichophyton tonsurans*, and occasionally by *Microsporum canis*. It is commonest in areas of socio-economic deprivation. Confluent patches of alopecia develop and there may be pruritis. Sometimes a severe inflammatory response produces an elevated boggy granulomatous mass (kerion), studded with sterile pustules. There may be fever and regional lymphadenopathy, and occasionally permanent scarring and alopecia may result. The crusted patches fluoresce dull green under Wood's light. Microscopic examination of a potassium hydroxide (KOH) preparation shows tiny spores and the fungi may be grown in Sabouraud medium with antibiotics. Oral griseofulvin for two to three months is required, or ketoconazole for resistant cases.

---

8. Pityriasis versicolor

Pityriasis versicolor, also called *tinea versicolor*, is a superficial cutaneous fungal infection caused by *Malassezia furfur*.

Features

◆ most commonly affects trunk
◆ patches may be hypopigmented, pink or brown (hence versicolor)
◆ scale is common
◆ mild pruritus

Predisposing factors

◆ occurs in healthy individuals
◆ immunosuppression
◆ malnutrition
◆ Cushing's

Management

+ topical antifungal, e.g. terbinafine or selenium sulphide

+ if extensive disease or failure to respond to topical treatment then consider oral itraconazole

9. Malignant melanoma

Diagnostic features for the early detection of malignant melanoma

A popular method for remembering the signs and symptoms of melanoma is the mnemonic **ABCDE**:

+ **A**symmetrical skin lesion

+ **B**order of the lesion is irregular

+ **C**olour: melanomas usually have multiple colours

+ **D**iameter: moles greater than 6 mm are more likely to be melanomas than smaller moles

+ **E**nlarging: enlarging or evolving

Prognostic factors

The invasion depth of a tumour (Breslow depth) is the single most important factor in determining prognosis of patients with malignant melanoma. Approximate 5-year survival times are provided in Table 2.3.

TABLE 2.3 Approximate 5-year survival times for malignant melanoma according to Breslow thickness

Breslow thickness	Approximate 5-year survival
<1 mm	95%–100%
1–2 mm	80%–96%
2.1–4 mm	60%–75%
>4 mm	50%

10. Actinic (solar) keratoses

Actinic, or solar, keratoses is a common premalignant skin lesion that develops as a consequence of chronic sun exposure.

Features

+ small, crusty or scaly, lesions
+ may be pink, red, brown or the same colour as the skin
+ typically on sun-exposed areas, e.g. temples of head
+ multiple lesions may be present

Management

+ prevention of further risk, e.g. sun avoidance, sun cream
+ fluorouracil cream: typically a 2–3 week course; the skin will become red and inflamed – sometimes topical hydrocortisone is given following fluorouracil to help settle the inflammation
+ topical diclofenac: may be used for mild actinic keratoses; moderate efficacy but much fewer side effects
+ topical imiquimod: trials have shown good efficacy
+ cryotherapy
+ curettage and cautery

11. Vitiligo

Vitiligo is an acquired pigmentary disorder of the skin and mucous membranes, and it is characterised by circumscribed depigmented macules and patches.

It is a progressive disorder in which some or all of the melanocytes in the affected skin are selectively destroyed.

The disease manifests itself as white or hypopigmented macules or patches. The lesions are usually well demarcated, and they are round, oval or linear in shape. The borders may be convex.

Lesions enlarge centrifugally over time at an unpredictable rate. Lesions range from millimetres to centimetres in size. Initial lesions occur most frequently on the hands, forearms, feet and face, favouring a perioral and periocular distribution.

Vitiligo is associated with numerous autoimmune conditions including, in order of frequency:

✤ autoimmune hypothyroidism

✤ pernicious anaemia

✤ alopecia areata

✤ Addison's disease

It is associated with both type 1 and 2 autoimmune polyendocrine syndromes but these are much rarer than the former diagnoses.

Lesions may be localised or generalised, with the latter being more common than the former. Localised vitiligo is restricted to one general area with a segmental or quasidermatomal distribution. Generalised vitiligo implies more than one general area of involvement. In this situation, the macules are usually found on both sides of the trunk, either symmetrically or asymmetrically arrayed.

The most common sites of involvement are the face, neck and scalp.

No single therapy for vitiligo produces predictably good results in all patients; the response to therapy is highly variable.

12. Bullous disorders: Pemphigus and pemphigoid

Pemphigus: lesions in mouth common. Autoantibodies against desmosomes which bridge adjacent epidermal cells. Bullae tend to break easily and even rubbing of normal skin causes sloughing of the epidermis (Nikolsky's sign). Widespread crusting and erosions. Bullous eruption on the trunk and flexor surfaces. Treat with steroids and immunomodulatory drugs.

BOX 2.4   A note on Nikolsky's sign

Increased skin fragility is seen in a number of disorders and is used as a clinical test in bullous disorders (Nikolsky's sign).

Other causes include pemphigus vulgaris, porphyria cutanea tarda, and drug reactions (especially pseudoporphyria).

Other causes of increased skin fragility (not associated with bullae) include long-term corticosteroid therapy, Ehlers-Danlos syndrome and scurvy (vitamin C deficiency).

Pemphigoid: mucosal ulceration rare. Autoantibodies present at the dermo-epidermal border. Tense bullae present with erythematous plaques. Many burst, leaving red, exuding, tender patches. Tends to affect the elderly. Treat with steroids.

Management of bullous pemphigoid

> You are advised to read the current evidence and the BNF section on skin disorders.

It is acknowledged that bullous pemphigoid (BP) is a common disease of the elderly. With our ageing population it will become increasingly frequent, and the age of the patients will add to the complexity of treatment.

There is a clear need to determine how to stratify patients clinically, and to ascertain the optimum regimens for treating mild, moderate and severe BP. Systemic corticosteroids are the best established treatment.

For localised bullous pemphigoid, very potent topical corticosteroids are perhaps worth trying first. For mild to moderate disease, tetracycline and nicotinamide should be considered.

Immunosuppressants cannot be recommended routinely from the outset but should only be considered if the corticosteroid dose cannot be reduced to an acceptable level.

Azathioprine is the best established; methotrexate may be considered in patients with additional psoriasis.

13. Leprosy

Leprosy is a chronic granulomatous disease principally affecting the skin and peripheral nervous system. It is caused by infection with *Mycobacterium leprae*.

The skin lesions and deformities were historically responsible for the stigma attached to the disease. However, even with proper multidrug therapy, the consequent sensory and motor damage results in the deformities and disabilities associated with leprosy.

The management of leprosy includes early pharmacotherapy and physical, social and psychological rehabilitation. The length of treatment ranges from 6 months to 2 years.

14. Genital warts

Genital warts (also known as *condylomata accuminata*) are a common cause of attendance at genitourinary clinics.

They are caused by the many varieties of the human papilloma virus HPV, especially types 6 and 11. It is now well established that HPV (primarily types 16, 18 and 33) predisposes to cervical cancer.

Features

◆ small (2–5 mm) fleshy protuberances which are slightly pigmented
◆ may bleed or itch

Management

◆ Topical podophyllum or cryotherapy are commonly used as first-line treatments depending on the location and type of lesion. Multiple, non-keratinised warts are generally best treated with topical agents, whereas solitary, keratinised warts respond better to cryotherapy.
◆ Imiquimod is a topical cream which is generally used second-line.
◆ Genital warts are often resistant to treatment and recurrence is common although the majority of anogenital infections with HPV clear without intervention within 1–2 years.

15. Seborrhoeic dermatitis

Seborrhoeic dermatitis in adults is a chronic dermatitis thought to be caused by an inflammatory reaction related to a proliferation of a normal skin inhabitant, a fungus called *Malassezia*.

It is common, affecting around 2% of the general population. Seborrhoeic dermatitis is more common in patients with Parkinson's disease.

Features

◆ eczematous lesions on the sebum-rich areas: scalp (may cause dandruff), periorbital, auricular and nasolabial folds
◆ otitis externa and blepharitis may develop

Associated conditions

◆ HIV
◆ Parkinson's disease

Scalp disease management

♦ Over-the-counter preparations containing zinc pyrithione ('Head & Shoulders') and tar ('Neutrogena T/Gel') are first-line.

♦ The preferred second-line agent is ketoconazole.

Face and body management

♦ topical antifungals: e.g. ketoconazole

♦ topical steroids: best used for short periods

♦ difficult to treat – recurrences are common

16. *Erythema ab igne*

Erythema ab igne is a skin disorder caused by overexposure to infrared radiation. Characteristic features include erythematous patches with hyperpigmentation and telangiectasia. A typical history would be an elderly woman who always sits next to an open fire.

If the cause is not treated then patients may go on to develop squamous cell skin cancer.

17. Acne vulgaris

Acne vulgaris is a common skin disorder which usually occurs in adolescence. It typically affects the face, neck and upper trunk and is characterised by the obstruction of the pilosebaceous follicle with keratin plugs which results in comedones, inflammation and pustules.

Epidemiology

♦ affects around 80%–90% of teenagers, 60% of whom seek medical advice

♦ acne may also persist beyond adolescence, with 10%–15% of females and 5% of males over 25 years old being affected

Pathophysiology

This is currently considered to be multifactorial, consisting of:

♦ follicular epidermal hyperproliferation resulting in the formation of a keratin plug, which in turn causes obstruction of the pilosebaceous follicle; activity of sebaceous glands may be controlled by androgen, although levels are often normal in patients with acne

◈ colonisation by the anaerobic bacterium *Propionibacterium acnes*

◈ inflammation

Management
First-line drugs for acne vulgaris include benzoyl peroxide, isoretinoin, erythro-mycin, tetracycline or clindamycin.

A very important drug in this repertoire is *isoretinoin*; however, the drug is contra-indicated in patients with hypervitaminosis A, uncontrolled hyperlipidae-mia, and during pregnancy or lactation. It should be used with caution in patients with renal and liver disease. Oral isotretinoin side effects include teratogenicity, hyperlipidaemia, dryness and irritation of skin and mucous membranes.

18. Acne rosacea
This is a chronic skin disease of unknown aetiology.

Features
◈ typically affects nose, cheeks and forehead

◈ flushing is often first symptom

◈ telangiectasia are common

◈ later develops into persistent erythema with papules and pustules

◈ rhinophyma

◈ ocular involvement: blepharitis

Management
◈ topical metronidazole may be used for mild symptoms (i.e. limited number of papules and pustules, no plaques)

◈ more severe disease is treated with systemic antibiotics, e.g. oxytetracycline

◈ recommend daily application of a high-factor sunscreen

◈ camouflage creams may help conceal redness

◈ laser therapy may be appropriate for patients with prominent telangiectasia

19. Skin disorders associated with malignancy

Paraneoplastic syndromes associated with internal malignancies:

+ acanthosis nigricans – gastric cancer
+ acquired ichthyosis – lymphoma
+ acquired hypertrichosis lanuginosa – gastrointestinal and lung cancer
+ dermatomyositis – bronchial and breast cancer
+ erythema gyratum repens – lung cancer
+ erythroderma: lymphoma
+ migratory thrombophlebitis – pancreatic cancer
+ necrolytic migratory erythema – glucagonoma
+ pyoderma gangrenosum (bullous and non-bullous forms) – myeloproliferative disorders
+ Sweet's syndrome – haematological malignancy, e.g. myelodysplasia – tender, purple plaques
+ tylosis – oesophageal cancer

20. Acanthosis nigricans

This term describes symmetrical, brown, velvety plaques that are often found on the neck, axilla and groin.

Common causes

+ internal malignancy (especially gastrointestinal)
+ insulin-resistant diabetes mellitus
+ obesity
+ acromegaly
+ Cushing's disease
+ hypothyroidism
+ polycystic ovarian syndrome
+ familial
+ Prader-Willi syndrome
+ drugs: oral contraceptive pill, nicotinic acid

21. Pretibial myxoedema

◆ symmetrical, erythematous lesions seen in Graves' disease

◆ shiny, orange-peel skin

22. Pyoderma gangrenosum

Features and causes

Pyoderma gangrenosum may begin as a nodular erythema or a sterile pustule, but develops often into large areas of painful, necrotic ulceration. There are large necrotic ulcers with ragged bluish-red overhanging edges together with areas containing erythematous plaques with pustules. They are situated on the legs. The appearances are suggestive of pyoderma gangrenosum. The patient may have Crohn's disease or ulcerative colitis.

Other causes: gastrointestinal (ulcerative colitis, Crohn's disease), rheumatological (rheumatoid disease, ankylosing spondylitis), liver (chronic active hepatitis, primary biliary cirrhosis, sclerosing cholangitis), haematological (lymphoproliferative and myeloproliferative disorders), others (diabetes mellitus, thyroid disease, sarcoidosis, Wegener's granulomatosis).

It is frequently an indicator of severity of the disease. Systemic steroids often help. The adjunctive use of minocycline may reduce corticosteroid requirements. Other causes of leg ulcers include venous ulceration, ischaemic arterial ulceration, diabetes mellitus, vasculitis, infection, Charcot's joints, tumour, haematological (sickle cell, thalassaemia, paroxysmal nocturnal haemoglobulinuria), neurological (diabetes, tabes dorsalis, leprosy, syringomyelia).

23. Necrobiosis lipoidica diabeticorum

Features

◆ shiny, painless areas of yellow/red skin typically on the shin of diabetics

◆ often associated with telangiectasia

24. Granuloma annulare

Granuloma annulare is a benign inflammatory condition of unknown aetiology with dermal papules and annular plaques. Histology reveals foci of degenerative collagen with palisaded granulomatous inflammation. It may be associated with diabetes but association with systemic disease is rare.

Localised lesions are usually groups of papules, about 1–2 mm in diameter with possible erythema. They tend to form an arc or a ring 1–5 cm in diameter. The centre of lesions may be slightly depressed and hyperpigmented. They are usually on the dorsal surfaces of hands, feet and fingers and the extensor surface of arms and legs.

The generalised variety has a similar appearance to the lesions but they are more numerous and more diffuse. They may coalesce into annular plaques 3–6 cm in diameter and these can expand over weeks or months. They tend to be on limbs or trunk.

Subcutaneous lesions are firm, skin-coloured or pink, not tender and the overlying skin looks normal. They are usually solitary lesions but can occur in clusters. The lower limb, especially the pretibial surface, is the most common area. Lesions are mobile, except on the scalp.

25. Dermatitis herpetiformis

A patient might typically present with a history of several months' duration of pruritic papules, vesicles and excoriations on the elbows, knees, buttocks and scalp.

Dermatitis hermetiformis is one of the immunobullous conditions and characteristically has very intensely pruritic vesicles. It is not usually responsive to topical steroids, but would respond well to dapsone.

It is associated with gluten sensitivity and coeliac disease.

26. Lichen planus and lichenoic drug eruptions

Lichen planus is a skin disorder of unknown aetiology, most probably being immune mediated.

Features of lichen planus

◆ itchy, papular rash most common on the palms, soles, genitalia and flexor surfaces of arms

◆ rash often polygonal in shape, 'white-lace' pattern on the surface ('Wickham's striae')

◆ Koebner phenomenon seen

◆ mucous membrane involvement

◆ nails: thinning of nail plate, longitudinal ridging

Causes of lichenoid drug eruptions

These include gold and quinine.

27. Features of skin disorders associated with pregnancy

Polymorphic eruption of pregnancy

◆ pruritic condition associated with last trimester

◆ lesions often first appear in abdominal striae

◆ management depends on severity: emollients, mild potency topical steroids and oral steroids may be used

Pemphigoid gestationis

◆ pruritic blistering lesions

◆ often develop in peri-umbilical region, later spreading to the trunk, back, buttocks and arms

◆ usually presents 2nd or 3rd trimester and is rarely seen in the first pregnancy

◆ oral corticosteroids are usually required

28. Neurofibromatosis

Neurofibromatosis is a neurocutaneous condition that can involve almost any organ system. Thus, the presenting signs and symptoms may vary widely.

Two major subtypes exist: type 1 neurofibromatosis, also known as von Recklinghausen neurofibromatosis, which is the most common subtype and is referred to as peripheral neurofibromatosis, and type 2 neurofibromatosis, which is referred to as central neurofibromatosis. These descriptions are not especially accurate because type 1 neurofibromatosis often has central features.

Neurofibromatosis is an autosomal dominant disorder that affects the bone, the nervous system, soft tissue, and the skin. NF1 is one of the most common autosomal dominant conditions. However almost half of all cases give no family history and are new mutations. The mutation rate is estimated to be 1 : 10 000 gametes.

Neurofibromatosis is often diagnosed because of unusual pigmentary patterns. The diagnosis is suggested by six or more café au lait macules (spots), each over 5 mm in diameter in prepubescent individuals and over 15 mm in post-pubertal individuals. Café au lait spots are irregularly shaped, evenly pigmented, brown macules. Most individuals with neurofibromatosis have six or more spots that are 1.5 cm or greater in diameter. In young children, five or more café au lait macules greater than 0.5 cm in diameter are suggestive of neurofibromatosis and further diagnostic workup should be pursued. Less than 1% of healthy children have three or more such spots, although one or two café au lait macules are commonly encountered in healthy individuals without disease.

Lisch nodules are hamartomas of the iris that appear dome shaped and are found superficially around the eyes on slit lamp examination. They are asymptomatic, but they help in confirming the diagnosis of neurofibromatosis. Lisch nodules of the iris are present in more than 90% of patients with neurofibromatosis type 1.

Axillary freckling (as well as freckling on the perineum), known as *the Crowe sign*, is a helpful diagnostic feature in neurofibromatosis. Both axillary freckling and inguinal freckling often develop during puberty. The development of freckles often follows the development of café au lait macules, but this precedes the development of neurofibromas.

Eighty per cent of type 1 neurofibromatosis patients have freckling of the axillae. Areas of freckling and regions of hypertrichosis occasionally overlay plexiform neurofibromas.

Neurofibromas are the most common benign tumour of type 1 neurofibromatosis. These tumours are composed of Schwann cells, fibroblasts, mast cells, and vascular components. They can develop at any point along a nerve.

Three subtypes of neurofibroma exist:

✦ cutaneous

✦ subcutaneous, and

✦ plexiform

Both cutaneous lesions and subcutaneous lesions are circumscribed; neither is specific for type 1 neurofibromatosis. These nodules may be brown, pink or skin coloured. They may be soft or firm to the touch, and they may have the pathognomonic buttonhole invagination when pressed with a finger.

Plexiform neurofibromas are non-circumscribed, thick and irregular, and they can cause disfigurement by entwining important supportive structures. The plexiform subtype is specific for type 1 neurofibromatosis.

29. CREST syndrome

Features

CREST syndrome consists of:

✦ **C**alcinosis

✦ **R**aynaud's phenomenon

✦ (o)**E**sophageal dysmotility

✦ **S**clerodactyly

✦ **T**elangiectasia

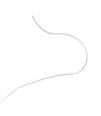

Investigations

ANAs: Limited scleroderma is associated with an early rise in ANA levels, particularly of the immunoglobulin G3 subclass. The overall sensitivity of ANA in systemic sclerosis is 85%, while the specificity is approximately 54%. Serial testing of ANAs to monitor the progress of disease is not currently recommended.

Anticentromere antibodies are found in approximately 50%–90% of patients with limited forms of scleroderma and 82%–96% of patients with the CREST variant. The specificity of this test is 95%.

Anti-Scl-70 (anti-topoisomerase I) antibody is associated with diffuse scleroderma, early internal organ involvement, and a worse prognosis. Perform this laboratory test early in the course of the patient's presentation to determine if the patient is at risk for this type of scleroderma.

Non-specific indicators of inflammation (e.g. mild leucocytosis, normocytic-normochromic anaemia, thrombocytosis, elevated erythrocyte sedimentation rate, elevated C-reactive protein) are rare but may be present in persons with limited scleroderma.

Calcinosis: Evaluate serum calcium and phosphorus levels to exclude a metabolic disturbance; however, calcinosis resulting from limited scleroderma is not associated with calcium or phosphorus abnormalities.

Raynaud's phenomenon: The presence of ANA predicts the development of connective-tissue disease. The positive and negative predictive values of ANA values by immunofluorescence are 65% and 93%, respectively.

Oesophageal dysmotility: Patients who are positive for ANAs and anticentromere antibodies while also being negative for anti-Scl70 antibody appear to have more oesophageal involvement.

Sclerodactyly: A thyrotropin level may help exclude the presence of thyroid disease as another potential cause of edematous or thickened skin.

C. 'Skin failure'

You will not be expected to have a detailed knowledge of the treatment of skin diseases or dermatoses. However, you should know the drugs which cause life-threatening skin conditions.

1. Erythroderma

Erythroderma (*exfoliative dermatitis*) is an erythematous dermatitis characterised by generalised or nearly generalised skin erythema, oedema, scaling, pruritus, and often loss of hair and nail dystrophy.

Causes
Cutaneous

- psoriasis
- atopic dermatitis
- contact dermatitis
- cutaneous T-cell lymphoma (including mycosis fungoides, Sézary syndrome)
- bullous pemphigoid
- pemphigus

Infectious

- dermatophytosis
- toxoplasmosis
- histoplasmosis
- leishmaniasis
- HIV
- Norwegian scabies

Haematology

- Hodgkin and other lymphomas
- leukaemia
- myelodysplasia

Systemic

- sarcoidosis
- SLE
- dermatomyositis
- histiocytosis
- thyrotoxicosis
- acute graft-versus-host disease (acute 'GVHD')
- post-transfusion

Neoplastic

- cancer of thyroid
- lung
- liver
- breast
- ovary and fallopian tube
- prostate
- stomach, oesophagus and rectum
- malignant melanoma

2. Angioedema

Angioedema is characterised by well-circumscribed areas of oedema caused by increased vascular permeability; this condition affects mostly the skin, and the gastrointestinal and respiratory tracts. Patients typically present with acute subcutaneous swelling, usually of the face, extremities or genitalia.

A **generalised anaphylactic reaction** may occur, which is potentially fatal if the upper airway is compromised. Urticaria can be associated with angioedema in 50% of cases; the angioedema is usually non-pruritic but burning. Although often idiopathic, angioedema can be induced by medications, allergens (e.g. food) or physical agents (e.g. vibration, cold).

Typically, 10%–25% of cases are due to angiotensin-converting-enzyme (ACE) inhibitor therapy, occurring in 1–2 per 1000 new users. Penicillins, NSAIDs and radiographic contrast media are other potential triggers.

Angioedema can occur as a result of C1 esterase inhibitor (C1INH) deficiency. Two rare but well-described categories exist: hereditary angioedema, which is transmitted in autosomal-dominant fashion, and acquired angioedema, which can be associated with autoimmune disorders and B-cell lymphoproliferative malignant disease.

Management

Treatment is largely supportive.

Airway patency must be ensured if the respiratory system is involved. Cool, moist compresses and antihistamines can be used to control local burning. Referral to an allergy specialist for appropriate investigations should be considered.

Avoidance of known triggers, such as associated medications, is paramount.

ACE inhibitors are contraindicated in patients with C1INH deficiency. Attenuated androgens danazol and stanozolol increase the amount of active C1INH and are used for the prevention of hereditary angioedema.

3. Stevens-Johnson syndrome/Toxic epidermal necrolysis (TEN)

Signs and symptoms

Toxic epidermal necrolysis (TEN) affects many parts of the body, but it most severely affects the mucous membranes. The severe findings of TEN are often preceded by 1–2 weeks of fever.

These symptoms may mimic those of a common upper respiratory tract infection.

When the rash appears it may be over large and varied parts of the body, and it is usually warm and appears red. The dermal layer fills with fluid being deposited there by the body's immune system, usually as a result of a negative reaction to an antibiotic. The skin then begins to sag from the body and can be peeled off in vast amounts. The mouth can become blistered and eroded.

Causes

Toxic epidermal necrolysis is a rare and usually severe adverse reaction to certain drugs. History of medication use exists in over 95% of patients with TEN.

The drugs most often implicated in TEN are antibiotics, including the following:

* sulphonamides
* NSAIDs
* allopurinol
* antimetabolites (e.g. methotrexate)
* anticonvulsants

The condition might also result from infection with agents such as Mycoplasma pneumonia.

Treatment

The first line of treatment is early withdrawal of culprit drugs, early referral and management in an intensive care unit, supportive management, and nutritional support.

The second line is IVIG. Uncontrolled trials showed promising effect of IVIG on treatment of TEN.

It is currently considered that systemic steroids are unlikely to offer any benefits.

D. Dermatological investigations

(Please also refer to section Q on immunology in Chapter 5.)

You should know the principles but not details of dermatological investigations such as patch testing.

1. Contact allergic dermatitis

There are **two** main types of contact dermatitis:

✦ **Irritant contact dermatitis:** common – non-allergic reaction due to weak acids or alkalis (e.g. detergents). Often seen on the hands. The erythema has a typical appearance, crusting and vesicles are rare.

✦ **Allergic contact dermatitis:** type IV hypersensitivity reaction. Uncommon – often seen on the head following hair dyes. Presents as an acute weeping eczema which predominately affects the margins of the hairline rather than the hairy scalp itself. Topical treatment with a potent steroid is indicated.

Cement is a frequent cause of contact dermatitis. The alkaline nature of cement may cause an irritant contact dermatitis whilst the dichromates in cement also can cause an allergic contact dermatitis.

Hair dye also contains substances which may induce contact allergic dermatitis. This type of reaction is typical for this sort of time scale, and is an example of a type IV, or delayed, hypersensitivity reaction. Sensitisation occurs on initial exposure to the allergen and 'memory' T-cells proliferate in lymphoid tissue. Subsequent exposure to allergen induces activation of the T-lymphocytes and an inflammatory response. Hairdressing chemicals are a very common cause of contact allergic dermatitis, a disorder which is very common amongst the hairdressing community.

You might be expected to know some sketchy details of the dermatology allergy tests (*see* Table 2.4).

TABLE 2.4 Dermatology allergy tests

Skin prick test	Most commonly used test as easy to perform and inexpensive. Drops of diluted allergen are placed on the skin after which the skin is pierced using a needle. A large number of allergens can be tested in one session. Normally includes a histamine (positive) and sterile water (negative) control. A wheal will typically develop if a patient has an allergy. Can be interpreted after 10-15 minutes.
	This method is particularly useful for food allergies and also pollen and wasp/bee venom.
Skin patch testing	Useful for contact dermatitis. Around 30-40 allergens are placed on the back. Irritants may also be tested for. The results are read 48 hours later by a dermatologist.

References

Grattan CEH, Humphreys F. Guidelines for evaluation and management of urticaria in adults and children. *Br J Dermatol.* 2007; **157**(6): 1116–23.

Hanifin JM, Rajka G. Diagnostic features of atopic eczema. *Acta Dermatol Venereol (Stockh).* 1980; **92**: 44–7.

MacDonald Hull SP, Wood ML, Hutchinson PE, *et al.* Guidelines for the management of alopecia areata. *Br J Dermatol.* 2003; **149**(4): 692–9.

Williams HC, Burney PGJ, Strachan D, *et al.* The UK Working Party's diagnostic criteria for atopic dermatitis II: observer variation of clinical diagnosis and signs of atopic dermatitis. *Br J Dermatol.* 1994; **131**(3): 397–405.

Chapter 3

Endocrinology and diabetes

The Foundation Programme and MRCP(UK) Part 1 syllabus (from the JRCPMTB) specify what is required in terms of competencies, skills and knowledge from junior physicians in core medical training in endocrine and diabetes. You are advised to consult carefully this syllabus, which emphasises the importance of basic medical sciences as well as a competent level of applied clinical practice.

ENDOCRINOLOGY

A. Thyroid

> Since thyroid disease is common, you are expected to have a broad knowledge of the mechanisms of thyroid disease, its clinical presentation and treatment.

1. Thyroid hormone biosynthesis and its control

Thyroid hormones contain iodine. Terrestrial vertebrates do not get much, so the thyroid is adapted to trap it. Iodide is trapped and transported into follicular cells, then excreted into the lumen of the follicle. The cell also makes thyroglobulin and exocytoses this into the lumen. The iodide is oxidised by a peroxidase on the luminal surface of the cell. The resulting free iodine reacts non-enzymatically with tyrosine residues of the thyroglobulin in the follicle, a process called iodination.

This forms mono- and diiodotyrosine residues (MIT, DIT), which are coupled together, possibly by the same peroxidase, to form mainly thyroxine (T_4) and some 3,5,3'-triiodothyronine (T_3). This process may be catalysed by the peroxidase, but is certainly helped by the structure of the thyroglobulin molecule.

The follicles may be used to store thyroid hormones. Next, the colloid is pinocytosed back into the cell and the thyroglobulin is split off by proteolysis to leave the free hormone in vesicles that may be exocytosed into the circulation. MIT and DIT that is taken up is recycled within the cell.

Thyroid hormones are water-insoluble, like steroids, so they require specific carrier/binding proteins in the plasma (and in the cell cytosol, to gain access to the nucleus).

Thyroxine binds to thyroxine-binding prealbumin (TBPA) and thyroxine-binding globulin (TBG), especially the latter, which carries 75% of all T_4 and T_3. It also binds to albumin; though the affinity is very low, there's so much albumin around that it carries a fair amount of thyroid hormone. Only about 0.5% of the serum T_4 and 0.3% of the T_3 is in the free state, but this is the physiologically active form (see below).

Iodine deficiency causes thyroid hypertrophy and goitre. Certain drugs can inhibit iodide transport (e.g. thiocyanates). After a while, this causes thyroid hypertrophy and goitre. Some plants contain cyanogenic glucosides (apricots, cherries, almonds, cassava, sweet potato) or thioglucosides (the Brassica family – cabbages, Brussels sprouts, cauliflowers, etc.), both of which are metabolised to thiocyanates.

These plants are therefore dietary goitrogens, and may be responsible for endemic goitre in parts of the world (especially where cassava is a staple food). Other drugs can inhibit different synthetic steps. Even iodine is transiently inhibitory to thyroid function in large doses – mechanism unknown.

2. Auto-immunity and thyroid disease

Graves' disease is an autoimmune disease, in which antibodies are made to the TSH receptor. The antibodies have the property of mimicking the action of TSH, so stimulate the thyroid and cause hyperthyroidism. The exophthalmos (protrusion of the eyes) is not a feature of the hyperthyroidism, but a feature instead of an autoimmune-mediated infiltration behind the eye.

B. Hyperthyroidism

1. De Quervain's thyroiditis

Also called subacute thyroiditis, this is thought to occur following viral infection and typically presents with acute painful thyroid swelling, *thyrotoxicosis*, hypothyroidism followed by return to normal thyroid function.

Features

- hyperthyroidism
- painful goitre
- raised ESR
- globally reduced uptake on iodine-131 scan

Management

- usually self-limiting – most patients do not require treatment
- thyroid pain may respond to aspirin or other NSAIDs. *A short course of non-selective beta-blockers such as propranolol may be used to reduce early symptoms of thyrotoxicosis*
- in more severe cases steroids are used *to shorten the painful, thyrotoxic phase*

[*The steroids may reduce occurrence of hypo, but are no use after the toxic phase.*]

2. Graves' disease

This is the most common cause of thyrotoxicosis in pregnancy. It is also recognised that activation of the TSH receptor by BHCG may also occur – often termed transient gestational hyperthyroidism. HCG levels will fall in second and third trimester.

Features

Features seen in Graves' disease, but not in other causes of thyrotoxicosis:

- eye signs: exophthalmos, ophthalmoplegia
- pretibial myxoedema
- thyroid acropachy

Autoantibodies

◆ anti-TSH receptor stimulating antibodies (90%)

◆ anti-thyroid peroxidase antibodies (50%)

Management

◆ Propylthiouracil has traditionally been the antithyroid drug of choice. This approach was supported by the **2007 UK Endocrine Society consensus guidelines in pregnancy thyrotoxicosis**; more recent alerts from 2009 and 2010 about acute liver dysfunction with propylthiouracil have raised concern about routine use in pregnancy.

◆ Carbimazole/methimazole is still the first-line treatment; treatment courses last 12–18 months after which recrudescence of thyrotoxicosis occurs in 50%–60%; long-term options in relapsing Graves' disease are radioiodine therapy, long-term antithyroid drugs or thyroid surgery.

◆ Maternal free thyroxine levels should be kept in the upper third of the normal reference range to avoid foetal hypothyroidism.

◆ Thyrotrophin receptor stimulating antibodies should be checked at 30–36 weeks' gestation – helps to determine risk of neonatal thyroid problems.

◆ Block-and-replace regimes should not be used routinely in pregnancy; however TSH receptor antibodies can cross the placenta and induce foetal hyperthyroidism and this is the only circumstance that block and replacement therapy is used in pregnancy.

◆ Radioiodine therapy is relatively contraindicated in active thyroid eye disease but may be used if it is quiescent (most cases are after 2–3 years after onset); however oral steroid therapy given with radioiodine therapy while thyroid eye disease is active does reduce exacerbation dramatically.

Despite many trials there is no clear guidance on the optimal management of Graves' disease.

Treatment options include titration of anti-thyroid drugs (for example carbimazole as a first-line and propythiouracil as a second-line), block-and-replace regimes, radioiodine treatment and surgery. Propranolol is often given initially to block adrenergic effects.

Anti-thyroid drug titration

◆ Carbimazole is started at 40 mg and reduced gradually to maintain euthyroidism.

◆ It is typically continued for 12–18 months.

Block-and-replace

◆ Carbimazole is started at 40 mg.

◆ Thyroxine is added when the patient is biochemically euthyroid.

◆ Treatment typically lasts for 12–18 months.

The major complication of carbimazole therapy is agranulocytosis. This occurs in approximately 0.3% of cases, usually within the first 3 months of therapy. It resolves quickly with discontinuation of antithyroid drugs. Patients must be warned to stop therapy and arrange a white cell count check if they have symptoms of sore throat, mouth ulcers or are unwell, particularly with a 'flu-like illness'.

Radioiodine treatment (RAI)

◆ Contraindications include pregnancy (should be avoided for 4–6 months following treatment) and age <16 years. Thyroid eye disease is a relative contraindication, as it may worsen the condition (but can be given with steroid cover).

◆ The proportion of patients who become hypothyroid depends on the dose given, but as a rule the majority of patients will require thyroxine supplementation after 5 years.

◆ It is associated with the induction of hypothyroidism in the majority of subjects by 3 months (70%) with 10% failing at the first dose at about 18 months.

◆ It may precipitate deterioration in ophthalmopathy in patients with Graves' disease.

◆ There is no evidence of either increased risk of infertility or lymphoma after RAI with evidence suggesting that it is quite safe.

◆ Withdrawing amiodarone is the preferred treatment in amiodarone-induced thyrotoxicosis and often the iodine uptake would be low in these patients, making 131-I therapy unhelpful.

3. Amiodarone-induced hyperthyroidism

Despite stopping the amiodarone, thyrotoxicosis may persist for many months and so additional treatment is often required.

Two types of **amiodarone-induced hyperthyroidism** are recognised; the first being a consequence of iodine overload contained within the amiodarone of which the above is a typical example, and the second type is due to an acute thyroiditis with thyroid cell destruction and increased parameters of inflammation. The former is best treated with carbimazole, the latter with prednisolone. Quite often it is not clear at onset which type is present and a mixed aetiology thyrotoxicosis is common. Therefore, concurrent treatment with both steroids and antithyroid drugs are often necessary with revision depending on the response.

C. Hypothyroidism

1. Key points

- Thyroxine is safe during pregnancy.
- Serum thyroid-stimulating hormone measured in each trimester and 6–8 weeks post-partum.
- Approximately 30% of women require an increased dose of thyroxine during pregnancy.
- TSH above 2.0mU/L at conception *or* in the first trimester and >2.6 in the second and third trimesters is associated with reduced foetal cognitive scores. There is no evidence at present to prove that optimisation of TSH prevents reduced foetal cognitive development, but it is common practice to optimise therapy prior to conception in women of child-bearing age.
- Breastfeeding is safe whilst on thyroxine.

Management

- The initial starting dose of levothyroxine should be lower in elderly patients and those with ischaemic heart disease (e.g. starting with 25 mcg/day).
- Following a change in thyroxine dose, thyroid function tests should be checked after 6–8 weeks.
- The therapeutic goal is 'normalisation' of the thyroid-stimulating hormone (TSH) level. As the majority of unaffected people have a TSH value 0.5–2.5 mU/l it is now thought preferable to aim for a TSH in this range.

◆ There is no evidence to support combination therapy with levothyroxine and liothyronine.

Side effects of thyroxine therapy

◆ hyperthyroidism: due to overtreatment

◆ reduced bone mineral density

◆ worsening of angina

◆ atrial fibrillation

D. Thyroid neoplasia

1. Features of hyperthyroidism or hypothyroidism

These features are not commonly seen in patients with thyroid malignancies as they rarely secrete thyroid hormones. These are shown in Table 3.1.

TABLE 3.1 Types of thyroid neoplasia

Type	Percentage	
Papillary	70%	Often young females – excellent prognosis
Follicular	20%	
Medullary	5%	Cancer of parafollicular cells, secrete calcitonin, part of MEN-2
Anaplastic	1%	Not responsive to treatment, can cause pressure symptoms
Lymphoma	Rare	Associated with Hashimoto's disease

Management of papillary and follicular cancer

◆ total thyroidectomy

◆ followed by ablative radioiodine (I-131) to kill residual cells

◆ long-term levothyroxine suppression therapy to keep TSH <0.1mU/L to prevent stimulation of growth of residual thyroid tissue

◆ levothyroxine withdrawal/recombinant human TSH stimulated I-131 whole body uptake scan and thyroglobulin to confirm successful thyroid ablation

◆ yearly thyroglobulin levels while on suppressive levothyroxine to detect early recurrent disease

E. Miscellaneous thyroid syndromes

1. Hashimoto's thyroiditis

Hashimoto's thyroiditis is an autoimmune disorder of the thyroid gland. It is typically associated with hypothyroidism although there may be a transient thyrotoxicosis in the acute phase. It is 10 times more common in women.

Features

◈ features of hypothyroidism

◈ goitre: firm, non-tender

◈ anti-thyroid peroxidase and also anti-thyroglobulin antibodies

2. Sick euthyroid syndrome

In **sick euthyroid syndrome** (now referred to as non-thyroidal illness), it is often said that everything (TSH, thyroxine and T_3) is low. In some cases the TSH level may be normal.

Changes are reversible upon recovery from the systemic illness.

3. Pregnancy and the thyroid gland

In pregnancy, there is an increase in the levels of thyroxine-binding globulin (TBG). This causes an increase in the levels of total thyroxine but does not affect the free thyroxine level.

F. Thyroid investigations

1. Interpretation

The interpretation of thyroid function tests is usually straightforward. A brief guide is given in Table 3.2.

TABLE 3.2 Overview of interpretation of thyroid function tests

	TSH	Free T$_4$	
Thyrotoxicosis (e.g. Graves' disease)	Low	High	In T$_3$ thyrotoxicosis the free T$_4$ will be normal
Primary hypothyroidism (primary atrophic hypothyroidism)	High	Low or normal	
Secondary hypothyroidism	Low or normal	Low	Replacement steroid therapy is required prior to thyroxine
Sick euthyroid syndrome	Low	Low	Common in hospital in-patients
Poor compliance with thyroxine	High	Normal/high	
Steroid therapy	Low	Normal	

G. Hypothalamus/Pituitary/Adrenal axis

[*Detailed knowledge of the structure of the pituitary and hypothalamic hormones is unnecessary.*]

1. The control of pituitary hormone secretion

Growth hormone usually decreases following an elevation in blood glucose after a meal. It is usually increased during sleep or during starvation. It causes both retention of sodium and potassium which are required for growth metabolism. Elevated GH levels increase IGF-1 blood levels. Because IGF-1 levels are much more stable over the course of the day, they are often a more practical and reliable measure than GH levels. Elevated IGF-1 levels almost always indicate acromegaly.

The oral glucose tolerance test is also used to diagnose acromegaly, because ingestion of 75 g of glucose lowers blood GH levels less than 2 ng/ml in healthy people. In patients with acromegaly, this reduction does not occur.

The mechanisms of maintaining plasma osmolality

Vasopressin (anti-diuretic hormone) acts on the distal tubule and collecting ducts to increase permeability to free water. Deficiency of this hormone in diabetes insipidus results in the excretion of dilute urine (increased water clearance) and hypernatraemia.

In a normal response to the water deprivation test the maximum urine osmolality exceeds plasma osmolality and the urine osmolality does not increase >**50%** after administration of vasopressin. The plasma osmolality normal range is 278–300 mOsmol/kg and urine osmolality normal range is 350–1000 mOsmol/kg.

In true *central* diabetes insipidus, patients are unable to concentrate their urine to greater than plasma osmolality but after administration of vasopressin the urine osmolality increases by >50%. Patients with nephrogenic diabetes insipidus are unable to concentrate their urine and they show no response to vasopressin.

In psychogenic diabetes insipidus or compulsive water drinking, fluid deprivation would stop the polyuria. Plasma and urine osmolality (<300 mOsm/kg) should be low in psychogenic diabetes insipidus.

SIADH is confirmed by *a low serum sodium and serum osmolality with an inappropriately* elevated urine osmolality (often above 300 mOsm/kg) and urine sodium concentration (usually above 40 mEq/litre). *Normal renal, liver, thyroid and adrenal function should be confirmed before making this diagnosis.*

2. Acromegaly

Features

In acromegaly there is excess growth hormone secondary to a pituitary adenoma in over 95% of cases. A minority of cases are caused by ectopic GHRH or GH production by tumours, e.g. pancreatic.

- coarse, oily skin, large tongue, prognathism, increased interdental spaces
- spade-like hands, increase in shoe size
- features of pituitary tumour: hypopituitarism, headaches, bitemporal hemianopia
- raised prolactin in ⅓ of cases indicates galactorrhoea
- 6% of patients have MEN-1
- excessive sweating (it appears that the increased sweating relates to sweat gland hyperplasia)

Complications

◆ hypertension

◆ diabetes (>10%)

◆ cardiomyopathy

Investigations

Growth hormone (GH) levels vary during the day and are therefore not diagnostic. The definitive test is the oral glucose tolerance (OGTT) with serial GH measurements. Serum IGF-1 may also be used as a screening test and is sometimes used to monitor disease.

Oral glucose tolerance test

◆ in normal patients GH is suppressed to <2 mu/L with hyperglycaemia

◆ in acromegaly there is no suppression of GH

◆ may also demonstrate impaired glucose tolerance which is associated with acromegaly

A pituitary MRI may demonstrate a pituitary tumour.

Management

Trans-sphenoidal surgery is first-line treatment for acromegaly in the majority of patients.

Dopamine agonists

◆ e.g. bromocriptine

◆ the first effective medical treatment for acromegaly, however now superseded by somatostatin analogues

◆ effective only in a minority of patients

Somatostatin analogue

◆ e.g. octreotide

◆ effective in 50%–70% of patients and may control both GH oversecretion and reduce tumour size and growth

◆ may be used as an adjunct to surgery

Pegvisomant

+ GH receptor antagonist – prevents dimerisation of the GH receptor

+ once daily s/c administration

+ very effective – decreases IGF-1 levels in 90% of patients to normal

+ does not reduce tumour volume therefore surgery still needed if mass effect

External irradiation is sometimes used for older patients or following failed surgical/medical treatment.

3. Hyperprolactinaemia

Prolactin secretion is inhibited by dopaminergic pathway.

Hyperprolactinaemia can be caused by dopamine receptor antagonists (many antipsychotic drugs, e.g. phenothiazines, risperidone, metoclopramide), hypothyroidism, liver or renal failure, pituitary adenoma/acromegaly. It leads to galactorrhoea, oligomenorrhoea, reduced fertility and osteoporosis/osteopenia.

Treatment is with dopamine receptor agonists (bromocriptine, cabergoline). These agents reduce prolactin oversecretion and reduce the size of the tumour mass.

Microprolactinoma: The most frequent symptoms at onset are oligoamenor-rhoea (60%), galactorrhoea (50%) and headaches. Treatment is with dopamine agonists, such as a low dose of bromocriptine.

4. Non-functional pituitary adenoma

May present with headache, visual disturbance (bitemporal hemianopia is classic), or symptoms of pituitary failure.

A minority occur in the context of previously unsuspected MEN-1.

A small rise in prolactin may occur due to disconnection hyperprolactinaemia (interruption of the dopamine signal from the hypothalamus to the anterior pituitary). It may be difficult to distinguish this from a prolactinoma, so surveillance scanning is necessary in either case; non-functional adenomata will not shrink in size with dopamine agonist therapy.

May grow very slowly over years and decades or enlarge aggressively. Monitoring by clinical assessment and surveillance scanning is therefore necessary. If encroaching on the optic chiasm then decompression surgery, usually by the transphenoidal route, may be necessary.

Medical care consists of hormone replacement as appropriate and treatment of the underlying cause.

◆ Glucocorticoids are required if the ACTH-adrenal axis is impaired. This is particularly important in sudden collapse due to pituitary apoplexy or acute obstetric haemorrhage with pituitary insufficiency. In such circumstances, doctors are advised not to delay initiation of a possibly life-saving treatment pending a definitive diagnosis. Treat secondary hypothyroidism with thyroid hormone replacement.

◆ Treat gonadotropin deficiency with sex-appropriate hormones. In men, testosterone replacement is used and modified if the patient desires fertility. In women, oestrogen replacement is used with or without progesterone as appropriate.

◆ GH is replaced in children as appropriate. GH is not routinely replaced in adults unless the patient is symptomatic.

BOX 3.1   A note on pituitary apoplexy

A patient will typically have an acute onset of headache secondary to haemorrhage into the pituitary gland. Biochemically, the patient may have evidence of hypopituitarism given his low random cortisol, with consistent biochemical results of hyponatraemia and hyperkalaemia. A third cranial nerve palsy may be present, due to enlargement of the pituitary causing compression of the third cranial nerve. This is clearly a medical emergency, and requires, under specialists, resuscitation and steroid replacement, urgent imaging of the pituitary gland and consideration of neurosurgical decompression.

You should also refer to acute adrenal insufficiency, p. 136.

H. Adrenal

A detailed knowledge of mechanisms of steroid biosynthesis is not required, but you are expected to have some knowledge of those parts which are clinically important.

1. Corticosteroid synthesis

Glucocorticoids are 21-carbon steroids. You should know that cholesterol (27-carbon, 'C27') is converted to progesterone (C21), which can be converted to adrenocorticosteroids (C21) or androgens (C19). Androgens can be aromatised (by aromatase) to oestrogens.

2. Cushing's syndrome

Causes
ACTH dependent causes

+ Cushing's disease (80%): pituitary tumour secreting ACTH-producing adrenal hyperplasia
+ ectopic ACTH production (5%–10%): e.g. small cell lung cancer
+ carcinoid (Carcinoid tumours of the foregut (such as lung), unlike tumours of the midgut, are not associated with carcinoid syndrome, but may secrete corticotropin-releasing hormone/adrenocorticotropic hormone (CRF/ACTH) resulting in ectopic Cushing's syndrome.)

ACTH independent causes

+ iatrogenic: steroids
+ adrenal adenoma (5%–10%)
+ adrenal carcinoma (*rare*)
+ Carney complex: syndrome including cardiac myxoma
+ micronodular adrenal dysplasia (*very rare*)

Pseudo-Cushing's

+ mimics Cushing's
+ often due to alcohol excess or severe depression
+ causes false positive dexamethasone suppression test or 24-hour urinary-free cortisol

◆ insulin stress test may be used to differentiate but is arguably not reliable as a similar normal rise of cortisol to hypoglycaemia may occur in patients with Cushing's disease; a 48-hour low-dose dexametasone suppression test is more reliable (2 mg/24 h).

Investigations

Investigations are divided into confirming Cushing's syndrome and then localising the lesion. A hypokalaemic metabolic alkalosis may be seen, along with impaired glucose tolerance. Ectopic ACTH secretion (e.g. secondary to small cell lung cancer) is characteristically associated with very low potassium levels. The two most commonly used tests are:

◆ overnight dexamethasone suppression test (most sensitive)

◆ 24-hour urinary-free cortisol

Localisation tests

The first-line localisation is 9 a.m. and midnight plasma ACTH (and cortisol) levels.

If ACTH is suppressed then a non-ACTH dependent cause is likely such as primary adrenal adenoma.

High-dose dexamethasone suppression test

◆ if pituitary source, then cortisol *is usually* suppressed

◆ if ectopic/adrenal, then *usually* no change in cortisol

CRH stimulation

◆ if pituitary source then cortisol rises

◆ if ectopic/adrenal then no change in cortisol

Petrosal sinus sampling of ACTH may be needed to differentiate between pituitary and ectopic ACTH secretion.

3. Hypokalaemia and hypertension

For exams, it is useful to be able to classify the causes of hypokalaemia in to those associated with hypertension, and those which are not.

Hypokalaemia with hypertension

+ Cushing's syndrome
+ Conn's syndrome (primary hyperaldosteronism)
+ Liddle's syndrome

Liddle's syndrome is a rare autosomal dominant condition that causes hypertension and hypokalaemic alkalosis. It is thought to be caused by a disorder of sodium channels in the distal tubules leading to increased re-absorption of sodium.

Treatment is with either amiloride or triamterene.

Carbenoxolone, an anti-ulcer drug, and liquorice excess can potentially cause hypokalaemia associated with hypertension.

4. Hypokalaemia without hypertension

+ diuretics
+ gastrointestinal loss (e.g. diarrhoea, vomiting)
+ renal tubular acidosis (type 1 and 2)
+ Bartter's syndrome
+ Gitelman's syndrome

5. Addison's disease

Autoimmune destruction of the adrenal glands is the commonest cause of hypo-adrenalism in the UK, accounting for 80% of cases.

Features

+ lethargy, weakness, anorexia, nausea and vomiting, weight loss
+ abdominal pain
+ hyperpigmentation, vitiligo, loss of pubic hair in women
+ crisis: collapse, shock, pyrexia

Investigations

In a patient with suspected Addison's disease the definite investigation is a short

ACTH test. Plasma cortisol is measured before and 30 minutes after giving synacthen 250ug i/m or i/v; adrenal autoantibodies such as anti-21-hydroxylase may also be demonstrated.

Associated electrolyte abnormalities:

◈ hyperkalaemia

◈ hyponatraemia

◈ hypoglycaemia

◈ metabolic acidosis

6. Phaeochromocytoma

In a patient with phaeochromocytoma, the history of episodic headaches *associated with paroxysmal sweating and palpitations* may be a key presenting feature. Often the symptoms are vague and rarely is the classical presentation encountered.

A recent review of the histories of 100 patients with proven phaeochromocytoma seen at the Mayo Clinic found that episodic headache was present in 80%. It was usually of rapid onset, bilateral, severe, throbbing, and associated with nausea in about half of the cases.

Phaeochromocytoma is a rare catecholamine-secreting tumour. About 10% are familial and may be associated with MEN type II, neurofibromatosis and von Hippel-Lindau syndrome.

◈ bilateral in 10%

◈ malignant in 10%

◈ extra-adrenal in 10% (most common site = organ of Zuckerkandl, adjacent to the bifurcation of the aorta)

Tests

◈ 24-hour urinary collection of catecholamines (*adrenaline, noradrenaline and dopamine, or catecholamine metabolites depending on the laboratory*)

Treatment

Surgery is the definitive mode of management. The patient must first however be stabilised with medical management:

◈ alpha-blocker (e.g. phenoxybenzamine), given before a

◈ beta-blocker (e.g. propranolol)

I. Ovary, testis and penis

You are expected to be conversant with the physiology of ovarian function and with the conditions presenting to a physician.

1. Hormonal changes across the menstrual cycle

One ovarian cycle is the time between successive ovulations. In humans it is 24–32 days long. (The menstrual cycle begins on the first day of menstruation, so ovulation occurs in the middle of the menstrual cycle, on day ~12.)

The oestrogen-dominated period prior to ovulation is called the follicular phase, since the oestrogens are made by follicles. This lasts 10–14 days.

The progestogen-dominated period after ovulation is called the luteal phase, as progesterone comes from the corpus luteum. This lasts 12–15 days.

Lactotrophs in the anterior pituitary secrete prolactin. Gonadotrophs in the anterior pituitary secrete the glycoprotein gonadotrophic hormones, LH and FSH. Their synthesis and secretion depend on gonadotrophin hormone releasing hormone (GnRH) from the hypothalamus.

Oestradiol normally suppresses LH/FSH secretion (negative feedback). However, if oestradiol levels increase greatly (e.g. 200%–400% more than in the early follicular phase) and remain high for ~48 hours, then LH/FSH secretion is enhanced (positive feedback).

Progesterone, at high concentrations, enhances the negative feedback effects of oestradiol to keep LH/FSH very low. It also prevents the positive feedback effects of oestradiol. Oestradiol and progesterone can act at the pituitary, but also at the hypothalamus. The positive feedback effect of oestradiol occurs because it increases the number of pituitary GnRH receptors.

Follicular phase

At the start of the menstrual cycle, luteal levels of oestrogen and progesterone fall, so negative feedback is relaxed and FSH/LH levels rise. (At this time, the antral phase of follicular growth is occurring and FSH/LH prevents follicular atresia.)

Follicular growth causes the production of oestrogens and inhibin. Oestrogen, androgen, LH and inhibin levels increase; FSH levels fall. In the second half of this phase there is an oestradiol surge, which initiates positive feedback.

This triggers a surge of LH/FSH, which in turn triggers the pre-ovulatory phase. Oestrogen levels then fall precipitously and progesterone levels start to rise. Lacking a continuing positive feedback stimulus, LH/FSH levels drop.

Luteal phase

Progesterone (from the corpus luteum) rises. Oestrogens and androgens are still being made in significant quantities, but the presence of progesterone prevents any positive feedback effect, and enhances the negative feedback effects of oestrogens, so LH and FSH levels reach their lowest point. When luteolysis occurs, both oestrogens and progesterone decline again and LH/FSH levels rise once more.

2. Physiological changes in pregnancy

Human chorionic gonadotrophin (βhCG)

Made by the conceptus within two weeks of fertilisation.

Maintains corpus luteum (immunising against βhCG prevents pregnancy).

Most is made by the syncytiotrophoblast; some from the cytotrophoblast.

Luteinising hormone (LH)

Pituitary LH supports the corpus luteum in (very) early pregnancy. Recall that βhCG is structurally like LH –βhCG supplements the low LH levels.

Transfer of endocrine support. The corpus luteum remains active for the whole of pregnancy, but is not required after 4–5 weeks, because by this time the conceptus is also synthesising all the steroidal hormones required for pregnancy.

After 8 weeks, βhCG levels fall – it is no longer needed.

Oestrogens

The primary oestrogen in pregnancy is oestriol (less potent than oestradiol 17β). The placenta makes progesterone; the foetal adrenal converts this to androgens (notably DHA); the placenta aromatises these to oestrogens.

The 'foeto-placental unit'

- priming agents – for example, induce progesterone receptors
- assist in causing the growth of breasts and uterus
- behavioural effects
- feedback on hypothalamus
- increase uterine blood flow

Progesterone

The trophoblast makes progesterone, and is autonomous. Acts together with oestrogens.

◆ endometrial and myometrial growth

◆ growth of mammary gland, though it prevents secretion

◆ smooth muscle inhibitor – myometrium, vascular smooth muscle, GI smooth muscle. Inhibition of uterine contraction is obviously important in maintaining pregnancy

◆ behavioural effects

◆ negative feedback

◆ stimulates respiratory centre

Prolactin
Pituitary prolactin stimulates breast development and inhibits ovulation. Release is stimulated by oestrogens.

3. The differential diagnosis of virilism
When hirsutism in women is accompanied by other signs of virilism, it may be a manifestation of a more serious underlying disorder causing hyperandrogenism, such as an ovarian tumour or adrenal neoplasm.

The most common causes of clinical hyperandrogenism are:

◆ polycystic ovary syndrome (PCOS)

◆ idiopathic (no other clinical or biochemical abnormalities)

◆ hyperandrogenism

◆ non-classic (late onset) adrenal hyperplasia

◆ androgen-secreting tumours (*of the ovary or adrenal glands*)

4. Causes of amenorrhoea and anovulation
Amenorrhoea can result because of an abnormality in the hypothalamic-pituitary-ovarian axis, anatomical abnormalities of the genital tract, or functional causes.

Hypothalamic causes
◆ craniopharyngioma

◆ teratoma

◆ sarcoidosis

◆ Kallmann syndrome

Nutritional deficiency

◆ low body weight

Pituitary causes

◆ hyperprolactinaemia

◆ other pituitary tumours

◆ post-partum pituitary necrosis (*Sheehan's syndrome*)

◆ autoimmune (*lymphocytic*) hypophysitis

◆ pituitary radiation

◆ sarcoidosis

Ovarian causes

◆ anovulation

◆ hyperandrogenemia

◆ polycystic ovary syndrome

◆ premature ovarian failure

◆ Turner syndrome

◆ pure gonadal dysgenesis

◆ fragile X

◆ radiation or chemotherapy

◆ galactosaemia

◆ anatomical abnormalities of the genital tract

◆ intrauterine adhesions

◆ transverse vaginal septum

◆ aplasia

Functional causes

◆ eating disorders

◆ chronic diseases (e.g. tuberculosis)

◆ excessive weight gain or weight loss

◆ malnutrition

◆ depression or other psychiatric disorders

◆ recreational drug abuse

- psychotropic drug use
- excessive stress
- excessive exercise

5. Causes of anovulation
Hormonal or chemical imbalance

- this is the most common cause of anovulation and is thought to account for about 70% of all cases
- about half the women with hormonal imbalances do not produce enough follicles to ensure the development of an ovule
- in 10% of the cases, alterations in the chemical signals from the hypothalamus can seriously affect the ovaries
- there are other hormonal anomalies with no direct link to the ones mentioned above that can affect ovulation
- functional problem (this accounts for around 10%–15% of all cases of anovulation)
- the ovaries can simply stop working in about 5% of cases
- a significant emotional shock
- luteinised unruptured follicle syndrome
- physical damage to the ovaries
- weight loss or anorexia

6. Polycystic ovarian syndrome
Features and investigations
Features

Polycystic ovary syndrome (PCOS) is a complex condition of ovarian dysfunction thought to affect between 5% and 20% of women of reproductive age.

The aetiology of PCOS is not fully understood.

Both hyperinsulinaemia and high levels of luteinising hormone are seen in PCOS and there appears to be some overlap with the metabolic syndrome.

- subfertility and infertility
- menstrual disturbances: oligomenorrhea and amenorrhoea
- hirsuitism, acne (due to hyperandrogenism)
- obesity
- *acanthosis nigricans* (due to insulin resistance)

Investigations

+ pelvic ultrasound

+ FSH, LH, prolactin, TSH and testosterone are useful investigations: raised LH:FSH ratio is a 'classical' feature but is no longer thought to be useful in diagnosis. Prolactin may be normal or mildly elevated. Testosterone may be normal or mildly elevated – however, if markedly raised consider other causes.

+ Check for impaired glucose tolerance.

Management

Polycystic ovarian syndrome (PCOS) is a complex condition of ovarian dysfunction thought to affect between 5% and 20% of women of reproductive age. Management is complicated and problem based.

General

+ weight reduction if appropriate

+ if a woman requires contraception then a combined oral contraceptive pill (OCP) may help regulate her cycle and induce a monthly bleed (see below)

+ metformin can improve the regularity of the menstrual cycle and improve oligomenorrhoea; it increases fertility in PCOS and increases the chances not only of successful conception but also that of a successful pregnancy

Differential diagnosis of hirsutism and acne

+ An oral contraceptive pill (OCP) may be used to manage hirsutism. Possible options include a third generation OCP which has fewer androgenic effects or cyproterone acetate, which has an anti-androgen action. Both of these types of OCP may carry an increased risk of venous thromboembolism.

+ If this does not respond to OCP then topical eflornithine may be tried.

+ (*Spironolactone, flutamide and finasteride may be used under specialist supervision only.*)

7. Female infertility

Causes of female infertility

Ovulation disorders account for infertility in ¼ of infertile couples.

These can be caused by flaws in the regulation of reproductive hormones by the hypothalamus or the pituitary gland, or by problems in the ovary itself.

It is possible to have an ovulation disorder if you ovulate infrequently or not at all.

- **Abnormal FSH and LH secretion.** The two hormones responsible for stimulating ovulation each month – follicle-stimulating hormone (FSH) and luteinising hormone (LH) – are produced by the pituitary gland in a specific pattern during the menstrual cycle. Excess physical or emotional stress or a very high or very low body weight can disrupt this pattern and affect ovulation. The main sign of this problem is irregular or absent periods. Much less commonly, specific diseases of the pituitary, usually associated with other hormone deficiencies, may be the cause.

- **Polycystic ovarian syndrome (PCOS).** In PCOS, complex changes occur in the hypothalamus, pituitary and ovary, resulting in overproduction of male hormones (androgens), which affects ovulation. PCOS can also be associated with insulin resistance and obesity. Metformin improves fertility in PCOS.

- **Luteal phase defect.** Luteal phase defect happens when the ovaries do not produce enough of the hormone progesterone after ovulation. Progesterone is vital in preparing the uterine lining for a fertilised egg.

- **Premature ovarian failure.** This disorder is usually caused by an autoimmune response, where your body mistakenly attacks ovarian tissues. It results in the loss of the eggs in the ovary, as well as in decreased oestrogen production.

- **Turner's syndrome** with streak ovaries: may be mosaic and the phenotype subtle.

Management

- weight reduction if appropriate
- the management of infertility in patients with PCOS should be supervised by a specialist (there is an ongoing debate as to whether metformin, clomifene or a combination should be used to stimulate ovulation)
- a 2007 trial published in the *New England Journal of Medicine* suggested

clomifene was the most effective treatment (there is a potential risk of multiple pregnancies with anti-oestrogen therapies such as clomifene)

◆ metformin is also used, either combined with clomifene or alone, particularly in patients who are obese

◆ gonadotrophins

The guidelines in the UK for female infertility are currently under review. They include a section on in vitro fertilisation.

Another point of interest is the suggestion that before undergoing uterine instrumentation women should be offered screening for *Chlamydia trachomatis* using an appropriately sensitive technique.

Also, women who are not known to have co-morbidities (such as pelvic inflammatory disease, previous ectopic pregnancy or endometriosis) should be offered hysterosalpingography (HSG) to screen for tubal occlusion because this is a reliable test for ruling out tubal occlusion, and it is less invasive and makes more efficient use of resources than laparoscopy.

8. Testis

> You are not expected to have a detailed knowledge of the urological investigation of infertility but some concept of relevant investigations and of the endocrine aspects of testicular function is required.

The aetiology of hypogonadism both primary and secondary

Male hypogonadism means the testicles don't produce enough of the male sex hormone testosterone. There are two basic types of hypogonadism:

◆ **Primary.** This type of hypogonadism – also known as primary testicular failure – originates from a problem in the testicles. *LH and FSH will be raised with low testosterone.*

◆ **Secondary.** This type of hypogonadism indicates a problem in the hypothalamus or the pituitary gland – parts of the brain that signal the testicles to produce testosterone. The hypothalamus produces gonadotropin-releasing hormone, which signals the pituitary gland to make follicle-stimulating hormone (FSH) and luteinising hormone. Luteinising hormone then signals the testes to produce testosterone. *LH and FSH will be inappropriately low or normal with low testosterone.*

Either type of hypogonadism may be caused by an inherited (congenital) trait or something that happens later in life (acquired), such as an injury or an infection.

9. Primary hypogonadism

Common causes of primary hypogonadism include:

◆ **Klinefelter's syndrome.** This condition results from a congenital abnormality of the sex chromosomes, X and Y. A male normally has one X and one Y chromosome. In Klinefelter's syndrome, two or more X chromosomes are present in addition to one Y chromosome. The Y chromosome contains the genetic material that determines the sex of a child and related development. The extra X chromosome that occurs in Klinefelter syndrome causes abnormal development of the testicles, which in turn results in underproduction of testosterone.

◆ **Mumps orchitis.** If a mumps infection involving the testicles in addition to the salivary glands ('*the mumps orchitis complex*') occurs during adolescence or adulthood, long-term testicular damage may occur. This may affect normal testicular function and testosterone production.

◆ haemochromatosis

◆ injury to the testicles

◆ treatment for cancer

◆ ageing

BOX 3.2   A note on haemochromatosis

Iron deposition can occur in the testes causing primary failure (high LH and FSH). Iron overload may also cause pituitary infiltration and secondary hypo-gonadism (normal or low LH and FSH).

---

10. Secondary hypogonadism

In secondary hypogonadism, the testicles are normal but function improperly due to a problem with the pituitary or hypothalamus. A number of conditions can cause secondary hypogonadism, including:

◆ Kallmann's syndrome. Abnormal development of the hypothalamus – the area of the brain that controls the secretion of pituitary hormones – can cause hypogonadism. This abnormality is also associated with impaired development of the ability to smell (anosmia).

◆ pituitary disorders

◆ inflammatory disease

◆ HIV/AIDS

◆ drugs

◆ obesity

Idiopathic hypogonadotrophic hypogonadism: isolated secondary gonadal failure, a diagnosis of exclusion. Genetic causes can be identified in some cases.

11. Causes of male infertility related to general medical disease and its treatment

◆ impaired production or function of sperm

◆ testosterone deficiency (male hypogonadism)

◆ chromosome defects

◆ infections

◆ hormonal disorders

◆ impaired delivery of sperm. Examples of problems that can interfere with sperm delivery include:

  ● sexual issues

  ● blockage of epididymis or vas deferens

  ● retrograde ejaculation

  ● no sperm in the ejaculate

  ● misplaced urinary opening (hypospadias)

  ● anti-sperm antibodies

  ● cystic fibrosis (men with cystic fibrosis often have a missing or obstructed vas deferens)

- general health and lifestyle
- excessive alcohol and drugs
- tobacco smoking
- emotional stress

Other medical conditions

A severe injury, major surgery or cancer can affect male fertility. Certain diseases or conditions, such as kidney disease, cirrhosis, sickle cell anaemia and coeliac disease can interfere with normal sperm production.

- age (a gradual decline in fertility is common in men older than 35)
- malnutrition
- obesity
- environmental exposure
- cancer and its treatment
- steroid misuse or steroid-induced hypogonadism

BOX 3.3 A note on steroid misuse

Body builders may be involved in the illicit use of anabolic and androgenic steroids. These results are consistent with ongoing use of androgens. The hypogonadism if persistent may be treated with human chorionic gonadotropin. In the event of a non-functioning pituitary tumour, the testosterone would be low together with the luteinising hormone (LH) and follicle-stimulating hormone (FSH) and an MRI of the pituitary would not miss this diagnosis. The growth hormone axis would also be likely to be suppressed, and a low IGF-1 would result.

---

12. Causes of erectile dysfunction and its investigation

Common causes

◆ cardiac disease

◆ atherosclerosis

◆ high blood pressure

◆ diabetes

◆ obesity

◆ metabolic syndrome

Other causes of erectile dysfunction include:

◆ certain prescription medications

◆ tobacco use

◆ alcoholism and other forms of drug abuse

◆ treatments for prostate cancer

◆ Parkinson's disease

◆ multiple sclerosis

◆ hormonal disorders such as low testosterone (hypogonadism)

◆ Peyronie's disease

◆ surgeries or injuries that affect the pelvic area or spinal cord

In some cases, erectile dysfunction is one of the first signs of an underlying medical problem, but in other cases it is a sign of an underlying psychological disturbance.

Investigations

◆ ultrasound

◆ neurological evaluation

◆ dynamic infusion cavernosometry and cavernosography (DICC).

◆ nocturnal tumescence test

J. Growth

1. Importance of growth

Growth is a very important topic in relation to general medicine as well as endocrinology.

Short stature refers to any person who is significantly below the average height for a person of the same age and sex.

The term often refers to children or adolescents who are significantly below the average height of their peers.

Considerations

A **growth chart** is used to compare a child's current height and how fast he or she is growing to other children of the same age and gender (male or female). A measurement called standard deviation (SD) is used. If a child's height is more than 2 SDs below the average height, the child is thought to have short stature.

Many parents become worried if their children are shorter than most or all of the children around them. However, short stature is not necessarily a symptom or sign of a health problem. Two relatively short but healthy parents may have an entirely healthy child who is in the shortest 5%.

On the other hand, short stature may be a symptom caused by a medical condition. Because many of these conditions are treatable, the person should be examined by a healthcare provider. The rate of growth over time is important in determining the cause.

Causes

Short stature may be due to a number of medical conditions or problems, including:

- growth hormone deficiency
- chronic diseases such as congenital heart disease, kidney diseases, asthma, sickle cell anaemia, thalassaemia, juvenile rheumatoid arthritis, inflammatory bowel disease, coeliac disease, Cushing's disease, hypothyroidism and diabetes
- genetic conditions such as Down's syndrome, Turner's syndrome and Noonan syndrome
- bone or skeletal disorders such as rickets or achondroplasia
- problems related to pregnancy, such as infections of the foetus before birth, poor growth of a baby while in the womb (intrauterine growth restriction), or born small for gestational age

- panhypopituitarism
- delayed puberty (causes temporary short stature, but children eventually grow to normal height)
- precocious puberty
- malnutrition
- psychological deprivation

Short stature that has no medical cause (idiopathic short stature) can be due to a family history of short stature (children are short but are expected to reach the height of one or both parents).

Constitutional growth delay is an important cause, however (this is normal growth until close to 12 months of age that slows afterward, puberty is delayed, adult height will eventually be in the expected range calculated from the parents' height).

Differential diagnosis of tall stature

1. Familial tall stature
2. Syndromes associated with tall stature:
   - Klinefelter's syndrome
   - XXXY, XYY syndromes overgrowth syndromes
   - hyperinsulinism
   - Marfan's syndrome
   - MEN 2B
   - ACTH resistance
   - homocystinuria
3. Tall stature of endocrine origin
   - GH secreting pituitary tumour
   - precocious puberty
   - hyperthyroidism
4. Simple obesity

2. Complications of growth hormone therapy

Known risks of GH therapy overall are few and rare. Most of the complications have been reported in children over 10 years of age or in adults. Though rare, the following harmful side effects have been reported during GH treatment often enough to be assumed:

◆ 'slipped capital femoral epiphysis' (SCFE)

◆ pseudotumour cerebri (also known as benign intracranial hypertension)

◆ pancreatitis

◆ joint pains

◆ carpal tunnel syndrome

K. Calcium

1. Control of calcium metabolism

Parathyroid hormone (PTH) acts to increase plasma Ca^{2+} concentration.

The only control mechanism is plasma Ca^{2+}. High levels depress PTH secretion, low levels stimulate it. There is a 'calcium sensor' on the chief cells (G-protein-coupled receptor).

Calcitonin is a 32-amino acid peptide hormone made by parafollicular cells ('C cells') of the thyroid gland. Calcitonin acts to decrease plasma Ca^{2+}. It is not essential.

No diseases are attributable to deficiency or excess. Its role is to 'prevent hypercalcaemia' – without calcitonin, experimental animals given a calcium infusion cannot bring calcium levels down to normal as fast as normal animals can. It inhibits osteoclasts, directly, thus lowering blood Ca^{2+}. Its effects are via the cAMP pathway.

Bone is the only important target site. Calcitonin is released in response to elevated plasma Ca^{2+}, and release is also stimulated by gut hormones (including gastrin, CCK) – this may help to lower blood Ca^{2+} in anticipation of Ca^{2+} absorption. Calcitonin assists in moving calcium into bone after a meal, preventing postprandial hypercalcaemia.

2. Causes of hypercalcaemia

These include:

◆ Overactivity of parathyroid glands. The primary cause of hypercalcaemia is overactivity in one or more of your four parathyroid glands (primary hyperparathyroidism).

◆ Cancer. Certain types of cancer, particularly lung cancer and breast cancer, as well as some cancers of the blood, such as multiple myeloma, increase the risk of hypercalcaemia.

◆ Other diseases. Some diseases that produce areas of inflammation due to tissue injury (granulomas) may raise blood levels of vitamin D (calcitriol). Granulomatous diseases including tuberculosis and sarcoidosis are also well-known causes.

◆ Medications. Certain drugs, such as lithium, which is used to treat bipolar disorder, may increase the release of parathyroid hormone and cause hypercalcaemia. Thiazide diuretics can cause elevated calcium levels in the blood by decreasing the amount of calcium lost in the urine.

◆ Supplements. Excessive intake of calcium or vitamin D supplements over time can raise calcium levels in the blood above normal.

◆ Dehydration. A common cause of mild or transient hypercalcaemia is dehydration, because when there is less fluid in your blood, calcium concentrations rise.

3. Primary hyperparathyroidism

In exams, **primary hyperparathyroidism** is stereotypically seen in elderly females with an unquenchable thirst and an inappropriately normal or raised parathyroid hormone level. It is most commonly due to a solitary adenoma.

Causes

◆ 80%: solitary adenoma

◆ 15%: hyperplasia

◆ 4%: multiple adenoma

◆ 1%: carcinoma

Features

'bones, stones, abdominal groans and psychic moans'

- polydipsia, polyuria
- peptic ulceration/constipation/pancreatitis
- bone pain/fracture
- renal stones
- depression
- hypertension

Associations

- hypertension
- multiple endocrine neoplasia: MEN I and II

Investigations

- raised calcium, low phosphate
- PTH may be raised or normal
- 24-hour urine calcium output (to exclude familial hypocalciuric hypercalcaemia)
- technetium-MIBI subtraction scan

Treatment

- total parathyroidectomy is indicated if: severe hypercalcaemia, osteoporosis, renal calculi or if 24-hour urine calcium is >10mmol/24h

4. Multiple endocrine neoplasia

Table 3.3 summarises the three main types of multiple endocrine neoplasia (MEN).

TABLE 3.3 The MEN syndromes

MEN type I	MEN type IIa	MEN type IIb
Mnemonic *'three P's'*: • parathyroid (95%): hyperparathyroidism due to parathyroid hyperplasia • pituitary (70%) • pancreas (50%, e.g. insulinoma, gastrinoma) • also: adrenal and thyroid	• phaeochromocytoma (95%) • medullary thyroid cancer (70%) • parathyroid (60%)	• medullary thyroid cancer • phaeochromocytoma • marfanoid body habitus • neuromas
MEN1 gene	RET oncogene	RET oncogene
Most common presentation = hypercalcaemia		

The presence of hyperprolactinaemia with hypogonadotrophic hypogonadism suggests a diagnosis of a microprolactinoma and in combination with the recurrent dyspepsia a diagnosis of multiple endocrine neoplasia (MEN) type 1 should be considered.

5. Osteopetrosis

Osteopetrosis is a clinical syndrome characterised by the failure of osteoclasts to resorb bone. As a consequence, bone modelling and remodelling are impaired. The defect in bone turnover characteristically results in skeletal fragility despite increased bone mass, and it may also cause haematopoietic insufficiency, disturbed tooth eruption, nerve entrapment syndromes, and growth impairment.

The primary underlying defect in all types of osteopetrosis is failure of the osteoclasts to reabsorb bone. A number of heterogeneous molecular or genetic defects can result in impaired osteoclastic function. The exact molecular defects or sites of these mutations are largely unknown.

History

Approximately one half of patients are asymptomatic, and the diagnosis is made incidentally, often in late adolescence because radiologic abnormalities start appearing only in childhood. In other patients, the diagnosis is based on family history. Still other patients might present with osteomyelitis or fractures.

Many patients have bone pains. Bony defects are common and include neuropathies due to cranial nerve entrapment (e.g. with deafness, with facial palsy), carpal tunnel syndrome and osteoarthritis. Bones are fragile and might fracture easily. Approximately 40% of patients have recurrent fractures.

Other manifestations include visual impairment due to retinal degeneration and psychomotor retardation.

Management
The goals of pharmacotherapy are to reduce morbidity and to prevent complications. Some of the medications include vitamin-D supplements, corticosteroids, interferon and erythropoietin. However, other treatment modalities may be useful. For example, in adult osteopetrosis, surgical treatment may be needed for aesthetic or for functional reasons. Severe, related degenerative joint disease may warrant surgical intervention as well.

6. The mechanisms of osteomalacia
Osteomalacia results from inadequate mineralisation of osteoid. The biochemical features are: elevated alkaline phosphatase, hypocalcaemia, and hypophosphataemia. The childhood equivalent is rickets. It is usually caused by a lack of vitamin D availability or metabolism.

Vitamin D deficiency
+ dietary
+ lack of sun exposure
+ malabsorption
+ gastrectomy
+ small bowel disease
+ pancreatic insufficiency

Defective 25-hydroxylation
+ liver disease
+ anticonvulsant treatment

Loss of vitamin D binding protein

◆ nephrotic syndrome

Defective 1 α-hydroxylation

◆ hypoparathyroidism
◆ chronic renal failure

Defective target-organ resistance

◆ Vitamin D-dependent rickets (type I)

Mineralisation defects

◆ abnormal matrix
◆ *osteogenesis imperfecta*
◆ chronic renal failure
◆ enzyme deficiencies
◆ hypophosphatasia

Inhibitors of mineralisation

◆ aluminium
◆ fluoride
◆ bisphosphonates

Phosphate deficiency

◆ decreased GI intake
◆ antacids
◆ impaired renal absorption
◆ Fanconi syndrome
◆ X-linked phosphatemic rickets

7. Hyperparathyroidism, both primary and secondary

Signs

Primary hyperparathyroidism

* signs of dehydration due to hypercalcaemia, such as tenting of skin, prolonged capillary refill time and dry mucous membranes
* bradycardia, with or without irregular heartbeat
* decreased muscle tone and somnolence

Secondary hyperparathyroidism

* skeletal deformity
* decreased muscle tone
* bone pain on palpation
* short stature

Causes

Primary hyperparathyroidism has an underlying genetic basis.

Secondary hyperparathyroidism may develop as a response to hypocalcaemia caused by intestinal disease resulting in calcium and vitamin D malabsorption.

* chronic renal insufficiency
* insufficient vitamin D and calcium intake: insufficient intake in children may cause rickets
* iatrogenic causes such as lithium administration, may decrease the ability of circulating levels of calcium that are within the reference range to suppress PTH secretion (the mechanism for this is currently unclear)

8. Hypoparathyroidism
Primary hypoparathyroidism

◆ decrease PTH secretion

◆ e.g. secondary to thyroid surgery

◆ low calcium, high phosphate

◆ treat with alphacalcidol

Pseudohypoparathyroidism

◆ target cells being insensitive to PTH

◆ due to abnormality in a G protein

◆ associated with low IQ, short stature, shortened 4th and 5th metacarpals

◆ low calcium, high phosphate, high PTH

◆ diagnosis is made by measuring urinary cAMP and phosphate levels
following an infusion of PTH

In hypoparathyroidism this will cause an increase in both cAMP and phosphate levels. In pseudohypoparathyroidism type I neither cAMP nor phosphate levels are increased whilst in pseudohypoparathyroidism type II only cAMP rises.

Pseudopseudohypoparathyroidism

◆ similar phenotype to pseudohypoparathyroidism but normal biochemistry

9. Autoimmune polyendocrinopathy syndrome
There are two distinct types of **autoimmune polyendocrinopathy syndrome** (APS), with type 2 (sometimes referred to as *Schmidt's syndrome*) being much more common.

APS type 2 has a polygenic inheritance and is linked to HLA DR3/DR4. Patients have Addison's disease plus either:

◆ type 1 diabetes mellitus

◆ autoimmune thyroid disease

APS type 1 is occasionally referred to as Multiple Endocrine Deficiency Autoimmune Candidiasis (MEDAC).

It is a very rare autosomal recessive disorder caused by mutation of AIRE1 gene on chromosome 21.

Features of APS type 1 (two out of three needed)

✦ chronic mucocutaneous candidiasis (typically first feature as young child)

✦ Addison's disease

✦ primary hypoparathyroidism

Vitiligo can occur in both types.

10. The prophylaxis and treatment of osteoporosis

> The NICE practice guidance, for the primary and secondary prevention of osteo-porosis, has been in a continual state of evolution between 2008 and 2011. You should note, also, that the SIGN publication number 71 (2003) provides useful details too.

Some key points are as follows.

Risk factors for osteoporosis

✦ Patients who have suffered one or more fragility fractures should be priority targets for investigation and treatment of osteoporosis.

✦ Use of family history in assessing risk of osteoporosis should include maternal, paternal and sister history.

✦ Smokers should be considered at greater risk of osteoporosis than non-smokers, and advised to stop, for this and other reasons.

Measurement, diagnosis and monitoring

✦ Conventional radiographs should not be used for the diagnosis or exclusion of osteoporosis.

✦ When plain films are interpreted as 'severe osteopaenia' it is appropriate to suggest referral for dual-energy X-ray absorptiometry (DEXA).

✦ Bone mineral density (BMD) should normally be measured by DEXA scanning performed on two sites, preferably anteroposterior spine and hip.

✦ Repeat measurements should only be performed if they influence treatment.

✦ Evidence of existing vertebral deformity should be used to modify the hip fracture risk estimated from age, sex and BMD.

◈ Biochemical markers of bone turnover should have no role in the diagnosis of osteoporosis or in the selection of patients for BMD measurement.

Non-pharmacological interventions

◈ High-intensity strength training is recommended as part of a management strategy for osteoporosis.

◈ Low-impact weight-bearing exercise is recommended as part of a management strategy for osteoporosis.

◈ Postmenopausal women should aim for a dietary intake of 1000 mg calcium per day.

Pharmacological management

For postmenopausal women with osteoporosis determined by axial DEXA, with or without previous non-vertebral fracture

To reduce fracture risk at all sites: treatment with either oral alendronate (10 mg daily or 70 mg once weekly + calcium $\pm$ vitamin D) or oral risedronate (5 mg daily or 35 mg once weekly + calcium $\pm$ vitamin D). Parenteral long-acting bisphosphonates are sometime used.

DIABETES

L. Background to diabetes

1. Introduction to diabetes mellitus

Aetiology and genetics of diabetes

The aetiological types designate defects, disorders or processes which often result in diabetes mellitus.

Type 1

Type 1 indicates the processes of beta-cell destruction that may ultimately lead to diabetes mellitus in which insulin is required for survival to prevent the development of ketoacidosis, coma and death. An individual with a Type 1 process may be metabolically normal before the disease is clinically manifest, but the process of beta-cell destruction can be detected. Type 1 is usually characterised by the presence of anti-GAD, islet cell or insulin antibodies which identify the autoimmune processes that lead to beta-cell destruction. In some subjects with this clinical form of diabetes, particularly non-Caucasians, no evidence of an auto-immune disorder is demonstrable and these are classified as 'Type 1 idiopathic'.

In general, Type 1 diabetes is considered as a complex genetic trait, i.e. not only do multiple genetic loci contribute to susceptibility, but environmental factors also play a major role in determining risk. A large body of evidence indicates that inherited genetic factors influence both susceptibility and resistance to the disease.

The armed forces, working offshore or aboard ships, air piloting, jobs which require an HGV/PSV license, policing, fire fighting or driving in the post office are career paths closed to subjects with Type 1 diabetes mellitus. Some local authorities do permit licenses to taxi drivers with insulin-treated diabetes whilst others do not.

BOX 3.4   A note on adhesive capsulitis

Adhesive capsulitis (frozen shoulder) is strongly associated with diabetes with as many as 40% of patients developing this problem at some stage. The restricted active and passive movements confirm that this patient's problems are either capsular or articular in origin rather than periarticular tendon problems where active movements are generally more restricted than passive movements. The shoulder joint is rarely affected by primary osteoarthritis.

Type 2

Type 2 is the most common form of diabetes and is characterised by disorders of insulin action and insulin secretion, either of which may be the predominant feature. Both are usually present at the time that this form of diabetes is clinically manifest. By definition, the specific reasons for the development of these abnormalities are not yet known. *In contrast to type 1 diabetes, a positive family history is very common.*

Maturity-onset diabetes of the young ('MODY') is characterised by the development of type 2 diabetes mellitus in patients <25 years old. It is typically inherited as an autosomal dominant condition. Over six different genetic mutations have so far been identified as leading to MODY. Ketosis is not a feature at presentation.

MODY 3

◆ 60% of cases

◆ due to a defect in the HNF-1α gene

MODY 2

◆ 20% of cases

Other specific types

These are currently less common causes of diabetes mellitus, but are those in which the underlying defect or disease process can be identified in a relatively specific manner. They include, for example, fibrocalculous pancreatopathy, a form of diabetes which was formerly classified as one type of malnutrition-related diabetes mellitus.

M. Key issues in diabetes

1. Diabetes and pregnancy

Diabetes mellitus may be a pre-existing problem or develop during pregnancy (gestational diabetes). It complicates around 1 in 40 pregnancies.

Risk factors for gestational diabetes

◆ BMI of >30 kg/m^2

◆ previous macrosomic baby weighing 4.5 kg or above

◆ previous gestational diabetes

◆ first-degree relative with diabetes

◆ family origin with a high prevalence of diabetes (South Asian, black Caribbean and Middle Eastern)

Screening for gestational diabetes

◆ If a woman has had gestational diabetes previously an oral glucose tolerance test (OGTT) should be performed at 16–18 weeks and at 28 weeks if the first test is normal.

◆ Women with any of the other risk factors should be offered an OGTT at 24–28 weeks.

Management

NICE has issued guidelines (2008) on the management of diabetes mellitus in pregnancy that includes weight loss for women with BMI of >27 kg/m^2

- stop oral hypoglycaemic agents, apart from metformin, and commence insulin
- folic acid 5 mg/day from pre-conception to 12 weeks' gestation
- detailed anomaly scan at 18–20 weeks including four-chamber view of the heart and outflow tracts
- tight glycaemic control reduces complication rates
- treat retinopathy as can worsen during pregnancy

Women who develop gestational diabetes should stop taking hypoglycaemic medication following delivery. A fasting glucose should be checked at the 6-week post-natal check.

Diagnosis

The following information is based on the **World Health Organisation 2006 guidelines**. If the patient is symptomatic:

◆ fasting glucose greater than or equal to 7.0 mmol/L

◆ random glucose greater than or equal to 11.1 mmol/L (or after 75 g oral glucose tolerance test)

In an asymptomatic individual, a single sample alone is not sufficient for diagnosis.

◆ Diabetes can be diagnosed if separate fasting samples read above 7 mmol/L.

◆ 75 gram oral glucose test (OGT) is still the gold standard for diagnosing diabetes, although fasting glucose can be used, provided adequate fast is ensured.

◆ Fasting glucose of above 6.1 but below 6.9 is classed as impaired fasting glycaemia, which is a new category of glycaemia. IGT = 7.8 – 11.1.

2. Long-term complications of diabetes

Glycosylated haemoglobin

Glycosylated haemoglobin (HbA1c) is the most widely used measure of long-term glycaemic control in diabetes mellitus. HbA1c is produced by the glycosylation of haemoglobin at a rate proportional to the glucose concentration. The level of HbA1c therefore is dependent on:

◆ red blood cell lifespan

◆ average blood glucose concentration

HbA1c is generally thought to reflect the blood glucose over the previous '2–3 months' although there is some evidence it is weighed more strongly to glucose levels of the past 2–4 weeks.

The relationship between HbA1c and average blood glucose is complex but has been studied by the **Diabetes Control and Complications Trial (DCCT).** A new internationally standardised method for reporting HbA1c has been developed by the International Federation of Clinical Chemistry (IFCC). This reports HbA1c in mmol per mol of haemoglobin without glucose attached and has been introduced from mid-2009. This is shown in Table 3.4.

TABLE 3.4 The new standardised method of reporting the HbA1c

HbA1c (%)	Average plasma glucose (mmol/L)	IFCC-HbA1c (mmol/mol)
5	5.5	
6	7.5	42
7	9.5	53
8	11.5	64
9	15	75
10	15.5	
11	17.5	
12	19.5	

From the above one may deduce that average plasma glucose = $(2 \times \text{HbA1c}) - 4.5$.

Diabetic nephropathy
Screening

◈ all patients should be screened annually

◈ albumin : creatinine ratio (ACR) in early morning specimen

◈ ACR >2.5 = microalbuminuria

Management

◈ dietary protein restriction

◈ tight glycaemic control

◈ BP control: aim for <130/80 mmHg

◈ benefits independent of blood pressure control have been demonstrated for ACE inhibitors and angiotensin II receptor blockers – these may be used alone or in combination

◈ control dyslipidaemia, e.g. statins

◈ aspirin

Diabetic neuropathy
NICE gives the following guidance for the management of neuropathic pain in diabetes:

◈ first-line: tricyclic antidepressants

◈ second-line: duloxetine, gabapentin or pregabalin

◈ other options: opioid analgesia, pain management clinic

Gastroparesis

◆ symptoms include erratic blood glucose control, bloating and vomiting

◆ management options include metoclopramide, domperidone or erythromycin (prokinetic agents)

Diabetic retinopathy

Diabetic retinopathy is the most common cause of blindness in adults aged 35–65 years old. Hyperglycaemia is thought to cause increased retinal blood flow and abnormal metabolism in the retinal vessel walls. This precipitates damage to endothelial cells and pericytes.

Endothelial dysfunction leads to increased vascular permeability which causes the characteristic exudates seen on fundoscopy. Pericyte dysfunction predisposes to the formation of microaneurysms. Neovasculisation is thought to be caused by the production of growth factors in response to retinal ischaemia.

In exams, you are most likely to be asked about the characteristic features of the various stages/types of diabetic retinopathy. Recently a new classification system has been proposed, dividing patients into those with non-proliferative diabetic retinopathy (NPDR) and those with proliferative retinopathy (PDR) (*see* Table 3.5).

TABLE 3.5 Types of retinopathy

Traditional classification	New classification
Background retinopathy	**Mild NPDR**
• microaneurysms (dots)	• 1 or more microaneurysm
• blot haemorrhages (= 3)	
• hard exudates	
Pre-proliferative retinopathy	**Moderate NPDR**
• cotton wool spots (soft exudates; ischaemic nerve fibres)	• microaneurysms
• >3 blot haemorrhages	• blot haemorrhages
• venous beading/looping	• hard exudates
• deep/dark cluster haemorrhages	• cotton wool spots, venous beading/looping and intraretinal microvascular abnormalities (IRMA) less severe than in severe NPDR
• more common in Type I DM, treat with laser photocoagulation	

(*continued*)

Traditional classification	New classification
	Severe NPDR
	• blot haemorrhages and microaneurysms in 4 quadrants
	• venous beading in at least 2 quadrants
	• IRMA in at least 1 quadrant

Proliferative retinopathy

◆ retinal neovascularisation – may lead to vitrous haemorrhage

◆ fibrous tissue forming anterior to retinal disc

◆ more common in Type I DM, 50% blind in 5 years

Maculopathy

◆ based on location rather than severity, anything is potentially serious

◆ hard exudates and other 'background' changes on macula

◆ check visual acuity

◆ more common in Type II DM

3. Management of diabetic emergencies
Diabetic ketoacidosis

The most common precipitating factors of **diabetic ketoacidosis** (DKA) are infection, missed insulin doses and myocardial infarction.

  American Diabetes Association diagnostic criteria are as follows:

◆ blood glucose >18 mmol/L

◆ pH <7.30

◆ serum bicarbonate <18 mmol/L

◆ anion gap >10

◆ ketonaemia

Management

◆ fluid replacement: most patients with DKA are deplete around 5–8 litres; isotonic saline is used initially

◆ insulin: an intravenous infusion should be started at 6u/hour; once blood glucose is <15 mmol/L an infusion of 5% dextrose should be started

◆ correction of hypokalaemia

◆ bicarbonate infusion (the role of this is controversial in the management of DKA; however, most authorities agree that a bicarbonate infusion may be used in subjects with a severe metabolic acidosis (pH less than 7))

The typical fluid deficit associated with DKA is approximately 6 litres. The initial half of this amount is derived from intracellular fluid and precedes signs of dehydration, while the other half is from extracellular fluid and is responsible for clinical signs of dehydration.

Appropriate fluid replacement requires 1 litre of normal saline over the first ½ hour, then 1 litre over the next hour, then 1 litre over the next 2 hours followed by 1 litre every 4 hours depending on the degree of dehydration.

Current guidelines suggest continuing to use basal/long-acting insulin while patients are on sliding scale insulin – this helps to get patients off the sliding scale earlier.

There is a major national UK safety initiative to prevent cerebral oedema in younger patients with DKA. The occurrence of cerebral oedema in those under 18 is much higher than in older age groups. The mortality of this condition is high. Many units have either adapted their adult DKA protocols for those under 18, or advocate the use of the **British Society for Paediatric Endocrinology and Diabetes SKA guidelines** for those under 18 years old. The principles of this are to ensure that insulin is only commenced 1 hour after IV fluid is commenced, that IV fluid volumes are carefully controlled according to needs and more slowly replaced and that intensive monitoring is used to prevent too rapid correction of blood sugars.

Complications of DKA and its treatment
◆ gastric stasis
◆ cerebral oedema
◆ thromboembolism
◆ acute respiratory distress syndrome
◆ acute renal failure

4. Non-acidotic hyperosmolar coma/severe hyperglycaemia

Management of diabetes in obese type 2 diabetic patients

An obese type 2 diabetic patient is almost certain to be insulin resistant.

Current guidelines suggest that first-line therapy in obese, insulin-resistant patients should be an insulin-sensitising agent.

Metformin is the drug of choice in this patient therefore. In patients intolerant of metformin, pioglitazone is licensed for monotherapy for insulin-resistant patients. It should however be avoided in patients who have a history of heart failure, because of the risk of fluid retention, and is associated with increased risk of bone fracture.

Management of hyperglycaemia in type 2 diabetes mellitus

The ADA-EASD consensus algorithm and **NICE guidance** emphasise the value of early and intensive treatment with specialist input from the beginning. It proposes that an HbA1c >7% is a 'call to action' to initiate or change therapy.

Treatment should be individualised and holistic, aiming to bring glycaemic control as near to normal as possible (e.g. HbA1c 6.5–7.5%) where practical, appropriate and free from significant hypoglycaemia. Two recent studies suggest that mortality may rise with diabetes control to <6.5%.

The structure of the algorithm and selection of therapies is mindful of the long-term progressive nature of type 2 diabetes, the problem of weight control and attendant cardiovascular risk.

Initial intervention is recommended to include both lifestyle modification and metformin therapy, provided the latter is not contraindicated and titrated for optimum tolerability and efficacy.

If glycaemic control is not achieved (within 2–3 months) or sustained then move promptly to additional medication which is likely to be a sulphonylurea or a thiazolidinedione. Where oral therapy is inadequate, or hyperglycaemia is marked (e.g. HbA1c >8.5%) or causing symptoms, then basal insulin therapy is advised. Clear guidance for the initiation and intensification of insulin regimens is given along with opinion on cautions and monitoring.

Differential diagnosis and treatment of hypoglycaemia

Causes and features

Over-treating with anti-diabetes agents is by far the most significant cause, but also note the possibility of an insulinoma, where there is an increased ratio of pro-insulin to insulin of hypoglycaemia: typically early in morning or just before meal, e.g. diplopia, weakness, etc. A popular examination is the self-administration of insulin/sulphonylureas.

A patient with an insulinoma might present with a history of weight gain and intermittent sweating.

Note also these causes:

+ liver failure
+ Addison's disease
+ alcohol

Features include:

+ rapid weight gain may be seen
+ high insulin, raised proinsulin:insulin ratio
+ high C-peptide

Diagnosis

+ supervised, prolonged fasting (up to 72 hours)
+ endoscopic ultrasound
+ CT pancreas

(In MRCP(UK) Part 1, also look out for a patient who has features of spontaneous hypoglycaemia which is relieved by eating and precipitated by fasting and exercise. The most relevant investigation to prove or disprove this would be a 72-hour fast which has a virtual 99% sensitivity. If proven then further investigation for an insulinoma or factitious hypoglycaemia is warranted.)

Other possible causes in children: nesidioblastosis – beta cell hyperplasia.

General principles of type 2 diabetes management

NICE updated its guidance on the management of type 2 diabetes mellitus (T2DM) in 2009. Key points are listed below.

Dietary advice

+ encourage high-fibre, low glycaemic index sources of carbohydrates
+ include low-fat dairy products and oily fish
+ control the intake of foods containing saturated fats and trans fatty acids

♦ limited substitution of sucrose-containing foods for other carbohydrates is allowable, but care should be taken to avoid excess energy intake

♦ discourage use of foods marketed specifically at people with diabetes

♦ initial target weight loss in an overweight person is 5%–10%

HbA1c

♦ The general target for patients is 6.5%. HbA1c levels below 6.5% should not be pursued.

♦ However, individual targets should be agreed with patients to encourage motivation.

♦ HbA1c should be checked every 2–6 months until stable, then 6-monthly.

Blood pressure

♦ target is <140/80 mmHg (or <130/80 mmHg if end-organ damage is present)

♦ ACE inhibitors are first-line

The NICE treatment algorithm has become much more complicated following the introduction of new therapies for type 2 diabetes. Below is a very selected group of points from the algorithm:

♦ NICE still suggest a trial of lifestyle interventions first.

♦ Usually metformin is first-line, followed by a sulphonylurea if the HbA1c remains >6.5%.

♦ If the patient is at risk from hypoglycaemia (or the consequences of) then a DPP-4 inhibitor or thiazolidinedione should be considered rather than a sulphonylurea.

♦ Meglitinides (insulin secretagogues) should be considered for patients with an erratic lifestyle.

♦ If HbA1c >7.5% then consider human insulin.

♦ Metformin treatment should be continued after starting insulin.

♦ Exenatide should be used only when insulin would otherwise be started, obesity is a problem (BMI >35 kg/m²) and the need for high-dose insulin is likely. (Continue only if beneficial response occurs and is maintained (>1.0 percentage point HbA1c reduction in 6 months and weight loss >5% at 1 year).)

Starting insulin

+ usually commenced if HbA1c >7.5%
+ NICE recommend starting with human NPH insulin (isophane, intermediate acting) taken at bed-time or twice daily according to need

Other risk factor modification

+ aspirin to all patients >50 years and to younger patients with other significant risk factors
+ the management of blood lipids in T2DM has changed slightly in that previously all patients with T2DM >40 years old were prescribed statins; now patients >40 years old who have no obvious cardiovascular risk (e.g. non-smoker, not obese, normotensive, etc.) and have a cardiovascular risk <20%/10 years do not need to be given a statin
+ if serum cholesterol target not reached, consider increasing simvastatin to 80 mg
+ if target still not reached consider using a more effective statin (e.g. atorvastatin) or adding ezetimibe
+ target total cholesterol is <4.0 mmol/L
+ LDL <2 mmol/L and HDL >0.9 mmol/L
+ if serum triglyceride levels are >4.5 mmol/L prescribe fenofibrate

Metformin

Metformin is a biguanide used mainly in the treatment of type 2 diabetes mellitus. It has a number of actions which improves glucose tolerance (see below). Unlike sulphonylureas it does not cause hypoglycaemia and weight gain and is therefore first-line if the patient is overweight. Metformin is also used in polycystic ovarian syndrome and non-alcoholic fatty liver disease.

Mechanism of action

+ increases insulin sensitivity
+ decreases hepatic gluconeogenesis
+ may also reduce gastrointestinal absorption of carbohydrates

Adverse effects

+ gastrointestinal upsets are common (nausea, anorexia, diarrhoea), intolerable in 20%

◆ reduced vitamin B_{12} absorption – rarely a clinical problem

◆ lactic acidosis with severe liver disease or renal failure

Contraindications

◆ chronic kidney disease: NICE recommend reviewing metformin dose if the eGFR is <45ml/min/1.73m² and stopping metformin if eGFR <30 ml/min/1.73m²

◆ do not use during suspected episodes of tissue hypoxia (e.g. recent MI, sepsis)

◆ alcohol abuse is a relative contraindication

◆ stop 2 days before general anaesthetic, restart when renal function normal

◆ stop prior to IV contrast, e.g. angiography, restart when renal function normal

Thiazolidinediones

Thiazolidinediones are a new class of agents used in the treatment of type 2 diabetes mellitus. They are agonists to the PPAR-γ receptor and reduce peripheral insulin resistance. The PPAR-γ receptor is an intracellular nuclear receptor. Its natural ligands are free fatty acids and it is thought to control adipocyte differentiation and function.

Adverse effects

◆ weight gain

◆ liver impairment: monitor LFTs

◆ fluid retention – therefore contraindicated in heart failure (the risk of fluid retention is increased if the patient also takes insulin)

◆ recent studies have indicated an increased risk of fractures

◆ rosiglitazone is not recommended for use in patients with ischaemic heart disease or peripheral arterial disease. The risk of complications may be increased if rosiglitazone is combined with insulin. Rosiglitazone has, in fact, been recently withdrawn. Pioglitazone remains the only agent in this class licensed for use in the UK.

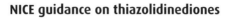

> ### NICE guidance on thiazolidinediones
>
> - Only continue if there is a reduction of >0.5 percentage points in HbA1c in 6 months.

Sulphonylureas

Sulphonylureas are oral hypoglycaemic drugs used in the management of type 2 diabetes mellitus. They work by increasing pancreatic insulin secretion and hence are only effective if functional ß-cells are present.

Common adverse effects

- hypoglycaemic episodes (more common with long-acting preparations such as chlorpropamide)
- increased appetite and weight gain

Rarer adverse effects

- syndrome of inappropriate ADH secretion
- bone marrow suppression
- liver damage (cholestasis)
- photosensitivity
- peripheral neuropathy

Sulphonylureas should be avoided in breastfeeding and pregnancy.

N. Disorders of lipid metabolism

Although a detailed knowledge of lipid metabolism is not required, you are expected to have an understanding of the importance of this group of disorders.

1. Hyperlipidaemia: management

In 2008, NICE issued guidelines on lipid modification. Key points are summarised below.

Primary prevention

A systematic strategy should be used to identify people aged 40–74 who are likely to be at high risk of cardiovascular disease (CVD), defined as a 10-year risk of 20% or greater.

The **1991 Framingham equations** are still recommended to assess 10-year CVD risk. It is, however, recommended that adjustments are made in the following situations:

◆ first-degree relative with a history of premature coronary heart disease (defined as <55 years in males and <65 years in females) – increase risk by 1.5 times if one relative affected or up to 2.0 times if more than one relative affected

◆ South Asian ethnicity – increase risk by 1.4 times

Along with lifestyle changes, drug treatment should be considered for patients with a 10-year CVD risk of 20% or greater

◆ simvastatin, 40 mg on is the first-line treatment

◆ there is no target level for total or LDL cholesterol for primary prevention

◆ liver function tests should be checked at baseline, within 3 months and at 12 months but not again unless clinically indicated

Secondary prevention

All patients with CVD should be taking a statin in the absence of any contraindication.

NICE recommend increasing to simvastatin 80 mg if a total cholesterol of less than 4 mmol/Litre or an LDL cholesterol of less than 2 mmol/Litre is not attained.

2. Causes of secondary hyperlipidaemia

Causes of predominantly hypertriglyceridaemia

+ diabetes mellitus (types 1 and 2)
+ obesity
+ alcohol
+ chronic renal failure
+ drugs: thiazides, non-selective beta-blockers, unopposed oestrogen
+ liver disease

Causes of predominantly hypercholesterolaemia

+ nephrotic syndrome
+ cholestasis
+ hypothyroidism (a mixed picture in this is equally common too)

O. Other endocrine emergencies

1. Myxoedema coma

Myxoedema coma is seen in severe hypothyroidism with decreased mental status and hypothermia. It is associated with high mortality, but is now rare owing to early diagnosis of hypothyroidism.

Myxoedema coma can be the first presentation of new hypothyroidism, often precipitated by infection, stroke, myocardial infarction, sedative drugs or exposure to cold.

Treatment is initiated on the basis of clinical suspicion, especially in unresponsive patients with a history of hypothyroidism, previous thyroidectomy or previous radioactive iodine treatment, although blood should be taken for thyroid function tests and cortisol first. Initially, the precipitating illness needs to be identified and treated and general supportive treatments instigated. Adrenal insufficiency should also be treated with intravenous hydrocortisone until it is excluded, as there may be adrenocorticotropic hormone (ACTH) deficiency along with thyroid-stimulating hormone deficiency in the pituitary.

The core temperature must be checked using a low reading thermometer, as the mortality of this condition is related to the severity of the hypothermia. The management of hypothermia is the same as that of any cause, with resuscitation, gradual re-warming and treatment of arrhythmias.

Management is ultimately through a specialist.

2. Thyroid storm

Thyroid storm is an extremely rare condition.

Thyroid storm is life-threatening and the features are usually those of thyrotoxicosis but more severe, and include fever (>38.5°C), tachycardia out of proportion to the fever, confusion, agitation, nausea and vomiting, hypertension, congestive cardiac failure, increased alanine transaminase, alkaline phosphatase and bilirubin, with biochemical evidence of thyrotoxicosis.

It is unusual for untreated hyperthyroidism to present as thyroid storm, as there are usually precipitating events such as surgery, sepsis, burns injury, DKA, cardiovascular accident, parturition, status epilepticus, I^{131} treatment or iodinated contrast dyes.

The treatment principles are to decrease the production and release of thyroid hormones, to block the effects of circulating T_4 and T_3, and to deal with the underlying precipitants.

Management is ultimately through a specialist.

3. Acute adrenal insufficiency

Acute adrenal insufficiency is a potentially life-threatening emergency that presents with shock and non-specific clinical features such as anorexia, nausea, vomiting, abdominal pain, fever and general lethargy.

Most crises occur in undiagnosed Addison's disease, in patients on steroid replacement with inter-current infection or acute stress with failure to increase the steroid dose.

The initial treatment is to resuscitate the patient with intravenous fluid (2–3 L 0.9% saline), with blood taken for random cortisol and ACTH levels (the sample must be placed on ice and must reach the laboratory within 30 minutes). Intravenous glucocorticoid (100 mg hydrocortisone 6-hourly) should be initiated immediately and not delayed, pending short synacthen test.

The precipitating causes of the adrenal crisis need to be identified and treated. Once patients are stable, the diagnosis can be confirmed by performing a short synacthen test. A long synacthen test may be required if ACTH level is equivocal to diagnose secondary adrenal failure. A steroid card needs to be carried or a medic-alert bracelet purchased to ensure notification of steroid replacement in case of incapacitation.

Management is ultimately through a specialist.

4. Pituitary failure

Acute hypopituitarism is very rare, and is due to either infarction of the pituitary gland or haemorrhage.

Infarction usually occurs after substantial loss of blood during childbirth in Sheehan's syndrome, and is usually suspected if at days or weeks after delivery there is lethargy, anorexia and failure to lactate.

Pituitary apoplexy results from haemorrhage into pituitary adenoma. The precise pathophysiology remains uncertain but is associated with trauma, hypertension, cardiac surgery, dynamic pituitary function test and a large number of other conditions.

Symptoms may evolve over several hours or days and include headaches, visual field defects, nausea and vomiting, focal neurology and altered consciousness.

Management is ultimately through a specialist.

5. Phaeochromocytoma crisis

The identification of patients with hypertension secondary to **phaeochromocytoma** is difficult. However, the classic triad of headache, palpitations and sweating in the presence of hypertension has high specificity (93.8%) and sensitivity (90.9%) for the diagnosis of phaeochromocytoma.

There is no arbitrary level of blood pressure at which hypertension becomes an emergency, rather than urgency, but systolic blood pressure >220 mmHg and diastolic blood pressure >120 mmHg are the generally accepted limiting values.

Patients with **phaeochromocytoma crisis** may present with clinical features of profound sweating, marked tachycardia, pallor, numbness, tingling and coldness of hands and feet.

Crisis can be precipitated by straining, exercise, pressure on the abdomen, and drugs such as anaesthesia. An episode can last for a few minutes to several hours and may occur as often as several times a day or once a month or less.

If phaeochromocytoma is suspected as the underlying cause of the hypertensive crisis, the treatment of choice should be intravenous α-blockers such as phentolamine or phenoxybenzamine.

Management is ultimately through a specialist.

References

Bailey CJ, Day C, Campbell IW. A consensus algorithm for treating hyperglycaemia in type 2 diabetes. *Brit J Diab Vasc Dis.* 2006; **6**: 147–8.

Scottish Intercollegiate Guidelines Network (SIGN). Management of osteoporosis: guideline number 71. Edinburgh: SIGN; June 2003 (updated April 2004). Available at: www.sign.ac.uk/guidelines/fulltext/71/index.html (accessed 10 September 2011).

Chapter 4

Gastroenterology and hepatology

The Foundation Programme and MRCP(UK) Part 1 syllabus (from the JRCPMTB) specify what is required in terms of competencies, skills and knowledge from junior physicians in core medical training in gastroenterology and hepatology. You are advised to consult carefully this syllabus, which emphasises the importance of basic medical sciences as well as a competent level of applied clinical practice.

A. The upper GI bleed

1. Management of the acute GI bleed

- Resuscitation is a priority.
- It has been demonstrated that early and aggressive resuscitation reduces mortality in an upper GI bleed.
- Maintain airway – remember vomitus can lead to airway obstruction.
- Provide high flow oxygen – this will aid tissue perfusion.
- Correct fluid losses (place two wide-bore cannulae and also send bloods at the same time). Initial fluid resuscitation may be with crystalloids or colloids; give intravenous blood when 30% of circulating volume is lost. Major haemorrhage protocols should be in place.

Once patient is more stable:

- Assess the patient, taking history and examining the patient as above – a collateral history might be needed.
- Identify and treat any co-morbid conditions.
- Estimate the severity of bleeding.

Rockall score – initial assessment or at admission

Calculate the initial Rockall score pre-endoscopy (Table 4.1).

TABLE 4.1 Rockall score pre-endoscopy

Initial Rockall score pre-endoscopy: total maximum score 7

Initial Rockall score (Clinical): (A)   (Maximum 7)

Age in yrs		Evidence of Shock		Co-morbidity	
<60	0	None	0	None	0
60–79	1	Pulse >100	1	CCF, IHD, or any other major concomitant disease	2
		Systolic BP >100			
>80	2	Systolic BP <100	2	Renal/liver failure, disseminated malignancy	3

If the Rockall score is zero, then consider patient for discharge or non-admission with out-patient follow-up. If the Rockall score >0 patients should be considered for admission and early endoscopy and should have a full Rockall score calculation. Patients who have a Rockall score >0 should have an early endoscopy which will allow calculation of their full Rockall score.

Endoscopy

Ideally, endoscopy should be performed within 24 hours. Endoscopy can be used both in diagnosis and therapy. Therapy might involve injection of adrenaline or other sclerosants, thermal coagulation or application of clips. Meta-analysis of trials has shown that endoscopic haemostatic techniques reduce bleeding, reduce the need for surgery and reduce mortality.

Endoscopic therapy should be applied to the following:

◆ actively bleeding lesion
◆ non-bleeding visible vessels
◆ ulcers with adherent clot

The preference is for dual therapy, e.g. injection of adrenaline with thermal coagulation. High-dose protein pump inhibitors should be given to those with major peptic ulcer bleeding, i.e. active bleeding or non-bleeding visible vessel. All other patients who do not receive endoscopic therapy should commence oral PPI post-procedure.

Post-initial endoscopy

Calculate the full (post-endoscopic) Rockall score (*see* Table 4.2).

TABLE 4.2 Rockall score post-endoscopy

Full Rockall Score after endoscopy: maximum score 11

Endoscopic diagnosis	
M-W tear or no lesion and no sign of bleeding	0
All other diagnoses	1
Malignancy of upper GI tract	2
Major stigmata of recent haemorrhage	
None or dark spot only	0
Blood in upper GI tract, adherent clot, visible or spurting vessel	2
BP= systolic blood pressure in mmHg	HR= heart rate in beats per minute

A score <3 is associated with low risk of re-bleeding or death and can be considered for early discharge.

A full Rockall score >3 indicates patients need further close observation as an inpatient. Careful monitoring is needed after endoscopy for upper GI bleed (pulse, blood pressure, urine output). It is imperative to identify re-bleeding or continuing bleeding.

Repeat endoscopy (within 24 hours) is needed if the initial endoscopy was sub-optimal, e.g. poor visualisation or in patients in whom re-bleeding is likely to be life-threatening.

Occasionally major re-bleeding may be an indication for surgical intervention without further endoscopy. If patients are stable 4–6 hours after endoscopy they should be put on a light diet, as there is no benefit in continued fasting.

Minor acute UGIB

- routine bloods
- observation on the general ward
- elective endoscopy
- early discharge from hospital

Re-bleeding post-endoscopy

This is associated with high mortality and need for urgent intervention.
Subsequent therapies may require:

+ further endoscopic treatment

+ surgery

+ angiography with selective arterial embolisation

+ surgical intervention

+ surgical intervention is required when endoscopic techniques fail or are contra-indicated; clinical judgement is required and consideration given to local expertise

In general, it is considered good practice to:

+ inform surgeons early of the possibility of surgery

+ use the most experienced personnel available

+ avoid operations in the middle of the night

The particular procedure required depends on a number of factors, not least the site of bleeding. Gastric ulcers are probably best excised. There are few studies comparing the different techniques.

Medical management post-endoscopy

All patients with bleeding peptic ulcer should be tested for *H. pylori*, e.g. urea breath test and biopsy specimen. Patients who test positive should receive a 1-week course of eradication therapy. This should be followed by 3 further weeks with ulcer healing treatment.

All therapy can be discontinued after successful healing of peptic ulcers provided patients are not taking NSAIDs.

A negative **urea breath test** should be confirmed on the initial biopsy specimen taken prior to diagnosis and before any PPI therapy was given.

Two weeks after successful therapy and stopping of all medication, a repeat urea breath test should be performed to confirm successful eradication.

Unsuccessful eradication should be treated with second-line therapy.

B. Disorders of the mouth, tongue and salivary glands

1. Causes of mouth ulcers and their management

The exact aetiology of **aphthous ulcers** has yet to be fully identified. Categorised as an idiopathic disease, aphthous ulcers are frequently misdiagnosed and treated incorrectly.

Factors predisposing patients to recurrent aphthous ulcers may include trauma, emotional stress, poor nutritional status, thiamine deficiency, vitamin B_{12} deficiency, malabsorption, coeliac disease, enteropathy, menstruation, food hypersensitivity, allergic reaction and exposure to toxins (e.g. nitrates in drinking water). Aphthous ulcers are more prevalent in non-smokers and in smokers who quit but are diminished with nicotine replacement therapy.

The primary goals of medical therapy in patients with aphthous ulcers are pain relief, maintenance of fluid and nutrition intake, early resolution, and prevention of recurrence. Most patients with minor or herpetiform aphthae should be treated empirically. Treatment of recurrent aphthous ulcers typically includes anti-inflammatory and/or symptomatic therapy, whereas immunomodulators are rarely used, except in severe, refractory cases.

Periodontal disorders

The accumulation of bacterial plaque on teeth induces a host response resulting in soft-tissue destruction and tooth loss. Although periodontal disease is common, affecting 30% of young adults and more than 80% of persons over 65 years of age, most cases are asymptomatic.

This chronic and progressive condition begins as inflammation of the gingiva (gingivitis) and may spread to the periodontal ligament and alveolar bone (periodontitis). Gingivitis may be suggested on physical examination by a darkening of the gingiva from their normal pink to bright red due to increased vascularity. As the inflammatory process spreads from the gingiva to the supporting tissues, the attachment of the gingiva moves down the root of the tooth. When the space between the tooth and soft-tissues becomes greater than 3 mm deep it is referred to as a periodontal '*pocket*'.

Symptoms of periodontitis include pain, looseness of a tooth, and bleeding from the gums during brushing or eating. Bacteria associated with periodontal disease include Gram-negative organisms such as *Porphyromonas gingivalis* and anaerobes such as *Actinobacillus actinomycetemcomitans* and *Bacteroides* species. Deposits of grey-yellow bacterial plaque on the teeth in conjunction with erythema, oedema and bleeding of the gingiva are seen in gingivitis.

In periodontitis, these symptoms and signs may be accompanied by halitosis and an unpleasant taste, but pain is not usually present. As the infectious and inflammatory process continues, the teeth may become loosened, and destruction of the periodontal ligament and supporting alveolar bone occurs. Spaces may develop between teeth, chewing may be difficult, and abscesses may occur.

Prevention, early recognition and treatment of periodontal disease are crucial to avoid the sequelae of inflammation and infection that lead to tooth loss. Local therapy to remove bacterial plaque and mineralised plaque or calculus includes regular dental visits, daily brushing and flossing of teeth, and the use of topical antibacterial rinses and mouthwashes that may help to prevent plaque accumulation. Reducing the bacterial load has been the mainstay of treatment for periodontal disease, but new treatments are being investigated.

Several groups of patients are at high risk for periodontal disease and may require aggressive personal hygiene and frequent dental visits. Patients with HIV infection or leukaemia may have rapidly progressive periodontitis, and those with inflammatory conditions such as rheumatoid arthritis and Crohn's disease may be severely affected. Individuals with uncontrolled type I and type II diabetes mellitus have a higher incidence of periodontal disease, and once established, the disease progresses more rapidly than in non-diabetic patients.

Pregnancy may exacerbate chronic gingivitis and cause proliferative responses in the soft-tissues that often regress after parturition. Certain medications such as nifedipine, cyclosporin, and phenytoin are well-described causes of gingival overgrowth and subsequent inflammation and plaque accumulation. In these cases, discontinuance of the causative medication is appropriate. Chronic alcoholism can also predispose individuals to periodontal disease.

C. Important upper GI conditions

1. Disorders of the oesophagus and stomach

 It can sometimes be helpful to consider these conditions as presenting complaints. They are extremely common in real life, and merit some careful consideration.

Dysphagia

Table 4.3 gives characteristic exam question features for conditions causing dysphagia.

TABLE 4.3 Causes of dysphagia

Oesophageal cancer	Dysphagia may be associated with weight loss, anorexia or vomiting during eating
	Past history may include Barrett's oesophagus, GORD, excessive smoking or alcohol use
Oesophagitis	May be history of heartburn or dyspepsia
	Odynophagia but no weight loss and systemically well
Oesophageal candidiasis	There may be a history of HIV, lymphoma or other risk factors such as steroid inhaler use
Achalasia	Dysphagia of both liquids and solids
	Heartburn
	Regurgitation of food – may lead to cough, aspiration pneumonia, etc.
Pharyngeal pouch	More common in older men
	Represents a posteromedial herniation between thyropharyngeus and cricopharyngeus muscles
	Usually not seen but if large then a midline lump in the neck that gurgles on palpation
	Typical symptoms are dysphagia, regurgitation, aspiration and chronic cough. Halitosis may occasionally be seen
Systemic sclerosis	Other features of CREST syndrome may be present, namely Calcinosis, Raynaud's phenomenon, oEsophageal dysmotility, Sclerodactyly, Telangiectasia
Myasthenia gravis	Other symptoms may include extraocular muscle weakness or ptosis
	Dysphagia with liquids as well as solids
Globus hystericus	May be history of anxiety
	Symptoms are often intermittent

The **World Gastroenterology Organisation** has recommended a very clear flowchart for the evaluation and management of oropharyngeal dysphagia.

2. Barrett's oesophagus

The 2005 British Society of Gastroenterology guidelines state that high-dose proton pump inhibitor therapy is first-line treatment in such patients. There is yet currently insufficient evidence to support the routine use of endoscopic ablation.

◆ Barrett's oesophagus refers to metaplasia of the lower oesophageal mucosa, with squamous epithelium being replaced by columnar epithelium. There is an increased risk of oesophageal adenocarcinoma, estimated at 50–100 fold.

Histological features

◆ The columnar epithelium may resemble that of either the cardiac region of the stomach or that of the small intestine (e.g. with goblet cells, brush border).

Management
Endoscopic surveillance with biopsies

One of the key aspects of the recommendations in the guidelines relates to the diagnosis of Barrett's oesophagus, with the UK guidelines stating that 'the presence of areas of intestinal metaplasia, although often present, is *not* a requirement for diagnosis'. In contrast guidelines from the US suggest that intestinal metaplasia is required to establish a diagnosis of Barrett's oesophagus. The rationale for the British guidelines is that sampling errors at initial endoscopy may miss areas affected with intestinal metaplasia.

Oesophageal strictures

Disease processes that can produce oesophageal strictures can be grouped into three general categories: (1) intrinsic diseases that narrow the oesophageal lumen through inflammation, fibrosis or neoplasia; (2) extrinsic diseases that compromise the oesophageal lumen by direct invasion or lymph node enlargement; and (3) diseases that disrupt oesophageal peristalsis and/or lower oesophageal sphincter (LES) function by their effects on oesophageal smooth muscle and its innervation.

Many diseases can cause oesophageal stricture formation. These include acid reflux or peptic, autoimmune, infectious, caustic, congenital, iatrogenic, medication-induced, radiation-induced, malignant and idiopathic disease processes.

History

♦ Patients may present with heartburn, dysphagia, odynophagia, food impaction, weight loss and chest pain.

♦ Progressive dysphagia for solids is the most common presenting symptom. This may progress to include liquids.

♦ Atypical presentations include chronic cough and wheeze secondary to aspiration of food or acid.

♦ The clinician cannot rely on the presence or absence of heartburn to determine definitely whether dysphagia is secondary to a peptic oesophageal stricture.

♦ Of patients with peptic oesophageal strictures, 25% have no previous history of heartburn.

♦ Heartburn may resolve with worsening of a peptic stricture.

♦ Approximately two-thirds of patients with adenocarcinoma in Barrett's oesophagus have a history of long-standing heartburn.

♦ The abnormal oesophageal motor activity in achalasia can produce a heartburn sensation.

Some important points regarding dysphagia to remember are:

♦ The obstruction usually is perceived at a point that is either above or at the level of the lesion.

♦ Dysphagia for solids and liquids simultaneously should alert the clinician to the possibility of a motility disorder such as achalasia.

♦ Dysphagia secondary to 'a Schatzki ring' usually is intermittent and nonprogressive.

♦ Dysphagia for solids and liquids early in the course of disease should alert the clinician to the possibility of achalasia as an aetiology.

♦ Benign oesophageal strictures usually produce dysphagia with slow and insidious progression (i.e. months to years) of frequency and severity with minimal weight loss.

♦ Malignant oesophageal strictures result in a rapid progression (i.e. weeks to months) of severity and frequency of dysphagia and are associated frequently with significant weight loss.

♦ Determining whether the patient takes any medications known to cause oesophagitis is important.

◆ Determining whether a history of collagen vascular disease or immunosuppression exists may provide clues to the underlying aetiology.

Traditionally, more emphasis has been placed on mechanical dilatation, and coexistent oesophagitis had been relatively ignored. However, several studies have demonstrated that aggressive acid suppression using PPIs is extremely beneficial in the initial treatment, as well as long-term management, and hence it is common practice to start these patients on protein-pump inhibitors.

3. Achalasia

Achalasia is a failure of oesophageal peristalsis and of relaxation of lower oesophageal sphincter (LOS) due to degenerative loss of ganglia from Auerbach's plexus, results in a contracted LOS, and oesophagus that is dilated above this. Achalasia typically presents in middle age and is more common in women.

Clinical features

◆ dysphagia of BOTH liquids and solids
◆ typically variation in severity of symptoms
◆ some heartburn
◆ regurgitation of food – may lead to cough, aspiration pneumonia, etc.
◆ malignant change in small number of patients

Investigations

◆ **Endoscopy** is usually performed to visual the LOS and exclude a stricture.
◆ **Manometry:** excessive LOS tone (>20 mmHg) which fails to relax on swallowing and lack of peristalsis in the body of the oesophagus. It is considered the most important and accurate diagnostic test.
◆ **Barium swallow** shows grossly expanded oesophagus, with a fluid level and the characteristic tapered narrowing of the lower end of the oesophagus ('rat tail appearance').
◆ **CXR:** wide mediastinum, with a fluid level.

Treatment

◆ intra-sphincteric injection of botulinum toxin
◆ Heller cardiomyotomy

- balloon dilation
- drug therapies (anti-cholingerics, nitrates and calcium channel blockers) have a role but are limited by side effects and a short lived effect

3. Pharyngeal pouch

A **pharyngeal pouch** is a posteromedial diverticulum through Killian's dehiscence. Killian's dehiscence is a triangular area in the wall of the pharynx between the thyropharyngeus and cricopharyngeus muscles. It is more common in older patients and is five times more common in men.

Features

- dysphagia
- regurgitation
- aspiration
- neck swelling which gurgles on palpation
- halitosis

4. Acute gastritis

Acute gastritis is a term covering a broad spectrum of entities that induce inflammatory changes in the gastric mucosa. The different aetiologies share the same general clinical presentation. However, they differ in their unique histologic characteristics.

Inflammation may involve the entire stomach (e.g. pangastritis) or a region of the stomach (e.g. antral gastritis). Acute gastritis can be broken down into two categories: erosive (e.g. superficial erosions, deep erosions, hemorrhagic erosions) and non-erosive (generally caused by *Helicobacter pylori*).

Acute erosive gastritis can result from the exposure to a variety of agents or factors. This is referred to as reactive gastritis.

These agents/factors include NSAIDs, alcohol, cocaine, stress, radiation, bile reflux and ischemia. The gastric mucosa exhibits haemorrhages, erosions and ulcers. NSAIDs, such as aspirin, ibuprofen, and naproxen, are the most common agents associated with acute erosive gastritis.

5. Chronic gastritis

Chronic gastritis is a histopathological entity characterised by chronic inflammation of the stomach mucosa.

Gastritides can be classified based on the underlying etiologic agent (e.g. *Helicobacter pylori*, bile reflux, non-steroidal anti-inflammatory drugs (NSAIDs), autoimmunity, allergic response) and the histopathological pattern, which may suggest the aetiological agent and clinical course (e.g. *H. pylori*–associated multifocal atrophic gastritis).

Treatment of chronic gastritis can be directed to a specific aetiological agent, when it is known. In other situations in which gastritis represents gastric involvement of a systemic disease, treatment is targeted to the primary disease.

6. The role of *Helicobacter*-associated gastritis in peptic ulcer disease

H. pylori is a Gram-negative bacteria associated with a variety of gastrointestinal conditions including peptic ulcer disease.

Associations

◈ peptic ulcer disease (95% of duodenal ulcers, 75% of gastric ulcers)

◈ gastric cancer

◈ B cell lymphoma of MALT tissue (eradication of *H. pylori* results causes regression in 80% of patients)

◈ atrophic gastritis

The role of *H. pylori* in gastro-oesophageal reflux disease (GORD) is currently unclear – there is currently no role in GORD for the eradication of *H. pylori*.

Management

Eradication may be achieved with a 7-day course of:

◈ a proton pump inhibitor + amoxicillin + clarithromycin

Tests
Urea breath test

◈ patient consumes a drink containing carbon isotope 13 (^{13}C) enriched urea

◈ urea is broken down by *H. pylori* urease

◈ after 30 minutes patient exhales into a glass tube

◈ mass spectrometry analysis calculates the amount of $^{13}C\ CO_2$

◈ sensitivity 95%–98%, specificity 97%–98%

Rapid urease test (e.g. CLO test)

◈ biopsy sample is mixed with urea and pH indicator

◈ colour change if *H. pylori* urease activity

◈ sensitivity 90%–95%, specificity 95%–98%

Serum antibody

◈ remains positive after eradication

◈ sensitivity 85%, specificity 80%

Culture of gastric biopsy

◈ provide information on antibiotic sensitivity

◈ sensitivity 70%, specificity 100%

Gastric biopsy

◈ histological evaluation alone, no culture

◈ sensitivity 95%–99%, specificity 95%–99%

Stool antigen test

◈ sensitivity 90%, specificity 95%

7. Gastric cancer

Epidemiology

◈ overall incidence is decreasing, but incidence of tumours arising from the cardia is increasing

◈ peak age = 70–80 years

◈ more common in Japan, China, Finland and Columbia than the West

◈ more common in males, 2 : 1

Associations

◈ *H. pylori* infection

◈ blood group A

- gastric adenomatous polyps
- pernicious anaemia
- smoking
- diet: salty, spicy, nitrates
- may be negatively associated with duodenal ulcer

Investigation

- **diagnosis:** endoscopy with biopsy
- **staging:** CT or endoscopic ultrasound – endoscopic ultrasound has recently been shown to be superior to CT

8. Gastric MALT lymphoma

Overview

- these are usually marginal zone B cell lymphomas and associated with an excellent prognosis
- associated with *H. pylori* infection in 95% of cases
- good prognosis
- if low grade then 80% respond to *H. pylori* eradication

Features

- paraproteinaemia may be present

Management

Low-grade gastric MALT tumours associated with *H. pylori* infection respond in over 80% to *H. pylori* eradiction as the primary mode of treatment. Radiotherapy is considered but generally unnecessary.

D. General upper GI topics

1. Oesophageal varices

Indications for an urgent referral following upper GI bleed

Acute treatment of variceal haemorrhage

- ABC: patients should ideally be resuscitated prior to endoscopy
- correct clotting: FFP, vitamin K
- vasoactive agents: terlipressin is currently the only licensed vasoactive agent; it has been shown to be of benefit in initial haemostasis and preventing re-bleeding
- prophylactic antibiotics have been shown in multiple meta-analyses to reduce mortality in patients with liver cirrhosis
- endoscopy: endoscopic variceal band ligation is superior to endoscopic sclerotherapy
- Sengstaken-Blakemore tube if uncontrolled haemorrhage
- Transjugular Intrahepatic Portosystemic Shunt (TIPSS) if above measures fail

Prophylaxis (secondary) of variceal haemorrhage

- Propranolol: reduced re-bleeding and mortality compared to placebo.
- Endoscopic variceal band ligation (EVL) is superior to endoscopic sclerotherapy. (It should be performed at two-weekly intervals until all varices have been eradicated. Proton pump inhibitor cover is given to prevent EVL-induced ulceration.)

2. Cancers

Associations

- smoking
- diabetes
- chronic pancreatitis
- hereditary pancreatitis
- hereditary non-polyposis colorectal carcinoma
- multiple endocrine neoplasia
- Peutz-Jeghers syndrome

+ BRCA2
+ dysplastic naevus syndrome

Management
+ Less than 20% are suitable for surgery at diagnosis.
+ Radio- and chemotherapy are ineffective.

E. Liver and biliary tract
1. Ascitic fluid analysis
+ cell count: leucocyte >500/cc or absolute neutrophil >250/cc suggests infection
+ protein <10 g/L in spontaneous peritonitis; >10 g/L in secondary peritonitis
+ fluid glucose <50 mg/dL or increased LDH in secondary peritonitis
+ albumin serum-ascites gradient = serum albumin – ascitic albumin. Gradient of >11 g/L suggests portal hypertension; seen in cirrhosis, alcoholic hepatitis, CHF, massive liver metastasis, fulminant liver failure, portal-vein thrombosis, Budd-Chiari syndrome, veno-occlusive disease, fatty liver of pregnancy, myxoedema. Gradient of <11 g/L seen in peritoneal carcinomatosis, TB, pancreatic ascites, biliary ascites, nephrotic syndrome, bowel obstruction or infarction, serositis
+ gram stain and culture/sensitivity
+ amylase in pancreatic or perforation
+ cytology or TB smear and culture prn

Transudative ascites (serum albumin – ascites albumin >11 g/L)
+ liver cirrhosis
+ congestive heart failure
+ hepatic vein obstruction (Budd-Chiari syndrome)
+ associated with tumours (hepatoma, hypernephroma, pancreatic Ca)
+ associated with haematological disorders (including the myeloproliferative conditions)
+ nephrotic syndrome
+ Meigs' ovarian tumour syndrome
+ constrictive pericarditis

- inferior vena cava obstruction
- viral hepatitis with sub-massive or massive hepatic necrosis

Exudative ascites (serum albumin – ascites albumin <11 g/L

- neoplastic diseases involving the peritoneum: peritoneal carcinomatosis, lymphomatous disorders
- tuberculous peritonitis
- pancreatitis
- post-surgery talc or starch powder peritonitis (rare)
- transected lymphatics following portal caval shunt surgery
- sarcoidosis
- lymphatic obstruction (e.g. intestinal lymphangiectasia, lymphoma)
- *pseudomyxoma peritonei*
- *struma ovarii*
- amyloidosis
- prior abdominal trauma with ruptured lymphatics
- haemodialysis CRF-related ascites

2. Sub-acute bacterial peritonitis (SBP)

Sub-acute bacterial peritonitis (SBP) is a frequent complication of the ascites of cirrhosis. It is diagnosed by ascitic fluid examination which reveals a PMN count of >250/ml. The high white cell count in the ascites makes spontaneous bacterial peritonitis (SBP) much more likely than Budd-Chiari syndrome (BCS), PVT, hepatocellular carcinoma (HCC), or a ruptured pancreatic pseudocyst.

SBP has poor prognostic significance with a one-year survival after a diagnosis of between 30% and 50%.

It is, as the name suggests, a spontaneous event that is not a consequence of intestinal perforation. It is speculated that the infective organism may leak into the ascitic fluid via the blood or from intestinal overgrowth.

Organisms should be cultured by directly collecting into blood culture bottles.

It is most commonly seen in alcoholic cirrhosis and the causative organism is usually *Escherichia coli, Klebsiella, S pneumoniae* or *Enterococci*. (Compare this with the mixed growth seen in other forms of peritonitis.) Hence cefotaxime is regarded as the drug of choice for treatment. Norfloxacin is recommended for short-term prophylaxis.

3. Hepatorenal syndrome (HRS)

Most individuals with cirrhosis who develop HRS have non-specific symptoms, such as fatigue, malaise or dysgeusia. Development of HRS is usually noticed when patients observe decreased urine output and when blood test results show a decline in renal function.

An abnormal urea and creatinine plus the low urine sodium might suggest a diagnosis of hepatorenal syndrome.

Fluid balance is very difficult in these patients but some respond to treatment with intravenous (IV) glypressin which improves kidney perfusion.

4. Acute and chronic hepatitis

[*See* Chapter 6: Infectious diseases.]

5. Autoimmune hepatitis

Autoimmune hepatitis is a condition of unknown aetiology which is most commonly seen in young females.

Recognised associations include other autoimmune disorders, hypergammaglobulinaemia and HLA-B8, DR3.

Three types of autoimmune hepatitis have been characterised according to the types of circulating antibodies present (Table 4.4).

TABLE 4.4 Three types of autoimmune hepatitis

Type I	Type II	Type III
Anti-nuclear antibodies (ANA) and/or anti-smooth muscle antibodies (SMA)	Anti-liver/kidney microsomal type I antibodies (LKM1)	Soluble liver-kidney antigen Affects adults in middle age
Affects both adults and children	Affects children only	

Features

⬥ fatigue and arthralgia

⬥ may present with signs of chronic liver disease

⬥ acute hepatitis: fever, jaundice, etc. (only 25% present in this way)

⬥ amenorrhoea (*common*)

⬥ ANA/SMA/LKM1 antibodies, raised IgG levels

⬥ liver biopsy: inflammation extending beyond limiting plate 'piecemeal necrosis', bridging necrosis

⬥ 60% are associated with HLA-B8, DR3 and Dw3

◆ the sicca syndrome (xerostomia/dry eyes, keratoconjunctivitis sicca) may occur

Management

◆ steroids, other immunosuppressants, e.g. azathioprine

◆ liver transplantation

6. Non-alcoholic fatty liver disease (NAFLD)

Non-alcoholic fatty liver disease (NAFLD) will arguably become the most common cause of liver disease in the developed world. It is largely caused by obesity and describes a spectrum of disease ranging from:

◆ steatosis – fat in the liver

◆ steatohepatitis – fat with inflammation, non-alcoholic steatohepatitis (NASH), see below

◆ progressive disease may cause fibrosis and liver cirrhosis

NAFLD is thought to represent the hepatic manifestation of the metabolic syndrome and hence insulin resistance is thought to be the key mechanism leading to steatosis.

It is a term used to describe liver changes similar to those seen in alcoholic hepatitis in the absence of a history of alcohol abuse. It is relatively common and thought to affect around 3%–4% of the general population. The progression of disease in patients with NAFLD may be responsible for a proportion of patients previously labelled as cryptogenic cirrhosis.

Associated factors

◆ obesity

◆ hyperlipidaemia

◆ type 2 diabetes mellitus

◆ jejunoileal bypass

◆ sudden weight loss/starvation

Features

◆ usually asymptomatic

◆ hepatomegaly

◆ ALT is typically greater than AST

NB The '**give-away**' for making the diagnosis is a '*bright echogenic structure in the ultrasound report*'.

The definitive diagnosis of this is made only by histology of liver biopsy which shows lesions suggestive of ethanol intake in a patient known to consume less than 40 g of alcohol per week.

7. Drugs, toxins, alcohol and the liver

Lactulose in encephalopathy

Lactulose, an osmotic diuretic which causes hypomagnesaemia associated with diarrhoea, is not absorbed, does not affect the absorption of spironolactone and may be used with diabetics.

It is used in patients with cirrhosis/hepatic encephalopathy to limit the proliferation of ammonia-forming gut organisms and increase the clearance of protein load in the gut.

Drug-induced liver disease

Drug-induced liver disease is generally divided into hepatocellular, cholestatic or mixed. There is however considerable overlap, with some drugs causing a range of changes to the liver.

The following drugs tend to cause a hepatocellular picture:

◆ paracetamol

◆ sodium valproate, phenytoin

◆ MAOIs

◆ halothane

◆ anti-tuberculosis: isoniazid, rifampicin, pyrazinamide

◆ statins

◆ alcohol

◆ amiodarone

◆ methyldopa

The following drugs tend to cause cholestasis (+/− hepatitis):

◆ oral contraceptive pill

◆ antibiotics: flucloxacillin, co-amoxiclav, erythromycin, nitrofurantoin

◆ anabolic steroids, testosterones

◆ phenothiazines: chlorpromazine, prochlorperazine

◆ sulphonylureas

◆ fibrates

◆ rare reported causes: nifedipine

Co-amoxiclav (Augmentin®) is notorious for causing drug-induced jaundice, often with a mixed hepatitic/cholestatic picture. A four-week delay in symptoms and signs is not unusual.

Liver fibrosis

◆ methotrexate

◆ methyldopa

◆ amiodarone

Wilson's disease (hepatolenticular degeneration)

Wilson's disease is an autosomal recessive disorder characterised by excessive copper deposition in the tissues. Metabolic abnormalities include increased copper absorption from the small intestine and decreased hepatic copper excretion. Wilson's disease is caused by a defect in the ATP7B gene located on chromosome 13.

The onset of symptoms is usually between 10 and 25 years. Children usually present with liver disease whereas the first sign of disease in young adults is often neurological disease.

Features result from excessive copper deposition in the tissues, especially the brain, liver and cornea:

◆ liver: hepatitis, cirrhosis

◆ neurological: speech and behavioural problems are often the first manifestations; also: excessive salivation, tremor, chorea, Parkinsonian syndrome/dementia

◆ Kayser-Fleischer rings

◆ renal tubular acidosis (especially Fanconi syndrome)

◆ haemolysis

◆ blue nails

Diagnosis

◆ reduced serum ceruloplasmin

◆ increased 24-hour urinary copper excretion

Management

+ D-penicillamine: chelates copper

Haemochromatosis

Haemochromatosis is the abnormal accumulation of iron in parenchymal organs, leading to organ toxicity. It is the most common inherited liver disease in whites and the most common autosomal recessive genetic disorder.

Features

Symptoms usually begin between age 30 years and age 50 years, but they may occur much earlier. Clinical manifestations include the following:

+ liver disease
+ skin pigmentation
+ diabetes mellitus
+ arthropathy
+ impotence in males
+ cardiac enlargement

Diagnosis

Homozygous mutation (C282Y mutation) of the human iron gene (HFE gene) accounts for over 80% of cases of hereditary haemochromatosis (HHC).

The diagnosis is made on DNA analysis.

A liver biopsy is not required to make the diagnosis of HHC although may be indicated for prognostic reasons if cirrhosis is suspected.

Treatment

If the diagnosis is confirmed, treatment with venesection to achieve and maintain a ferritin of 50–100 µg/l is currently recommended.

F. Anorectal disorders

1. Anal fistulas and fissures

An **anal fissure** is a superficial linear tear in the anoderm most commonly caused by passage of a large, hard stool. This tear is distal to the dentate line. Anal fissures are among the most common anorectal disorders in the paediatric population; however, adults also are affected. Paroxysms of pain, accompanied by episodes of bleeding are typical of anal fissure. The initiating factor for formation of an anal fissure is thought to be passage of a particularly hard motion which leads to trauma. In most people acute tears in the anal mucosa heal spontaneously but in some they lead to a chronic anal fissure. Stool softeners are the mainstay of therapy, with surgery reserved for those who fail medical intervention.

Fissures are defined as acute if present for less than six weeks, and they are defined as chronic if present for more than six weeks.

An **anal fistula** is an inflammatory tract between the anal canal and skin. The four categories of fistulas, based on the relationship of fistula to sphincter muscles, are inter-sphincteric, trans-sphincteric, supra-sphincteric, and extra-sphincteric.

Pathophysiology

In anal fissures, anus distal to dentate line is involved. About 90% of anal fissures occur in the posterior midline where skeletal muscle fibres that circle the anus are weakest. The remaining 10% are found in the anterior midline.

Most anal fistulas originate in anal crypts, which become infected with abscess formation. When the abscess is opened or ruptures, a fistula is formed.

Anal fistulas are a complication of anorectal abscesses, which are more common in men than in women (male-to-female ratio of 2 : 1 to 3 : 1).

Only 8% of anal fissures are anterior in men; 75%–90% of fissures in women are posteriorly located.

For reasons of intrinsic anatomy, rectovaginal fistulas are found only in women.

Clinical history

- rectal pain, usually described as burning, cutting, or tearing
- pain with bowel movements; spasm of the anus is very suspicious for an anal fissure
- bloody stools
- typically, bright-red blood appears on the surface of stools. Blood usually is not mixed into stool
- occasionally, blood is found on toilet paper after wiping
- patient may report no bleeding
- mucoid discharge
- pruritus
- a patient with an anal fistula may complain of recurrent malodorous perianal drainage, pruritus, recurrent abscesses, fever, or perianal pain due to an occluded tract

✦ pain occasionally resolves spontaneously with reopening of a tract or formation of a new outflow tract

✦ pain occurs with sitting, moving, defecating, and even coughing

✦ pain usually is throbbing in quality and is constant throughout the day

Causes

✦ passage of hard stool

✦ chronic diarrhoea

✦ childbirth (accounts for 10% of chronic anal fissures)

Causes of anal fistula also include opened perianal or ischiorectal abscesses, which drain spontaneously through these fistulous tracts.

Anal fissures can be observed in patients with syphilis and other sexually transmitted diseases, tuberculosis, leukaemia, inflammatory bowel disease such as Crohn's disease, previous anal surgery, HIV, and other conditions or diseases.

Anal fistulas also are associated with diverticulitis, foreign body reactions, actinomycosis, chlamydia, lymphogranuloma venereum, syphilis, tuberculosis, radiation exposure and HIV.

Approximately 30% of patients with HIV develop anorectal abscesses and fistulas.

2. Haemorrhoids

The term '**haemorrhoid**' is usually related to the symptoms caused by haemorrhoids. Haemorrhoids are present in healthy individuals. Haemorrhoids generally cause symptoms when they become enlarged, inflamed, thrombosed, or prolapsed.

Causes

✦ low-fibre diet

✦ pregnancy

✦ prolonged sitting on a toilet

✦ ageing

Presentation

Non-haemorrhoidal causes of symptoms (e.g. fissure, abscess, fistula, pruritus ani, condylomata, and viral or bacterial skin infection) need to be excluded.

Haemorrhoidal symptoms are divided into internal and external sources.

Internal haemorrhoids cannot cause cutaneous pain, because they are above the dentate line and are not innervated by cutaneous nerves.

However, they can bleed, prolapse, and, as a result of the deposition of an irritant onto the sensitive perianal skin, cause perianal itching and irritation. Internal haemorrhoids can produce perianal pain by prolapsing and causing spasm of the sphincter complex around the haemorrhoids. When these catastrophic events occur, the sphincter spasm often causes concomitant external thrombosis.

External thrombosis causes acute cutaneous pain. This set of symptoms is referred to as acute haemorrhoidal crisis. It usually requires emergent treatment. Internal haemorrhoids most commonly cause painless bleeding with bowel movements.

External haemorrhoids cause symptoms in two ways. First, acute thrombosis of the underlying external haemorrhoidal vein can occur. External haemorrhoids can also cause hygiene difficulties, with the excess, redundant skin left after an acute thrombosis (skin tags) being accountable for these problems. External haemorrhoidal veins found under the perianal skin obviously cannot cause hygiene problems; however, excess skin in the perianal area can mechanically interfere with cleansing.

Indications
Haemorrhoids are only treated when the patient complains of them.

Medical management
Treatment is divided by the cause of symptoms, into internal and external treatments. Internal haemorrhoids do not have cutaneous innervation and can therefore be destroyed without anaesthetic.

Because it is believed that straining and a low-fibre diet cause haemorrhoidal disease, conservative treatment includes increasing fibre and liquid intake and retraining in toilet habit.

Stool softeners play a limited role in the treatment of routine haemorrhoidal symptoms.

Many patients see improvement or complete resolution of their symptoms with the above conservative measures. Aggressive therapy is reserved for patients who have persistent symptoms after one month of conservative therapy. Treatment is directed solely at symptoms and not at the appearance of the haemorrhoids. Many patients have been referred for surgery because they have severely swollen prolapsed haemorrhoids or very large external skin tags.

Treatment of the underlying disease often relieves anal symptoms.

Numerous methods to destroy internal haemorrhoids are available; they include rubber band ligation, sclerotherapy injection, infrared photocoagulation, laser ablation, carbon dioxide freezing, '*Lord dilatation*', stapled haemorrhoidectomy and surgical resection.

Sclerotherapy can provide adequate treatment of early internal haemorrhoids. (*Note*: cryotherapy and sclerotherapy are infrequently used today.)

G. Functional disorders of gut

1. Irritable bowel syndrome

Diagnosis

NICE published clinical guidelines on the diagnosis and management of irritable bowel syndrome (IBS) in 2008.

You should have a look at the guidelines for yourself, as they do change periodically. At the time of writing, however, the 'conventional wisdom' is that the diagnosis of IBS should be considered, if the patient has had the following for at least six months:

+ abdominal pain, and/or

+ bloating, and/or

+ change in bowel habit

A positive diagnosis of IBS should be made if the patient has abdominal pain relieved by defaecation or associated with altered bowel frequency stool form, in addition to two of the following four symptoms:

+ altered stool passage (straining, urgency, incomplete evacuation)

+ abdominal bloating (more common in women than men), distension, tension or hardness

+ symptoms made worse by eating

+ passage of mucus

The ROME criteria for IBS are given in Table 4.5.

TABLE 4.5 ROME criteria for IBS

Recurrent abdominal pain or discomfort at least 3 days per month in the last 3 months associated with 2 or more of the following
(1) Improvement with defecation
(2) Onset associated with a change in frequency of stool
(3) Onset associated with a change in form (appearance) of stool

Features such as lethargy, nausea, backache and bladder symptoms may also support the diagnosis.

'Red flag' features of back pain

These features should be enquired about to exclude other pathology:

+ rectal bleeding

+ unexplained/unintentional weight loss

+ family history of bowel or ovarian cancer

+ onset after 60 years of age

Primary care investigations

Suggested primary care investigations should include:

+ full blood count

+ ESR/CRP

+ coeliac disease screen (tissue transglutaminase antibodies)

+ stool cultures if diarrhoea

Management

The management of irritable bowel syndrome (IBS) is often difficult and varies considerably between patients. NICE issued guidelines in 2008.

First-line pharmacological treatment – according to predominant symptom

+ pain: antispasmodic agents

+ constipation: laxatives but avoid lactulose

+ diarrhoea: loperamide is first-line

Second-line pharmacological treatment

+ Low-dose tricyclic antidepressants (e.g. amitriptyline 5–10 mg) are used in preference to selective serotonin reuptake inhibitors.

Other management options

◆ psychological interventions – if symptoms do not respond to pharmacological treatments after 12 months and patient develops a continuing symptom profile (refractory IBS), consider referring for cognitive behavioural therapy, hypnotherapy or psychological therapy

◆ complementary and alternative medicines: '*do not encourage use of acupuncture or reflexology for the treatment of IBS*'

General dietary advice

◆ Have regular meals and take time to eat.

◆ Avoid missing meals or leaving long gaps between eating.

◆ Drink at least eight cups of fluid per day, especially water or other non-caffeinated drinks such as herbal teas.

◆ Restrict tea and coffee to three cups per day.

◆ Reduce intake of alcohol and fizzy drinks.

◆ Consider limiting intake of high-fibre food (for example, wholemeal or high-fibre flour and breads, cereals high in bran, and whole grains such as brown rice).

◆ Reduce intake of 'resistant starch' often found in processed foods.

◆ Limit fresh fruit to three portions per day.

◆ For diarrhoea, avoid sorbitol.

◆ For wind and bloating consider increasing intake of oats (e.g. oat-based breakfast cereal or porridge) and linseeds (up to one tablespoon per day).

H. Infective causes of malabsorption
Infective gastroenteritis is described in full in Chapter 6.

1. Whipple's disease
Whipple's disease is a rare multi-system disorder caused by *Tropheryma whippelii* infection. It is more common in those who are HLA-B27 positive and in middle-aged men.

Features
+ malabsorption: diarrhoea, weight loss
+ large-joint arthralgia
+ lymphadenopathy
+ skin: hyperpigmentation and photosensitivity
+ pleurisy, pericarditis
+ neurological symptoms (rare): ophthalmoplegia, dementia, seizures, ataxia, myoclonus

Investigation
+ jejunal biopsy shows deposition of macrophages containing Periodic acid-Schiff (PAS) granules

Management
+ varies, e.g. IV penicillin then oral co-trimoxazole for a year

Bacterial overgrowth: investigation
The **gold standard investigation** of bacterial overgrowth is small bowel aspiration and culture.

Other possible investigations include:
+ hydrogen breath test
+ ^{14}C-xylose breath test
+ ^{14}C-glycocholate breath test: used increasingly less due to low specificity

In practice, many clinicians indeed give an empirical course of antibiotics as a trial.

I. Hormone-secreting tumour disorders of the small intestine

1. Zollinger-Ellison syndrome

Zollinger-Ellison syndrome is a condition characterised by excessive levels of gastrin, usually from a gastrin-secreting tumour of the duodenum or pancreas. Around 30% occur as part of MEN type I syndrome.

Features

+ multiple gastroduodenal ulcers

+ diarrhoea

+ malabsorption

Diagnosis

+ fasting gastrin levels: the single best screen test

+ secretin stimulation test

2. VIPoma

Possible source: small intestine, pancreas.

Actions: endocrine tumours secreting excessive amounts of VIP32, stimulating secretion by pancreas and intestines, and inhibiting acid and pepsinogen secretion.

Features

+ 90% arises from pancreas

+ large-volume watery diarrhoea

+ weight loss

+ dehydration

+ hypokalaemia, hypochlorhydia

The mean age of patients is 49 years; however it can occur in children and when it does is usually caused by a ganglioneuroma or ganglioneuroblastoma.

A stool volume of less than 700 mL/d excludes the diagnosis of VIPoma.

J. Coeliac disease

Coeliac disease is caused by sensitivity to the protein gluten. Repeated exposure leads to villous atrophy which in turn causes malabsorption. Conditions associated with coeliac disease include dermatitis herpetiformis (a vesicular, pruritic skin eruption) and autoimmune disorders (type 1 diabetes mellitus and autoimmune hepatitis). It is strongly associated with HLA-DQ2 (95% of patients) and HLA-B8 (80%) as well as HLA-DR3 and HLA-DR7.

In 2009 NICE issued guidelines on the investigation of coeliac disease. They suggest that the following patients should be screened for coeliac disease.

TABLE 4.6 NICE guidelines for a possible screening for coeliac disease

Queried signs and symptoms	Queried conditions
Chronic or intermittent diarrhoea	Type 1 diabetes
Prolonged fatigue ('*tired all the time*')	Autoimmune thyroid disease
Failure to thrive or faltering growth (in children)	Dermatitis herpetiformis
Persistent or unexplained gastrointestinal symptoms including nausea and vomiting	Irritable bowel syndrome
Sudden or unexpected weight loss	First-degree relatives (parents, siblings or children) with coeliac disease
Recurrent abdominal pain, cramping or distension	
Unexplained iron-deficiency anaemia, or other unspecified anaemia	

Complications

◆ anaemia: iron, folate and vitamin B_{12} deficiency (folate deficiency is more common than vitamin B_{12} deficiency in coeliac disease)

◆ hyposplenism

◆ osteoporosis

◆ lactose intolerance

◆ enteropathy-associated T-cell lymphoma of small intestine

◆ subfertility, unfavourable pregnancy outcomes

rare: oesophageal cancer, other malignancy

Investigations

Coeliac disease is caused by sensitivity to the protein gluten. Repeated exposure leads to villous atrophy which in turn causes malabsorption. Conditions associated with coeliac disease include dermatitis herpetiformis (a vesicular, pruritic skin eruption) and autoimmune disorders (type 1 diabetes mellitus and autoimmune hepatitis).

Diagnosis is made by a combination of immunology and small bowel biopsy via endoscopy. Villous atrophy and immunology normally reverse on a gluten-free diet.

According to the NICE guidelines, if patients are already taking a gluten-free diet they should be asked, if possible, to reintroduce gluten for at least 6 weeks prior to testing.

Patients may appear with a blood picture of hyposplenism, including target cells and Howell-Jolly bodies.

Immunology

- tissue transglutaminase (TGT) antibodies (IgA) are first-choice according to NICE
- endomyseal antibody (IgA)
- anti-gliadin antibody (IgA or IgG) tests are not recommended by NICE
- anti-casein antibodies are also found in some patients

Small bowel biopsy

- partial villous atrophy
- crypt hyperplasia
- increase in intraepithelial lymphocytes
- lamina propria infiltration with lymphocytes

Rectal gluten challenge has been described but is not widely used.

Management

The management of coeliac disease involves a gluten-free diet. Gluten-containing cereals include:

- wheat: bread, pasta, pastry
- barley: beer

◆ rye

◆ oats

Some notable foods which are gluten-free include:

◆ rice

◆ potatoes

◆ corn (maize)

K. Hyperbilirubinaemias

1. Gilbert's syndrome

Gilbert's syndrome is an autosomal recessive condition of defective bilirubin conjugation due to a deficiency of UDP glucuronyl transferase. The prevalence is approximately 1%–2% in the general population.

Features

◆ unconjugated hyperbilinemia (i.e. not in urine)

◆ jaundice may only be seen during an intercurrent illness

Investigation and management

◆ investigation: rise in bilirubin following prolonged fasting or IV nicotinic acid

◆ no treatment required

L. Disorders of the biliary tract and the pancreas

1. Primary biliary cirrhosis

Primary biliary cirrhosis is a chronic liver disorder typically seen in middle-aged females (female : male ratio of 9 : 1).

The aetiology is not fully understood although it is thought to be an autoimmune condition.

Pathology

Interlobular bile ducts become damaged by a chronic inflammatory process causing progressive cholestasis, which may eventually progress to cirrhosis. The classic presentation is itching in a middle-aged woman with xanthelasma.

Clinical features

- **early:** may be asymptomatic (e.g. raised ALP on routine LFTs) or fatigue, pruritus
- cholestatic jaundice
- hyperpigmentation, especially over pressure points
- xanthelasmas, xanthomata
- also: clubbing, hepatosplenomegaly
- **late:** may progress to liver failure

Complications

- malabsorption: osteomalacia, coagulopathy
- *sicca syndrome* occurs in 70% of cases
- portal hypertension: ascites, variceal haemorrhage
- hepatocellular cancer (20-fold increased risk)

2. Primary sclerosing cholangitis

Primary sclerosing cholangitis (PSC) is a biliary disease of unknown aetiology characterised by inflammation and fibrosis of intra and extra-hepatic bile ducts.

Associations

- ulcerative colitis: 4% of patients with UC have PSC, 80% of patients with PSC have UC
- Crohn's (much less common association than UC)
- HIV

Features

- cholestasis

Investigation

- MRCP(UK) and ERCP are the standard diagnostic tools, showing multiple biliary strictures giving a 'beaded' appearance
- ANCA may be positive
- there is a limited role for liver biopsy, which may show fibrous, obliterative cholangitis often described as '*onion skin*'

Complications

◈ cholangiocarcinoma (in 10%)

◈ increased risk of colorectal cancer

Common pancreatic disorders including carcinoma

3. Acute pancreatitis

Causes

The vast majority of cases in the UK are caused by gallstones and alcohol.
The popular, and very apt, mnemonic is '**GET SMASHED**'.

◈ **G**allstones

◈ **E**thanol

◈ **T**rauma

◈ **S**teroids

◈ **M**umps (other viruses include Coxsackie B)

◈ **A**utoimmune (e.g. polyarteritis nodosa), Ascaris infection

◈ **S**corpion venom

◈ **H**ypertriglyceridaemia, Hyperchylomicronaemia, Hypercalcaemia, Hypothermia

◈ **E**RCP

◈ **D**rugs (e.g. azathioprine, mesalazine, bendroflumethiazide, furosemide, steroids, sodium valproate)

4. Chronic pancreatitis

Chronic pancreatitis is an inflammatory condition which can ultimately affect both the exocrine and endocrine functions of the pancreas. Around 80% of cases are due to alcohol excess with up to 20% of cases being unexplained.

Features

◈ Pain is typically worse 15 to 30 minutes following a meal.

◈ Steatorrhoea: symptoms of pancreatic insufficiency usually develop between 5 and 25 years after the onset of pain.

◈ Diabetes mellitus develops in the majority of patients. It typically occurs more than 20 years after symptoms begin.

Investigation

◆ abdominal X-ray shows pancreatic calcification in 30% of cases

◆ CT is more sensitive at detecting pancreatic calcification

◆ functional tests: pancreolauryl and Lundh tests may be used to assess exocrine function if imaging inconclusive

Management

◆ pancreatic enzyme supplements

◆ analgesia

◆ antioxidants: limited evidence base – one study suggests benefit in early disease

M. The acute abdomen and surgical emergencies

1. General approach to the acute abdomen

The term **acute abdomen** refers to a sudden, severe abdominal pain that is less than 24 hours in duration. It is in many cases a medical emergency, requiring urgent and specific diagnosis. Several causes need surgical treatment.

Causes

The differential diagnoses of acute abdomen include but are not limited to:

◆ acute appendicitis

◆ acute peptic ulcer and its complications

◆ acute cholecystitis

◆ acute pancreatitis

◆ acute intestinal ischaemia

◆ diabetic ketoacidosis

◆ acute diverticulitis

◆ ectopic pregnancy with tubal rupture

◆ acute peritonitis

◆ bowel perforation with free air or bowel contents in the abdominal cavity

◆ acute ureteric colic

◆ bowel volvulus

◆ acute pyelonephritis

◆ peritonitis

Ischaemic acute abdomen

Vascular abdominal disorders are more likely to affect the small bowel than the large bowel. Arterial supply to the intestines is provided by the superior and inferior mesenteric arteries respectively, both of which are direct branches of the aorta.

Acute abdomen of the ischaemic variety is usually due to:

- A thromboembolism from the left side of the heart, such as may be generated during atrial fibrillation, occluding the SMA.

- Non-occlusive ischaemia, such as that seen in hypotension secondary to heart failure may also contribute, but usually results in a mucosal or mural infarct, as contrasted with the typically transmural infarct seen in thromboembolus of the SMA.

- Primary mesenteric vein thromboses may also cause ischaemic acute abdomen, usually precipitated by hypercoagulable states such as polycythaemia vera.

Presentation

Clinically, patients present with diffuse abdominal pain, bowel distention, and bloody diarrhoea. On physical examination, bowel sounds will be absent.

Investigations

Laboratory tests reveal a neutrophilic leucocytosis, sometimes with a left shift, and increased serum amylase. Abdominal radiography will show many air-fluid levels, as well as widespread oedema.

Acute ischaemic abdomen is a surgical emergency. Typically, treatment involves removal of the region of the bowel that has undergone infarction, and subsequent anastomosis of the remaining healthy tissue.

Preparation for surgery

Patients presenting to A&E with severe abdominal pain will almost always have an abdominal X-ray and/or a CT scan. These tests can provide a differential diagnosis between simple and complex pathologies. It can also provide evidence to the doctor whether surgical intervention is necessary.

Patients will also most likely receive a FBC, looking for characteristic findings such as neutrophilia in appendicitis, and a Group & Save.

Traditionally, the use of opiates or other painkillers in patients with an acute abdomen has been discouraged before the clinical examination, because these would alter the examination.

2. Perforated viscus and peritonitis

Characteristics

+ intra-abdominal infections result in two major clinical manifestations
+ early or diffuse infection results in localised or generalised peritonitis
+ late and localised infections produce an intra-abdominal abscess
+ pathophysiology depends on competing factors of bacterial virulence and host defences
+ bacterial peritonitis (primary or secondary (see below))

Primary peritonitis

+ diffuse bacterial infection without loss of integrity of GI tract
+ often occurs in adolescent girls
+ *Streptococcus* pneumonia is the commonest organism involved

Secondary peritonitis

+ peritoneal infection commonly due to spread of infection from elsewhere in the GI tract
+ gut perforation
+ infected pancreatic necrosis
+ foreign bodies like peritoneal dialysis catheter
+ often involves multiple organisms – both aerobes and anaerobes

Commonest organisms are *E. coli* and *Bacteroides fragilis.*

Surgical management

The management of secondary peritonitis primarily involves the following:

+ elimination of the source of infection
+ reduction of bacterial contamination of the peritoneal cavity
+ prevention of persistent or recurrent intra-abdominal infections

(Could be combined with fluid resuscitation, antibiotics and ITU/HDU management. Source control achieved by closure or exteriorisation of perforation. Bacterial contamination reduced by aspiration of faecal matter and pus.)

Recurrent infection is prevented by:

◆ drains

◆ planned re-operations

◆ leaving the wound open/laparostomy

◆ peritoneal lavage (evidence-base not clear)

◆ simple swabbing of pus from peritoneal cavity may be of some value

3. Intra-abdominal abscesses

An intra-abdominal abscess may arise following:

◆ localisation of peritonitis

◆ gastrointestinal perforation

◆ anastomotic leak

◆ haematogenous spread

They develop in sites of gravitational drainage:

◆ pelvis

◆ subhepatic spaces

◆ subphrenic spaces

◆ paracolic gutters

Management

◆ ultrasound scanning may reveal the diagnosis

◆ contrast-enhanced CT is probably the investigation of choice

◆ identifies collection and often allows percutaneous drainage

Operative drainage may be required if:

◆ multi-locular abscess

◆ no safe route for percutaneous drainage

◆ recollection after percutaneous drainage

◆ patients should receive antibiotic therapy guided by organism sensitivities

4. Large bowel obstruction

Features

◆ 15% colorectal cancers present with obstruction

◆ most patients are over 70 years old

◆ risk of obstruction greatest with left-sided lesions

◆ usually present at a more advanced stage

◆ 25% have distant metastases at presentation

◆ perforation can occur at site of tumour or in a dilated caecum

Clinical presentation

◆ caecal tumours often present as small bowel obstruction

◆ colicky central abdominal pain

◆ early vomiting

◆ late absolute constipation

◆ variable extent of distension

◆ left-sided tumours present with large bowel obstruction

◆ change in bowel habit

◆ abdominal distension

◆ late vomiting

Investigation

◆ plain supine abdominal X-ray will show dilated large bowel

◆ small bowel may also be dilated depending on competence of ileocaecal valve

◆ if doubt over diagnosis or site of obstruction, consider a water soluble contrast enema

Management

All patients require:

◆ adequate resuscitation

◆ prophylactic antibiotics

◆ consenting and marking for potential stoma formation at operation

Full laparotomy should be performed.

Liver should be palpated for metastases.

Colon should be inspected for synchronous tumours.

Appropriate operations include:

- right-sided lesions – right hemicolectomy
- transverse colonic lesion – extended right hemicolectomy
- left-sided lesions – various surgical options

N. Further important lower GI condition

1. Inflammatory bowel diseases

Overview

You should be familiar with the **inflammatory bowel diseases** (Crohn's disease and ulcerative colitis).

Histology

The histological differences between ulcerative colitis and Crohn's are summarised below.

Ulcerative colitis

- inflammation in mucosa and submucosa only (unless fulminant disease)
- widespread ulceration with preservation of adjacent mucosa which has the appearance of polyps ('*pseudopolyps*')
- inflammatory cell infiltrate in lamina propria
- crypt abscesses
- depletion of goblet cells and mucin from gland epithelium
- granulomas are infrequent

Crohn's disease

- inflammation occurs in all layers, down to the serosa predisposing to strictures, fistulas and adhesions
- oedema of mucosa and submucosa, combined with deep fissured ulcers ('rose-thorn') leads to a 'cobblestone' pattern
- lymphoid aggregates
- non-caseating granulomas

Management
Crohn's disease is a form of inflammatory bowel disease. It commonly affects the terminal ileum and colon but may be seen anywhere from the mouth to anus.

General points
✦ Patients should be strongly advised to stop smoking.
✦ Some studies suggest an increased risk of relapse secondary to NSAIDs and the combined oral contraceptive pill but the evidence is patchy.

Active disease
✦ imesalazine: whilst evidence base is limited widely used in active disease
✦ steroids (oral, topical or intravenous)
✦ azathioprine is used as a second-line or steroid sparing treatment in active disease
✦ methotrexate is used in patients intolerant of azathioprine or refractory disease (*usually given intramuscularly*)
✦ infliximab is useful in refractory disease and fistulating Crohn's disease; patients typically continue on azathioprine or methotrexate

Perianal disease
✦ metronidazole is first-line; ciprofloxacin has also been used

Ulcerative colitis
Treatment can be divided into inducing and maintaining remission.

Inducing remission
✦ treatment depends on the extent and severity of disease
✦ rectal aminosalicylates or steroids: for distal colitis rectal mesalazine has been shown to be superior to rectal steroids
✦ oral aminosalicylates or steroids
✦ severe colitis should be referred to hospital

Maintaining remission
✦ oral aminosalicylates, e.g. mesalazine

Aminosalicylate drugs

5-aminosalicyclic acid (5-ASA) is released in the colon and is not absorbed. It acts locally as an anti-inflammatory. The mechanism of action is not fully understood but 5-ASA may inhibit prostaglandin synthesis.

Sulphasalazine

◈ a combination of sulphapyridine (a sulphonamide) and 5-ASA

◈ many side effects are due to the sulphapyridine moiety: rashes, oligospermia, headache, Heinz body anaemia

◈ other side effects are common to 5-ASA drugs (*see* mesalazine)

Mesalazine

◈ a delayed release form of 5-ASA, and commonest first line 5-ASA

◈ sulphapyridine side effects seen in patients taking sulphasalazine are avoided

◈ mesalazine is still however associated with side-effects such as GI upset, headache, agranulocytosis, pancreatitis, interstitial nephritis

O. Laxative abuse

1. Melanosis coli

Melanosis coli is the result of prolonged laxative use.

Often the bowel mucosa looks dark and 'stained' during colonoscopy; officially, rectal biopsy shows normal epithelium and pigment-laden macrophages in the lamina propria.

It is generally considered to be harmless, although the question of whether the condition increases the risk of colorectal cancer has been raised without any clear-cut conclusions to date. Most gastroenterologists consider it to be harmless.

It may be seen as early as 4 months after regular use of herbal laxatives, but will disappear within 6 to 12 months after laxative abuse has stopped.

P. Colorectal disorders

1. Peutz-Jeghers syndrome

Peutz-Jeghers syndrome is an autosomal dominant condition characterised by numerous hamartomatous polyps in the gastrointestinal tract. It is also associated with pigmented freckles on the lips, face, palms and soles. Around 50% of patients will have died from a gastrointestinal tract cancer by the age of 60 years.

Genetics

+ autosomal dominant
+ responsible gene encodes serine threonine kinase LKB1 or STK11

Features

+ hamartomatous polyps in GI tract (mainly small bowel)
+ pigmented lesions on lips, oral mucosa, face, palms and soles
+ intestinal obstruction, e.g. intussusception
+ gastrointestinal bleeding

Management

+ conservative (unless complications develop)

2. Colorectal cancer

Familial adenomatous polyposis (FAP) is the most common adenomatous polyposis syndrome. It is an autosomal dominant inherited disorder characterised by the early onset of hundreds of adenomatous polyps throughout the colon. If left untreated, patients with this syndrome develop colon cancer by age 35–40 years. In addition, an increased risk exists for the development of other malignancies.

The genetic defect in FAP is a germline mutation in the adenomatous polyposis coli (*APC*) gene. Syndromes once thought to be distinct from FAP are now recognised to be, in reality, part of the phenotypic spectrum of FAP.

Chapter 5

Clinical haematology (and immunology and oncology)

HAEMATOLOGY

The Foundation Programme and MRCP(UK) Part 1 syllabus (from the JRCPMTB) specify what is required in terms of competencies, skills and knowledge from junior physicians in core medical training in clinical haematology, clinical immunology and oncology. You are advised to consult carefully this syllabus, which emphasises the importance of basic medical sciences as well as a competent level of applied clinical practice.

A. Iron

1. Physiology of iron, including its absorption

Muñoz *et al.* provide an excellent overview of the **physiology of iron** in a recent review.

Iron is an essential micronutrient, as it is required for satisfactory erythropoietic function, oxidative metabolism and cellular immune response.

Absorption of dietary iron (about 1 mg/day) is tightly regulated and just balanced against iron loss because there are no active iron excretory mechanisms. Dietary iron is found in haem (10%) and non-haem (ionic, 90%) forms, and their absorption occurs at the apical surface of duodenal enterocytes via different mechanisms.

Iron is exported by ferroportin 1 (the only putative iron exporter) across the basolateral membrane of the enterocyte into the circulation (absorbed iron), where it binds to transferrin and is transported to sites of use and storage. Transferrin-bound iron enters target cells (mainly erythroid cells, but also immune and hepatic cells) via receptor-mediated endocytosis. Senescent

183

erythrocytes are phagocytosed by reticuloendothelial system macrophages, haem is metabolised by haem oxygenase, and the released iron is stored as ferritin. Iron will be later exported from macrophages to transferrin.

This internal turnover of iron is essential to meet the requirements of erythropoiesis (c. 20–30 mg/day). As transferrin becomes saturated in iron-overload states, excess iron is transported to the liver, the other main storage organ for iron, carrying the risk of free radical formation and tissue damage.

Miscellaneous causes of iron overload, apart from hereditary haemochromatosis, include:

- vitamin C overuse
- blood transfusions
- iron supplements
- iron injections

2. Heriditary haemochromatosis

Haemochromatosis is an autosomal recessive disorder of iron absorption and metabolism resulting in iron accumulation. It is caused by inheritance of mutations in the HFE gene on both copies of chromosome 6.

The British Committee for Standards in Haematology (BCSH) published **guidelines for the investigation and management of genetic haemochromatosis** in 2000.

There is continued debate about the best investigation to screen for haemochromatosis. The 2000 BCSH guidelines suggest:

- in the general population, transferrin saturation is considered the most useful marker; ferritin should also be measured but is not usually abnormal in the early stages of iron accumulation
- testing family members: genetic testing for HFE mutation

These guidelines may change as HFE gene analysis becomes less expensive.

Clinical features

- presentation above the age of 40
- hepatomegaly preceding nodular cirrhoses
- chondrocalcinosis and pseudogout
- bronze skin pigmentation
- diabetes mellitus and exocrine pancreatic failure

◆ hypopituitarism, hypogonadism and testicular atrophy

◆ cardiomyopathy and arrhythmias

Diagnostic tests

◆ molecular genetic testing for the C282Y and H63D mutations

◆ liver biopsy: Perl's stain

Typical iron study profile in a patient with haemochromatosis reveals

◆ transferrin saturation >55% in men or >50% in women

◆ raised ferritin (e.g. >500 ug/l) and iron

◆ low TIBC

Monitoring adequacy of venesection

BSCH recommend *'transferrin saturation should be kept below 50% and the serum ferritin concentration below 50 ug/l'.*

Joint X-rays characteristically show chondrocalcinosis.

3. States of iron deficiency

Iron deficiency states including diagnosis, causes and treatment.

Features

◆ koilonychia

◆ atrophic glossitis

◆ post-cricoid webs

◆ angular stomatitis

Blood film

◆ target cells

◆ *'pencil'* poikilocytes

◆ if combined with B_{12}/folate deficiency a 'dimorphic' film occurs with mixed microcytic and macrocytic cells

4. Anaemia of chronic disease and sideroblastic anaemia

Anaemia of chronic disorders (ACD)

Anaemia of chronic disease (ACD) is a form of anaemia seen in chronic illness, e.g. from chronic infection, chronic immune activation or malignancy. It is often a mild normocytic anaemia, but can sometimes be more severe, and can sometimes be a microcytic anaemia; thus, it often closely resembles iron-deficiency anaemia. Indeed, many people with chronic disease can also be genuinely iron-deficient, and the combination of the two causes of anaemia can produce a more severe anaemia. As with iron deficiency, anaemia of chronic disease is a disorder of red cell production.

While no single test is always reliable to distinguish the two causes of disease, there are sometimes some suggestive data:

◆ In ACD *without* iron deficiency, ferritin levels should be normal or high, reflecting the fact that iron is stored within cells, and ferritin is being produced as an acute phase reactant but the cells are not releasing their iron. In iron deficiency anaemia ferritin should be low.

◆ TIBC should be high in genuine iron deficiency whereas TIBC should be low or normal in anaemia of chronic disease.

5. Sideroblastic anaemia

Sideroblastic anaemia is a condition where red cells fail to completely form haem, whose biosynthesis takes place partly in the mitochondrion. This leads to deposits of iron in the mitochondria that form a ring around the nucleus called a ring sideroblast. It may be congenital or acquired.

Congenital cause

◆ δ-aminolevulinate synthase-2 deficiency

Acquired causes

◆ myelodysplasia
◆ alcohol
◆ lead
◆ anti-TB medications

Investigations

- hypochromic microcytic anaemia (more so in congenital)
- bone marrow: sideroblasts and increased iron stores

Management

- supportive
- treat any underlying cause
- pyridoxine may help

6. Hereditary haemorrhagic telangiectasia

Also known as **Osler-Weber-Rendu syndrome**, hereditary haemorrhagic telangiectasia is an autosomal dominant condition characterised by multiple telangiectasia over the skin and mucous membranes. Twenty per cent of cases occur spontaneously without prior family history.

Features

- epistaxis
- telangiectasia often found in skin, mucous membranes and internal organs
- associated with pulmonary AV malformations and other AV malformations in 10%
- may present as iron-deficiency anaemia secondary to bleeding in the GI tract or nasal mucosa

B. Megaloblastic anaemias

You should understand the physiology of vitamin B_{12} and folic acid and the mechanisms and investigation of deficiencies and their management.

1. Vitamin B_{12} deficiency

Vitamin B_{12} is mainly used in the body for red blood cell development and also maintenance of the nervous system. It is absorbed after binding to intrinsic factor (secreted from parietal cells in the stomach) and is actively absorbed in the terminal ileum. A small amount of vitamin B_{12} is passively absorbed without being bound to intrinsic factor.

Causes of vitamin B_{12} deficiency

◆ pernicious anaemia

◆ post gastrectomy

◆ poor diet

◆ disorders of terminal ileum (site of absorption): Crohn's disease, Blind-Loop syndrome, etc.

Features of vitamin B_{12} deficiency

◆ macrocytic anaemia

◆ sore tongue and mouth

◆ neurological symptoms: e.g. ataxia, subacute degeneration of the cord

◆ neuropsychiatric symptoms: e.g. mood disturbances

Management

◆ If no neurological involvement 1 mg of IM hydroxocobalamin three times each week for 2 weeks, then once every 3 months.

◆ If a patient is also deficient in folic acid then it is important to treat the B_{12} deficiency first to avoid precipitating subacute combined degeneration of the cord.

2. Folate deficiency

In adults, blood cells are made by red bone marrow. Red blood cells live for around 120 days before they are broken down and replaced, as part of a normal renewal process. Folate (folic acid) is required for production of red blood cells.

Symptoms

People with **folate-deficiency anaemia** have symptoms caused by a low level of oxygen-carrying red blood cells in the body.

Causes

There are many different types of anaemia. Folate deficiency is just one possible cause.

◆ The most common cause of folate deficiency is a poor diet. This can be due to simply not eating enough, as with anorexia nervosa or poverty, or because the diet has very limited variety. This can be a problem for the elderly, teenagers and people with drug and alcohol problems. Fad diets, where food choice is limited, can also lack sufficient folate.

◆ Certain medicines, such as some anti-epileptics and the drug methotrexate used for rheumatoid arthritis, can interfere with folate levels.

◆ Excess alcohol intake can impair the body's ability to use folate.

◆ During pregnancy, women require extra folate to meet the needs of the baby. Women who are trying to conceive or are pregnant are advised to take a daily 400 microgram folate supplement.

◆ Certain conditions that affect the gut can cause poor absorption of folate, e.g. coeliac disease and Crohn's disease.

◆ Faster turnover of red blood cells can happen with certain blood conditions. These include thalassaemia, a genetic disorder in which haemoglobin is not correctly formed, and haemolytic anaemia, in which red blood cells are fragile and easily damaged in the bloodstream.

Diagnosis

Serum red cell folate (*low*) and MCV (*increased*).

Treatment

Folate deficiency is treated by taking daily folate tablets. The folate comes in the form of the synthetic form called folic acid. This is a water-soluble vitamin that the body can use instead of folate. The normal dose is 5 mg per day for four months.

Prevention

The best way to prevent folate-deficiency anaemia is to eat a balanced, varied diet containing plenty of folate. The recommended daily amount for adults is 200 micrograms per day. A normal diet that includes vegetables, fruit and grains contains about 200 to 300 micrograms. Folate is also found in small amounts in leafy green vegetables.

C. Haemolytic anaemias

1. Causes of haemolysis

Classification by site

In intravascular haemolysis free haemoglobin is released which binds to haptoglobin. As haptoglobin becomes saturated haemoglobin binds to albumin forming methemalbumin (detected by Schumm's test). Free haemoglobin is excreted in the urine as haemoglobinuria, haemosiderinuria.

Intravascular haemolysis: causes

- mismatched blood transfusion
- glucose-6 phosphate deficiency (G6PD deficiency) (Heinz bodies are found, which are bits of oxidised denatured Hb)
- red cell fragmentation: heart valves, TTP, DIC, HUS
- paroxysmal nocturnal haemoglobinuria
- cold autoimmune haemolytic anaemia

Extravascular haemolysis: causes

- haemoglobinopathies: sickle cell, thalassaemia
- hereditary spherocytosis
- haemolytic disease of newborn
- warm autoimmune haemolytic anaemia

2. Hereditary spherocytosis

Basics

◆ most common hereditary haemolytic anaemia in northern Europeans

◆ autosomal dominant defect of RBC cytoskeleton

◆ bi-concave disc – spherocyte

◆ red cell survival reduced, destroyed by spleen

Presentation

◆ e.g. failure to thrive

◆ jaundice, gallstones

◆ splenomegaly

◆ aplastic crisis precipitated by parvovirus infection

◆ degree of haemolysis variable

Diagnosis

◆ osmotic fragility test

Management

◆ folate replacement

◆ (*surgical*: splenectomy)

3. Autoimmune haemolytic anaemia

Autoimmune haemolytic anaemia (AIHA) may be divided in to 'warm' and 'cold' types, according to at what temperature the antibodies best cause haemolysis. It is most commonly idiopathic but may be secondary to a lympho-proliferative disorder, infection or drugs. AIHA is characterised by a positive direct antiglobulin test (Coombs' test).

Warm AIHA

In warm AIHA, the antibody (usually IgG) causes haemolysis best at body temperature and haemolysis tends to occur in extravascular sites, e.g. the spleen. Management options include steroids, immunosuppression and splenectomy.

Causes of warm AIHA

◆ autoimmune disease: e.g. systemic lupus erythematosus

◆ neoplasia: e.g. lymphoma, chronic lymphatic leukaemia

◆ drugs: e.g. methyldopa

Cold AIHA

The antibody in cold AIHA is usually IgM and causes haemolysis best at 4°C. Haemolysis is mediated by complement and is more commonly intravascular. Features may include symptoms of Raynaud's phenomenon and acrocynaosis. Patients respond less well to steroids.

Causes of cold AIHA

◆ neoplasia: e.g. lymphoma

◆ infections: e.g. mycoplasma, EBV

4. Sickle cell disease

Sickle cell disease is characterised by periods of good health with intervening crises.

Molecular basis

Sickle cell anaemia is caused by a point mutation in a globin chain of haemoglobin, causing the hydrophilic amino acid glutamic acid to be replaced with the hydrophobic amino acid valine at the sixth position. This globin gene is found on the short arm of chromosome 11. The association of two 'wild-type'-globin subunits with two mutant globin subunits forms haemoglobin S (HbS).

Under low-oxygen conditions (being at high altitude, for example), the absence of a polar amino acid at position six of the globin chain promotes the non-covalent polymerisation (aggregation) of haemoglobin, which distorts red blood cells into a sickle shape and decreases their elasticity.

A low partial pressure of oxygen (PO_2) causes HbS to polymerise and precipitate, resulting in sickling of the erythrocyte. HbSS patients sickle at PO_2 of 5–6 kPa and HbAS patients sickle at PO_2 of 2.5–4 kPa.

The loss of red blood cell elasticity is central to the pathophysiology of sickle cell disease. In sickle cell disease, low-oxygen tension promotes red blood cell sickling and repeated episodes of sickling damage the cell membrane and decrease the cell's elasticity. These cells fail to return to normal shape when normal oxygen tension is restored.

Consequently, these rigid blood cells are unable to deform as they pass through narrow capillaries, leading to vessel occlusion and ischaemia. The actual anaemia of the illness is caused by haemolysis, the destruction of the red cells inside the spleen, because of their misshape. Although the bone marrow attempts to compensate by creating new red cells, it does not match the rate of destruction.

Healthy red blood cells typically live 90–120 days, but sickle cells only survive 10–20 days.

A mild disease is produced when heterozygotes for HbS combine with other haemoglobins; for example, haemoglobin C, thus creating HbSC. Sickling occurs at around 4 kPa.

Investigation

Diagnosis of sickle cell disease requires the detection of HbS. The Sickledex test involves the addition of reagent to blood; turbidity of the mixture confirms the presence of HbS, but it gives no information on other haemoglobins. Haemoglobin electrophoresis is the only investigation that determines the nature of the haemoglobinopathy.

Crises

Four main types of crises are recognised:

◆ thrombotic, 'painful crises'

◆ sequestration

◆ aplastic

◆ haemolytic

Thrombotic crises

◆ also known as painful crises or vaso-occlusive crises

◆ precipitated by infection, dehydration, deoxygenation

◆ infarcts occur in various organs including the bones (e.g. avascular necrosis of hip, hand-foot syndrome in children, lungs, spleen and brain

Sequestration crises

◆ sickling within organs such as the spleen or lungs causes pooling of blood with worsening of the anaemia

◆ acute chest syndrome: dyspnoea, chest pain, pulmonary infiltrates, low pO_2 – the most common cause of death after childhood

Aplastic crises

◆ caused by infection with parvovirus

◆ sudden fall in haemoglobin

Haemolytic crises

+ rare
+ fall in haemoglobin due to an increased rate of haemolysis

5. Paroxysmal nocturnal haemoglobinuria

Paroxysmal nocturnal haemoglobinuria (PNH) is an acquired disorder leading to haemolysis (mainly intravascular) of haematological cells. It is thought to be caused by increased sensitivity of cell membranes to complement due to a lack of glycoprotein glycosyl-phosphatidylinositol (GPI). Patients are more prone to venous thrombosis.

Pathophysiology

+ GPI can be thought of as an anchor which attaches surface proteins to the cell membrane.
+ Complement-regulating surface proteins, e.g. decay-accelerating factor (DAF), are not properly bound to the cell membrane due to a lack of GPI.
+ Thrombosis is thought to be caused by a lack of CD59 on platelet membranes predisposing to platelet aggregation.
+ Post-translational modification by the GPI glycolipid anchor is essential for the surface expression of many membrane proteins.
+ Defect of GPI biosynthesis due to somatic mutation in the haematopoietic stem cell is the basis for an acquired genetic disease, paroxysmal nocturnal haemoglobinuria.

Features

+ haemolytic anaemia
+ red blood cells, white blood cells, platelets or stem cells may be affected therefore pancytopaenia may be present
+ haemoglobinuria: classically dark-coloured urine in the morning (although has been shown to occur throughout the day)
+ thrombosis, e.g. Budd-Chiari syndrome
+ aplastic anaemia may develop in some patients

Diagnosis

+ flow cytometry of blood to detect low levels of CD59 and CD55 has now replaced Ham's test as the gold standard investigation in PNH

+ Ham's test: acid-induced haemolysis (normal red cells would not)

Management

+ blood product replacement

+ anticoagulation

+ ?monoclonal antibodies

+ stem cell transplantation

6. Thalassaemia

Thalassaemia is an inherited autosomal co-dominant blood disease. In thalassaemia, the genetic defect results in reduced rate of synthesis of one of the globin chains that make up haemoglobin.

Reduced synthesis of one of the globin chains can cause the formation of abnormal haemoglobin molecules, thus causing anaemia, the characteristic presenting symptom of the thalassaemias.

Thalassaemia is a quantitative problem of too few globins synthesised. Thalassaemias usually result in underproduction of normal globin proteins, often through mutations in regulatory genes.

D. Bone marrow failure

1. Causes of bone marrow failure

The main causes of **bone marrow failure** are congenital in nature ('constitutional'), or bone marrow failure may be acquired. Acquired bone marrow failure syndromes include single cytopaenias and pancytopaenias.

Constitutional causes include the following:

+ Constitutional aplastic anaemia is associated with chronic bone marrow failure, congenital anomalies, familial incidence, or thrombocytopaenia at birth.

+ Fanconi anaemia is characterised by familial aplastic anaemia, chromosomal breaks, and in some cases, congenital anomalies of the thumb or kidneys.

Single cytopaenias include pure red cell aplasia, which may be secondary, caused by a thymoma. It may occur transiently, resulting from a viral infection such as with parvovirus B19. Pure red cell aplasia also may be permanent, as a result of viral hepatitis. It may also be the result of lymphoproliferative diseases (e.g. lymphomas, chronic lymphocytic leukaemia) or collagen vascular diseases (e.g. systemic lupus erythematosus, refractory anaemia), or it may occur during pregnancy.

Early forms of myelodysplastic syndrome initially can also manifest as a single cytopaenia or, more often, as a bicytopaenia. Pancytopaenia (decrease in all three cell lines) is the most common manifestation of bone marrow failure. Aplastic or hypoplastic anaemia can be idiopathic in nature, or it can develop from secondary causes. Myelodysplastic anaemia also can cause pancytopaenia.

2. Complications of bone marrow failure

Patients with bone marrow failure present with low blood counts.

Low platelet counts predispose patients to spontaneous bleeding in the skin and mucous membranes. Neutropaenia places the patient at risk for serious infections. Bleeding complications are usually the most alarming symptom, and infections prompt individuals to visit the emergency department.

Weakness and fatigue resulting from anaemia can develop slowly. Months may elapse before the patient seeks medical help with these symptoms.

Family and personal medical histories can help distinguish inherited causes from acquired causes. Inherited bone marrow failure is usually diagnosed in young adults but may be missed until their fifth or sixth decades of life. These diseases should be considered if any of the following are present: subtle but characteristic physical anomalies, haematologic cytopaenias, unexplained macrocytosis, myelodysplastic syndrome or acute myelogenous leukaemia, or squamous cell cancer even in the absence of pancytopaenia or a positive family history. Cases in which siblings of a patient with known Fanconi anaemia who developed abnormal blood counts should be investigated.

Exposure to toxins, drugs, environmental hazards and recent viral infections (e.g. hepatitis) should be noted.

E. Oral anticoagulation treatment

1. Indications for oral anti-coagulant treatment

According to current guidance (**SIGN 36**), recent overviews of such controlled trials have suggested that antithrombotic prophylaxis in appropriate people at increased risk of thrombosis, and antithrombotic treatment in appropriate patients with acute thrombosis, not only reduces disability and mortality, but is also cost-effective.

Warfarin is the oral anticoagulant of choice. Nicoumalone and phenindione are licensed in the UK but are potentially more toxic than warfarin and are seldom used.

All currently available oral anticoagulants act by antagonising the effect of vitamin K, resulting in reduced hepatic production of active coagulation factors II, VII, IX and X, and hence in prolongation of the prothrombin time and INR. This usually takes 48–72 hours to develop fully. Hence in acute thromboembolism anticoagulation should be commenced with heparin, which should be continued until the INR has been within the desired range of the target for at least two consecutive days. Heparin is not required when oral anticoagulants are started electively for prophylaxis of thromboembolism, except in certain thrombophilias.

The average daily dose of warfarin to achieve an INR within the desired range of the target (usually 2.0–3.0) is 5 mg, but with wide variation (range 1–15 mg). Warfarin sensitivity varies widely between individuals, and within the same person, due to variables such as age, diet, diseases and drugs. A well-stabilised patient may need an INR check only every 4–8 weeks; however, any change in clinical state or in medication should prompt more frequent checks.

2. Monitoring of oral anticoagulation treatment

When initiating warfarin therapy ('**warfarinisation**'), the doctor will decide how strong the anticoagulant therapy needs to be. The target INR level will vary from case to case depending on the clinical indicators, but tends to be 2–3 in most conditions. In particular, target INR may be 2.5–3.5 (or even 3.0–4.5) in patients with one or more mechanical heart valves.

Dosing of warfarin is complicated by the fact that it is known to interact with many commonly used medications and even with chemicals that may be present in certain foods. These interactions may enhance or reduce warfarin's anticoagulation effect. In order to optimise the therapeutic effect without risking dangerous side effects such as bleeding, close monitoring of the degree of anticoagulation is required by blood testing (INR).

During the initial stage of treatment, checking may be required daily; intervals between tests can be lengthened if the patient manages stable therapeutic INR levels on an unchanged warfarin dose.

3. Management of oral anti-coagulant over-treatment

Reversal of anticoagulation can be achieved by stopping warfarin, administering vitamin K1, or giving blood products containing the vitamin K-dependent clotting factors, i.e. factor IX complex concentrate (containing factors II, IX and X) and factor VII concentrate, or fresh frozen plasma.

This is, however, a complex area and specialist help should be sought.

The most common cause of fatal or disabling bleeding in patients receiving anticoagulant therapy is intracranial or intraspinal bleeding.

In the patient with active bleeding, as well as measuring the INR, it is important to perform a full coagulation screen (APTT, fibrinogen and platelet count) and a full blood count to ensure that the patient does not have any other abnormality predisposing to bleeding, e.g. thrombocytopaenia. Blood urea and liver function tests should be checked to assess the hepatic and renal status.

Immediate management should be directed towards arresting bleeding, even although in doing so it may temporarily increase the risk of thrombosis in individuals with continuing long term risk, e.g. in the presence of a prosthetic heart valve.

F. Transfusion reactions

1. Overview of transfusion reactions

Clear information about transfusion reactions is provided in the **UK Blood Transfusion and Tissue Transplantation Services**.

These are classified as:

⬧ acute haemolytic transfusion reaction

⬧ reaction to infusion of a bacterially contaminated unit

⬧ 'transfusion-related acute-lung injury' (TRALI)

⬧ acute fluid overload and severe allergic reaction or anaphylaxis

Serious or life-threatening acute reactions are rare but new symptoms or signs that appear while a patient is being transfused must be taken seriously as they may be the first warnings of a serious reaction. It can be difficult to determine the type of reaction in the early stages.

Recognition and management of transfusion reactions

Incompatible transfused red cells react with the patient's own anti-A or anti-B antibodies and cause an acute severe clinical reaction. Infusion of ABO-incompatible blood is most commonly due to errors in taking or labelling the sample, collecting the wrong blood from the fridge, or failure to carry out the required checks immediately before transfusion of the pack is started.

If red cells are mistakenly administered to the 'wrong' patient, the chance of ABO incompatibility is about one in three. The reaction is usually most severe if group A red cells are infused to a group O patient. Even a few millilitres of ABO incompatible blood may cause symptoms within a few minutes that will be noticed by a conscious patient. However, if the patient is unconscious or cannot communicate, the first signs of the reaction may be bleeding, tachycardia, hypotension or hypertension. Acute haemolysis may also occur following infusion of plasma-rich components, usually platelets or FFP, containing high-titre of anti-red-cell antibodies, usually anti-A or B.

Management

Stop the transfusion. Maintain venous access. Resuscitate with crystalloid fluid. Consider inotrope support if hypotension is prolonged. Take blood cultures and samples for culture from component pack. Inform the blood bank. Seek urgent critical care and haematology advice. Admit to ICU if possible.

G. Polycythaemia

1. Polycythaemia

Causes

Polycythaemia may be relative, primary (polycythaemia rubra vera) or secondary.

Relative causes

◆ dehydration

◆ stress: Gaisbock syndrome

Primary

◆ polycythaemia rubra vera

Secondary causes

◆ COPD

◆ altitude

◆ obstructive sleep apnoea

◆ excessive erythropoietin: cerebellar haemangioma, hypernephroma, hepatoma, uterine fibroids

To differentiate between true (primary or secondary) polycythaemia and relative polycythaemia red cell mass studies are sometimes used. In true polycythaemia the total red cell mass in males >35 ml/kg and in women >32 ml/kg.

2. Overview of myeloproliferative disorders

Myeloproliferative disorders is the name for a group of conditions that cause blood cell platelets, white blood cells, and red blood cells to grow abnormally in the bone marrow. Though myeloproliferative disorders are serious, and may pose certain health risks, people with these conditions often live for many years after diagnosis. The prognosis largely depends on the type of disorder.

Myeloproliferative disorders include:

◆ polycythaemia vera – occurs when the bone marrow produces too many blood cells, especially red blood cells

◆ essential thrombocytosis – occurs when the body produces too many platelet cells, which help blood to clot; clots can block blood vessels leading to heart attack or stroke

◆ primary or idiopathic myelofibrosis (also known as myelosclerosis) – occurs when the bone marrow produces too much collagen or fibrous tissue in the bone marrow; this reduces bone marrow's ability to produce blood cells

* chronic myeloid leukaemia (CML) – cancer of the bone marrow that produces abnormal granulocytes in the bone marrow

Diagnosis

A sign shared by all myeloproliferative disorders (with the exception of essential thrombocytosis) is an enlarged spleen, which can be detected during a routine physical examination. In addition to performing a physical exam, the doctor may also conduct the following tests:

* **Blood tests** – detect abnormal types or numbers of red or white blood cells. They can also detect anaemia and leukaemia.

* **Bone marrow biopsy** – sample of bone marrow may be taken after blood tests. It can show the presence of abnormal types or numbers of red or white blood cells and may detect certain types of anaemia and cancer in the marrow.

* **Cytogenetic analysis** – blood or bone marrow are viewed under a microscope to look for changes in the chromosomes.

3. Polycythaemia rubra vera

Polycythaemia rubra vera (PRV) is a myeloproliferative disorder caused by clonal proliferation of a marrow stem cell leading to an increase in red cell volume, often accompanied by overproduction of neutrophils and platelets. It has recently been established that a mutation in JAK2 is present in approximately 95% of patients with PRV and this has resulted in significant changes to the diagnostic criteria. The incidence of PRV peaks in the sixth decade.

Features

* hyperviscosity
* pruritus, typically after a hot bath
* splenomegaly
* haemorrhage (secondary to abnormal platelet function)
* plethoric appearance
* hypertension in a third of patients

Investigations

Following history and examination, the British Committee for Standards in Haematology (BCSH) recommend the following tests are performed.

◆ full blood count/film (raised haematocrit; neutrophils, basophils, platelets raised in half of patients)

◆ JAK2 mutation

◆ serum ferritin

◆ renal and liver function tests

If the JAK2 mutation is negative and there is no obvious secondary causes the BCSH suggest the following tests:

◆ red cell mass

◆ arterial oxygen saturation

◆ abdominal ultrasound

◆ serum erythropoietin level

◆ bone marrow aspirate and trephine

◆ cytogenetic analysis

◆ erythroid burst-forming unit (BFU-E) culture

Other features that may be seen in PRV include a low ESR and a raised leucocyte alkaline phosphatase.

 The diagnostic criteria for PRV have recently been updated by the BCSH. This replaces the previous PRV Study Group criteria.

◆ JAK2-positive PRV – diagnosis requires both criteria to be present

◆ A1 high haematocrit (>0.52 in men, >0.48 in women) OR raised red cell mass (>25% above predicted)

◆ A2 mutation in JAK2

◆ JAK2-negative PRV – diagnosis requires A1 + A2 + A3 + either another A or two B criteria

◆ A1 raised red cell mass (>25% above predicted) OR haematocrit >0.60 in men, >0.56 in women

◆ A2 absence of mutation in JAK2

◆ A3 no cause of secondary erythrocytosis

◆ A4 palpable splenomegaly

◆ A5 presence of an acquired genetic abnormality (excluding BCR-ABL) in the haematopoietic cells

◆ B1 thrombocytosis (platelet count >450 × 10^9/l)

◆ B2 neutrophil leucocytosis (neutrophil count >10 × 10^9/l in non-smokers; >12.5 × 10^9/l in smokers)

◆ B3 radiological evidence of splenomegaly

◆ B4 endogenous erythroid colonies or low serum erythropoietin

Management

Polycythaemia rubra vera is a myeloproliferative disorder caused by clonal proliferation of a marrow stem cell leading to an increase in red cell volume, often accompanied by overproduction of neutrophils and platelets. It has peak incidence in the sixth decade, with typical features including hyperviscosity, pruritus and splenomegaly.

◆ venesection – first-line treatment

◆ hydroxyurea – slight increased risk of secondary leukaemia

◆ phosphorus-32 therapy

Prognosis

◆ thrombotic events are a significant cause of morbidity and mortality

◆ 30% of patients progress to myelofibrosis

◆ 5%–15% of patients progress to acute leukaemia

H. Important leukaemias and lymphomas
1. Acute lymphocytic leukaemia (ALL)

Before treatment was available, most people who had **acute lymphocytic leukaemia** (ALL) died within 4 months of the diagnosis. Now, nearly 80% of children and 30%–40% of adults with ALL are cured. For most people, the first course of chemotherapy brings the disease under control (complete remission). Children between the ages of 3 and 7 have the best prognosis. Children younger than 2 and older adults fare least well. The white blood cell count and particular chromosome abnormalities in the leukaemia cells also influence outcome.

2. Associations with haematological malignancies and infections

Viruses

✦ EBV: Hodgkin's and Burkitt's lymphoma, nasopharyngeal carcinoma

✦ HTLV-1: adult T-cell leukaemia/lymphoma

✦ HIV-1: high-grade B-cell lymphoma

Bacteria

✦ *Helicobacter pylori*: gastric lymphoma (MALT)

Protozoa

✦ malaria: Burkitt's lymphoma

3. Haematological malignancies and genetics

Genetics

Below is a brief summary of the common translocations associated with haematological malignancies.

t(9;22) – Philadelphia chromosome

✦ present in >95% of patients with CML

✦ this results in part of the *Abelson* proto-oncogene being moved to the BCR gene on chromosome 22

✦ the resulting BCR-ABL gene codes for a fusion protein which has tyrosine kinase activity in excess of normal; the product of the bcr/abl gene that is seen in 97% cases of chronic myeloid leukaemia is a constitutively active tyrosine kinase – this is responsible for the leukaemic process

✦ poor prognostic indicator in ALL

t(15;17)

✦ seen in acute promyelocytic leukaemia (M3)

✦ fusion of PML and RAR-alpha genes

t(8;14)

✦ seen in Burkitt's lymphoma

✦ MYC oncogene is translocated to an immunoglobulin gene

t(11;14)

+ mantle cell lymphoma

+ deregulation of the cyclin D1 (BCL-1) gene

4. A note on proto-oncogenes

Oncogenes are endogenous human deoxyribonucleic acid (DNA) sequences that arise from normal genes called proto-oncogenes.

Proto-oncogenes are normally expressed in many cells, particularly during foetal development, and are thought to play an important regulatory role in cell growth and development.

Alterations in the proto-oncogene can activate an oncogene, which produces unregulated gene activity, contributing directly to tumourogenesis.

Oncogene alterations are also important causes of:

+ rhabdomyosarcomas (ras oncogene)

+ Burkitt's lymphoma (C-myc is translocated intact from its normal position on chromosome 8 to chromosome 14)

+ Neuroblastoma (N-myc proto-oncogene is seen in a proportion of patients with poor prognosis)

They should be contrasted with tumour suppressor genes. In this situation, the genes normally down-regulate cell growth, and require inactivation to allow malignant growth. Examples include retinoblastoma.

5. Hodgkin's disease

Lymphoproliferative diseases include **Hodgkin's disease, non-Hodgkin's lymphomas**, and **plasma cell dyscrasias**. Hodgkin's lymphoma is a malignant proliferation of lymphocytes characterised by the presence of the Reed-Sternberg cell. It has a bimodal age distribution being most common in the third and seventh decades.

Staging
Ann-Arbor staging of Hodgkin's lymphoma
   I: single lymph node
   II: two or more lymph nodes/regions on same side of diaphragm
   III: nodes on both sides of diaphragm
   IV: spread beyond lymph nodes

Each stage may be subdivided into A or B

A = no systemic symptoms other than pruritus

B = weight loss >10% in last 6 months, fever >38°C, night sweats (poor prognosis)

Histological classification

◆ nodular sclerosing: most common, good prognosis

◆ mixed cellularity: good prognosis

◆ lymphocyte predominant: best prognosis

◆ lymphocyte depleted: least common, worst prognosis

'B' symptoms also imply a poor prognosis

◆ weight loss >10% in last 6 months

◆ fever >38°C

◆ night sweats

Other factors associated with a poor prognosis identified in a 1998 *NEJM* paper included:

◆ age = 45 years

◆ stage IV disease

◆ haemoglobin <10.5 g/dl

◆ lymphocyte count <600/µl or <8%

◆ male

◆ albumin <40 g/L

◆ white blood count = 15 × 10⁹/l

6. Burkitt's lymphoma

Burkitt's lymphoma is a high-grade B-cell neoplasm. There are two major forms:

◆ endemic (African) form: typically involves maxilla or mandible

◆ sporadic form: abdominal (e.g. ileo-caecal) tumours are the most common form; more common in patients with HIV

Burkitt's lymphoma is associated with the c-myc gene translocation, usually t(8;14). The Epstein-Barr virus (EBV) is strongly implicated in the development of the African form but the link to sporadic Burkitt's is less clear.

Management is with chemotherapy. This tends to produce a rapid response which may cause '**tumour lysis syndrome**'.

Complications of tumour lysis syndrome include:

- hyperkalaemia
- hyperphosphataemia
- hypocalcaemia
- hyperuricaemia
- acute renal failure

7. Acute promyelocytic leukaemia

You are not normally expected to be able to differentiate the different subtypes of acute myeloid leukaemia (AML) for the MRCP(UK). An exception to this is **acute promyelocytic leukaemia** (APML, the M3 subtype of AML). The importance of identifying APML lies in both the presentation (classically disseminated intravascular coagulation) and management.

APML is associated with the t(15;17) translocation which causes fusion of the PML and RAR genes.

Features

- presents younger than other types of AML (average age 25 years)
- DIC or thrombocytopaenia often at presentation
- good prognosis

BOX 5.1   A note on dissesseminated intravascular coagulation (DIC)

DIC is caused by the enhanced and abnormally sustained generation of thrombin. Organ failure is a common finding, being as common as bleeding in DIC, and is likely to be due to fibrin deposition within the organ.

The presence of DIC significantly increases mortality rates in affected patients, and treatment of the underlying cause of the DIC, e.g. sepsis, does not always lead to resolution of the condition. Several clinical trials have been published to guide treatment in DIC, one of which confirms the improved mortality with recombinant human-activated protein C.

Secondary bursts of thrombin formation seen in DIC are instigated by the intrinsic pathway.

8. Acute myeloid leukaemia

Acute myeloid leukaemia is the more common form of acute leukaemia in adults. It may occur as a primary disease or following a secondary transformation of a myeloproliferative disorder.

Poor prognostic features

+ age >60 years
+ 20% blasts after first course of chemotherapy
+ cytogenics: deletions of chromosome 5 or 7

Acute promyelocytic leukaemia M3

+ associated with t(15;17)
+ fusion of PML and RAR-alpha genes
+ presents younger than other types of AML (average = 25 years old)
+ DIC or thrombocytopaenia often at presentation
+ good prognosis

Classification – French-American-British (FAB)

+ MO – undifferentiated
+ M1 – without maturation
+ M2 – with granulocytic maturation
+ M3 – acute promyelocytic
+ M4 – granulocytic and monocytic maturation
+ M5 – monocytic
+ M6 – erythroleukaemic
+ M7 – megakaryoblastic

9. Chronic lymphocytic leukaemia

Chronic lymphocytic leukaemia (CLL) is caused by a monoclonal proliferation of well-differentiated lymphocytes which are almost always B-cells (99%). A definitive diagnosis of CLL is based on the combination of a lymphocytosis and characteristic lymphocyte morphology and immunophenotype.

Features

◆ often none

◆ constitutional: anorexia, weight loss

◆ bleeding, infections

◆ lymphadenopathy more marked than CML

Complications

◆ pan-hypogammaglobulinaemia leading to recurrent infections (often, for example, recurrent bacterial infections)

◆ warm autoimmune haemolytic anaemia in 10–15% of patients

◆ transformation to high-grade lymphoma (Richter's transformation)

Investigations

◆ blood film: '*smudge cells*'

◆ immunophenotyping

Management
Indications for treatment

◆ progressive marrow failure: the development or worsening of anaemia and/or thrombocytopaenia

◆ massive (*>6 cm*) or progressive lymphadenopathy

◆ massive (*>10 cm*) or progressive splenomegaly

◆ progressive lymphocytosis: >50% increase over 2 months or lymphocyte doubling time <6 months

◆ systemic symptoms: weight loss >10% in previous 6 months, fever >38ºC for >2 weeks, extreme fatigue, night sweats

◆ autoimmune cytopaenias, e.g. ITP

◆ none early on

◆ chlorambucil to reduce lymphocyte count

◆ other options include fludarabine

10. Chronic myeloid leukaemia

The Philadelphia chromosome is present in more than 95% of patients with **chronic myeloid leukaemia** (CML). It is due to a translocation between the long arm of chromosome 9 and 22 – t(9;22)(q34; q11). This results in part of the ABL proto-oncogene from chromosome 9 being fused with the BCR gene from chromosome 22. The resulting BCR-ABL gene codes for a fusion protein which has tyrosine kinase activity in excess of normal.

Presentation

◆ middle age

◆ anaemia, weight loss, abdominal discomfort

◆ splenomegaly may be marked

◆ spectrum of myeloid cells seen in peripheral blood

◆ decreased neutrophil alkaline phosphatase

◆ may undergo blast transformation (AML in 80%, ALL in 20%)

Management

◆ hydroxyurea

◆ interferon

◆ imatinib

◆ allogenic bone marrow transplant

Imatinib

◆ inhibitor of the tyrosine kinase associated with the BCR-ABL defect

◆ very high response rate in chronic phase CML

I. Further important haematological malignancies

1. Myelodysplastic syndromes

The **myelodysplastic syndromes** are a diverse collection of haematological conditions united by ineffective production (or dysplasia) of myeloid blood cells and risk of transformation to acute myelogenous leukaemia (AML).

Myelodysplastic syndromes are bone marrow stem cell disorders resulting in disorderly and ineffective haematopoiesis manifested by irreversible quantitative and qualitative defects in haematopoietic cells. In a majority of cases, the course of disease is chronic with gradually worsening cytopaenias due to progressive bone marrow failure. Approximately ⅓ of patients with MDS progress to AML within months to a few years.

The median age at diagnosis of a MDS is between 60 and 75 years; a few patients are younger than 50; MDS diagnoses are rare in children. Males are slightly more commonly affected than females.

Signs and symptoms are non-specific and generally related to the blood cytopaenias. Although there is some risk for developing acute myelogenous leukaemia, about 50% of deaths occur as a result of bleeding or infection.

Investigations

⬥ FBC and examination of blood film. Blood tests to eliminate other common causes of cytopaenias, such as lupus, hepatitis, B12, folate or other vitamin deficiencies, renal failure or heart failure, HIV, haemolytic anaemia, monoclonal gammopathy. Bone marrow examination by a haematopathologist.

⬥ Cytogenetics or chromosomal studies.

⬥ Flow cytometry is helpful to establish the presence of any lymphoproliferative disorder in the marrow.

2. Causes of myelodysplastic syndromes

Myelodysplastic syndromes into two categories based on their cause:

⬥ **Myelodysplastic syndromes with no known cause.** Called *de novo* myelodysplastic syndromes; doctors do not know what causes these. *De novo* myelodysplastic syndromes are often more easily treated than are myelodysplastic syndromes with a known cause.

⬥ **Myelodysplastic syndromes caused by chemicals and radiation.** Myelodysplastic syndromes that occur in response to cancer treatments, such as chemotherapy and radiation, or in response to chemical exposure are called secondary myelodysplastic syndromes. Secondary myelodysplastic syndromes are often more difficult to treat.

Treatment – various treatment regimens exist, details of which are beyond the scope of the book (and probably the exam).

J. Disorders of clotting

1. Essential thrombocythaemia

Essential thrombocythaemia is characterised by an increased platelet count, megakaryocytic hyperplasia, and a haemorrhagic or thrombotic tendency.

Symptoms and signs may include weakness, headaches, paresthesias, bleeding, splenomegaly and digital ischaemia.

Diagnosis is based on a platelet count >500,000/µL, normal RBC mass or normal Hct in the presence of adequate iron stores, and absence of myelofibrosis, the Philadelphia chromosome (or ABL-BCR rearrangement) and any other disorder that could cause thrombocytosis.

Treatment is controversial but may include oral low dose aspirin. Patients >60 years and those with multiple co-morbidities require cytotoxic drugs to lower platelet counts.

2. Idiopathic thrombocytopaenic purpura

Idiopathic thrombocytopaenic purpura (ITP) is an immune-mediated reduction in the platelet count. Antibodies are directed against the glycoprotein IIb-IIIa or Ib complex ITP.

The condition can essentially be divided into acute and chronic forms.

Acute ITP

◈ more commonly seen in children

◈ equal sex incidence

◈ may follow an infection or vaccination

◈ usually runs a self-limiting course over 1–

Chronic ITP

◈ more common in young/middle-aged women

◈ tends to run a relapsing-remitting course

Evan's syndrome

+ ITP in association with autoimmune haemolytic anaemia (AIHA)

Investigations

+ antiplatelet autoantibodies (usually IgG)
+ bone marrow aspiration shows megakaryocytes in the marrow; this should be carried out prior to the commencement of steroids in order to rule out leukaemia

Management

+ oral prednisolone (80% of patients respond)
+ splenectomy if platelets <30 after 3 months of steroid therapy
+ IV immunoglobulins
+ immunosuppressive drugs, e.g. cyclophosphamide

3. Thrombophilia: causes
Inherited

+ activated protein C resistance (factor V Leiden)
+ antithrombin III deficiency
+ protein C deficiency
+ protein S deficiency

Acquired

+ antiphospholipid syndrome
+ the oral contraceptive pill

4. Protein C deficiency
Protein C deficiency is an autosomal dominant condition which causes an increased risk of thrombosis.

Features

+ venous thromboembolism
+ skin necrosis following the commencement of warfarin: when warfarin is first started biosynthesis of protein C is reduced

Thrombosis may occur in venules leading to skin necrosis.

5. Antithrombin III deficiency

Antithrombin III deficiency is an inherited cause of thrombophilia occurring in approximately 1 : 2000 of the population. Inheritance is autosomal dominant.

Antithrombin III inhibits several clotting factors, primarily thrombin, factor X and factor IX. It mediates the effects of heparin.

Antithrombin III deficiency comprises a heterogeneous group of disorders, with some patients having a deficiency of normal antithrombin III while others produce abnormal antithrombin III.

Features

+ recurrent venous thromboses
+ arterial thromboses do occur but are uncommon

Management

+ thromboembolic events are treated with lifelong warfarinisation
+ heparinisation during pregnancy
+ antithrombin III concentrates (often used during surgery or childbirth)

6. Activated protein C resistance

Activated protein C resistance is the most common inherited thrombophilia. It is due to a mutation in the Factor V Leiden gene. Heterozygotes have a five-fold risk of venous thrombosis whilst homozygotes have a 50-fold increased risk.

7. Haemophilia

Haemophilia is an X-linked recessive disorder of coagulation. Up to 30% of patients have no family history of the condition. Haemophilia A is due to a deficiency of factor VIII while in haemophilia B (Christmas disease) there is a lack of factor IX.

Features

+ haemoarthroses, haematomas
+ prolonged bleeding after surgery or trauma

Blood tests

+ prolonged APTT
+ bleeding time, thrombin time, prothrombin time normal

Up to 10%–15% of patients with haemophilia A develop antibodies to factor VIII treatment.

8. Von Willebrand's disease

Von Willebrand's disease is the most common inherited bleeding disorder. The majority of cases are inherited in an autosomal dominant fashion and characteristically behave like a platelet disorder, i.e. epistaxis and menorrhagia are common whilst haemoarthroses and muscle haematomas are rare.

Role of von Willebrand factor

+ large glycoprotein which forms massive multimers up to 1 000 000 Da in size
+ promotes platelet adhesion to damaged endothelium
+ carrier molecule for factor VIII

Types

+ type 1: partial reduction in vWF (80% of patients)
+ type 2: abnormal form of vWF
+ type 3: total lack of vWF (autosomal recessive)

Investigation

+ prolonged bleeding time (as a screening test)
+ APTT may be prolonged
+ factor VIII levels (FVIIIc) may be moderately reduced
+ defective platelet aggregation with ristocetin

In Type I vWF the prothrombin time (PT) and platelet aggregation will be normal. Bleeding time, APTT and FVIIIc are likely to be abnormal. The bleeding time would be a good screening test, but the most useful test in practice is to do the VWB antigen and activity (RICOF) test to get a quantitative measure.

Management

+ tranexamic acid for mild bleeding
+ desmopressin (DDAVP): raises levels of vWF by inducing release of vWF from endothelial cells
+ factor VIII concentrate

K. Aplastic anaemia

1. Causes

◆ high-dose radiation and chemotherapy treatments

◆ exposure to toxic chemicals, e.g. benzene

◆ use of certain drugs

◆ autoimmune disorders (e.g. Epstein Barr virus, HIV)

◆ pregnancy

◆ unknown factors

An **aplastic crisis** in also most commonly caused by infection with the parvovirus B19.

2. Outcome

The virus infects red cell progenitors in bone marrow, resulting in cessation of erythropoiesis and a very rapid drop in haemoglobin.

The condition is self-limiting, with bone marrow recovery occurring in 7–10 days, followed by brisk reticulocytosis.

L. Blood films

1. Typical pictures

Hyposplenism, e.g. post-splenectomy

◆ target cells

◆ Howell-Jolly bodies

◆ Cabot's rings

◆ siderotic granules

◆ acanthocytes

◆ schizocytes

Iron-deficiency anaemia

◆ target cells

◆ *'pencil'* poikilocytes

◆ if combined with B_{12}/folate deficiency, a 'dimorphic' film occurs with mixed microcytic and macrocytic cells

Myelofibrosis

◆ *'tear-drop'* poikilocytes

Intravascular haemolysis

◆ schistocytes

◆ hypersegmented neutrophils

M. Myeloma and related conditions

1. Myeloma

Clinical features

Myeloma is a neoplasm of the bone marrow plasma cells. The peak incidence is in patients aged 60–70 years. Clinical presentation is varied. Presenting features include:

◆ symptoms of bone disease: typically persistent, unexplained backache

◆ impaired renal function

◆ anaemia: typically normochromic, normocytic, and less frequently leucopenia and/or thrombocytopaenia

◆ hypercalcaemia

◆ recurrent or persistent bacterial infection

◆ hyperviscosity

◆ symptoms suggestive of spinal cord/nerve root compression

◆ features suggestive of amyloidosis, such as nephrotic syndrome and cardiac failure

◆ persistently raised erythrocyte sedimentation rate (ESR) or plasma viscosity as an incidental finding

Diagnosis is based on:

◆ monoclonal proteins in the serum and urine (Bence Jones proteins)

◆ increased plasma cells in the bone marrow

◆ bone lesions on the skeletal survey

Hypercalcaemia in myeloma

◆ due primarily to increased osteoclastic bone resorption caused by local cytokines released by the myeloma cells

✦ other contributing factors include impaired renal function, increased renal tubular calcium reabsorption and elevated PTH-rP levels

Smith *et al.* (2006) in the *British Journal of Haematology* for the management of multiple myeloma recommends the following:

✦ in mild hypercalcaemia, rehydrate with oral fluids

✦ in moderate–severe hypercalcaemia (corrected calcium) rehydrate with intravenous fluids and give furosemide if required

✦ if not already on a bisphosphonate, start bisphosphonate immediately

✦ if already on a bisphosphonate, consider changing to a more potent bisphosphonate or increasing the dose; additional therapy may be required in refractory patients

This paper also makes the following useful recommendations on pain control:

✦ an analgesic appropriate to the severity of the pain should be used

✦ non-steroidal anti-inflammatory drugs should be avoided

✦ analgesics should be given regularly

✦ oral analgesia is preferable where possible

✦ side effects should be actively managed

✦ analgesic requirements should be regularly recorded

✦ additional non-analgesic drugs should be considered in individual circumstances

Prognosis

$\beta2$-microglobulin is a useful marker of prognosis (it is recommended, overall, in preference to the *Salmon-Durie* index) – raised levels imply poor prognosis. Low levels of albumin are also associated with a poor prognosis (Table 5.1).

TABLE 5.1 International prognostic index

Stage	Criteria	Median survival (months)
I	B2 microglobulin <3.5 mg/l	62
	Albumin >35 g/L	
II	Not I or III	45
III	β2 microglobulin >5 mg/l	29

Management

Significant improvements in survival may be expected through the addition of thalidomide to standard chemotherapeutic regimes. Studies suggest a significant improvement at both two years and five years with thalidomide.

2. Waldenström's macroglobulinaemia

Waldenström's macroglobulinaemia is an uncommon condition seen in older men. It is a lymphoplasmacytoid malignancy characterised by the secretion of a monoclonal IgM paraprotein.

Features

* monoclonal IgM paraproteinaemia
* systemic upset: weight loss, lethargy
* hyperviscosity syndrome, e.g. visual disturbance
* hepatosplenomegaly
* lymphadenopathy
* cryoglobulinaemia, e.g. Raynaud's phenomenon

3. Monoclonal gammopathy of undetermined significance (MGUS)

Monoclonal gammopathy of undetermined significance (MGUS, also known as benign paraproteinaemia and monoclonal gammopathy) is a common condition that causes a paraproteinaemia and is often mistaken for myeloma. Differentiating features are listed below. Around 10% of patients eventually develop myeloma at 5 years, with 50% at 15 years.

Features

* usually asymptomatic
* no bone pain or increased risk of infections
* around 10%–30% of patients have a demyelinating neuropathy

Differentiating features from myeloma

* normal immune function
* normal $\beta 2$ microglobulin levels
* lower level of paraproteinaemia than myeloma (e.g. <30 g/l IgG, or <20 g/l IgA)
* stable level of paraproteinaemia
* no clinical features of myeloma (e.g. lytic lesions on X-rays or renal disease)

N. White cell disorders

1. Leukaemoid reaction

The leukaemoid reaction describes the presence of immature cells such as myeloblasts, promyelocytes and nucleated red cells in the peripheral blood. This may be due to infiltration of the bone marrow causing the immature cells to be 'pushed out' or sudden demand for new cells.

Causes

◆ severe infection

◆ severe haemolysis

◆ massive haemorrhage

◆ metastatic cancer with bone marrow infiltration

A relatively common clinical problem is differentiating chronic myeloid leukaemia from a leukaemoid reaction.

Leukaemoid reaction

◆ high leucocyte alkaline phosphatase score

◆ toxic granulation (*Döhle bodies*) in the white cells

◆ '*left shift*' of neutrophils, i.e. three or less segments of the nucleus

Chronic myeloid leukaemia

◆ low leucocyte alkaline phosphatase score

2. Leucocytosis

Leucocytosis is more accurately described by the term neutrophilia. The most common and important cause of neutrophilia is infection, and most infections cause neutrophilia. The degree of elevation often indicates the severity of the infection.

Tissue damage from other causes raises the white count for similar reasons. Burns, infarction (cutting off the blood supply to a region of the body so that it dies), crush injuries, inflammatory diseases, poisonings and severe diseases, like kidney failure and diabetic ketoacidosis, all cause neutrophilia.

Counts almost as high occur in leukaemoid (leukaemia-like) reactions caused by infection and non-infectious inflammation. Drugs can also cause leucocytosis. Cortisone-like drugs (such as prednisolone), lithium, and NSAIDs are the most common offenders.

Non-specific stresses also cause white blood cells to increase in the blood.

3. Leucopenia

Low white cell counts are associated with chemotherapy, radiation therapy, leukaemia (as malignant cells overwhelm the bone marrow), myelofibrosis and aplastic anaemia (failure of white and red cell creation, along with poor platelet production).

Other causes of low white blood cell count include influenza, systemic lupus erythematosus, Hodgkin's lymphoma, some types of cancer, typhoid, malaria, tuberculosis, dengue, rickettsial infections, enlargement of the spleen, folate deficiencies, psittacosis and sepsis. Many other causes exist, such as a deficiency in certain minerals, e.g. copper and zinc.

Some medications can have an impact on the number and function of white blood cells. Medications which can cause leucopenia include clozapine, an antipsychotic medication with a rare adverse effect leading to the total absence of all granulocytes (neutrophils, basophils, eosinophils). Other medications include immunosuppressive drugs, such as sirolimus, mycophenolate mofetil, tacrolimus and cyclosporine. Minocycline, a commonly prescribed antibiotic, is another drug known to cause leucopenia.

O. Pharmacology

You should understand the mechanisms by which drugs produce their pharmacological effects.

1. Monoclonal antibodies

Monoclonal antibodies have an increasing role in medicine. They are manufactured by a technique called *somatic cell hybridisation*. This involves the fusion of myeloma cells with spleen cells from a mouse that has been immunised with the desired antigen. The resulting fused cells are termed a hybridoma and act as a 'factory' for producing monoclonal antibodies.

The main limitation to this is that mouse antibodies are immunogenic, leading to the formation of human anti-mouse antibodies (HAMAs). This problem is overcome by combining the variable region from the mouse body with the constant region from a human antibody.

Clinical examples of monoclonal antibodies

- infliximab (anti-TNF): used in rheumatoid arthritis and Crohn's disease
- rituximab (anti-CD20): used in non-Hodgkin's lymphoma and rheumatoid arthritis

+ cetuximab (anti-epidermal growth factor receptor): used in metastatic colorectal cancer and head and neck cancer

+ trastuzumab (anti-HER2, an EGF receptor): used in metastatic breast cancer

+ alemtuzumab (anti-CD52): used in chronic lymphocytic leukaemia

+ abciximab (anti-glycoprotein IIb/IIIa receptor): prevention of ischaemic events in patients undergoing percutaneous coronary interventions

+ OKT3 (anti-CD3): used to prevent organ rejection

Monoclonal antibodies are also used for:

+ medical imaging when combined with a radioisotope

+ identification of cell surface markers in biopsied tissue

+ diagnosis of viral infections

BOX 5.2   A note on trastuzumab

Trastuzumab (*Herceptin*) is a monoclonal antibody directed against the HER2/neu receptor. It is used mainly in metastatic breast cancer, although some patients with early disease are now also given trastuzumab. Only 25% of breast cancers are HER2 positive. NICE approved this drug for use in the adjuvant setting as well as in metastatic disease. Echocardiogram is required every 3 months whilst on active treatment.

Adverse effects

+ '*Flu-like symptoms*' and diarrhoea are common.

+ Cardiotoxicity – more common when anthracyclines have also been used. An echo is usually performed before starting treatment.

2. Cytotoxic agents

Drugs can be conveniently divided by their mechanism of action.

+ alkylating agents (e.g. cyclophosphamide, ifosfamide, chlorambucil, cisplatin, carboplatin, oxaliplatin)

+ anthracyclines (e.g. doxorubicin, epirubicin, mitoxantrone)

+ antibiotics (e.g. bleomycin, mitomycin)

+ antimetabolites (e.g. gemcitabine, 5-FU, capecitabine, methotrexate, pemetrexed, cytarabine, fludarabine)

◆ mitotic inhibitors (e.g. vincristine, vinblastine, vinorelbine, paclitaxel, docetaxel)

◆ topoisomerase inhibitors (e.g. irinotecan, topotecan, etoposide)

Table 5.2 summarises the mechanism of action and major adverse effects of commonly used cytotoxic agents.

TABLE 5.2 Cytotoxic agents

Cytotoxic agent	Mechanism of action	Major adverse effects
Vincristine	Inhibits formation of microtubules	Peripheral neuropathy
Cisplatin	Causes cross-linking in DNA	Ototoxicity, peripheral neuropathy, hypomagnesaemia
Bleomycin	Degrades preformed DNA	Lung fibrosis
Doxorubicin	Stabilises DNA-topoisomerase II	Cardiomyopathy
	Complex inhibits DNA and RNA	
	Synthesis	
Methotrexate	Inhibits dihydrofolate reductase and thymidylate synthesis	Myelosuppression, mucositis
Cyclophosphamide	Alkylating agent – causes cross-linking in DNA	Haemorrhagic cystitis, TCC carcinoma, myelosuppression
Docetaxel	Decreases free tubulin	Neutropaenia

3. Drug-induced pancytopaenia

Causes

◆ cytotoxics

◆ antibiotics: trimethoprim, chloramphenicol

◆ rheumatoid disease medications: gold, penicillamine

◆ carbimazole

◆ anti-epileptics: carbamazepine

◆ sulphonylureas: tolbutamide

P. Important specific clotting scenarios

1. Pregnancy and the risk of DVT/PE

Overview

◈ pregnancy is a hypercoagulable state

◈ majority occur in last trimester

Pathophysiology

◈ increase in factors VII, VIII, X and fibrinogen

◈ decrease in protein S

◈ uterus presses on IVC causing venous stasis in legs

Management

◈ warfarin contraindicated

◈ S/C low molecular weight heparin preferred to IV heparin (less bleeding and thrombocytopaenia)

Q. Immunology

1. Acute anaphylactic shock

The guidance for this is given in *Emergency Treatment of Anaphylactic Reactions: guidelines for healthcare providers* by the Working Group of the Resuscitation Council (UK) from January 2008.

A diagnosis of anaphylactic reaction is likely if a patient who is exposed to a trigger (allergen) develops a sudden illness (usually within minutes of exposure) with rapidly progressing skin changes and life-threatening airway and/or breathing and/or circulation problems. The reaction is usually unexpected.

> The European Academy of Allergology and Clinical Immunology Nomenclature Committee proposed the following broad definition:
> *'Anaphylaxis is a severe, life-threatening, generalised or systemic hypersensitivity reaction. This is characterised by rapidly developing life-threatening airway and/or breathing and/or circulation problems usually associated with skin and mucosal changes.'*

Anaphylaxis can be triggered by any of a very broad range of triggers, but those most commonly identified include food, drugs and venom.

The relative importance of these varies very considerably with age, with medicinal products being much more common triggers in older people. Virtually any food or class of drug can be implicated, although the classes of foods and drugs responsible for the majority of reactions are well described. Of foods, nuts are the most common cause; muscle relaxants, antibiotics, NSAIDs and aspirin are the most commonly implicated drugs. It is important to note that, in many cases, no cause can be identified. A significant number of cases of anaphylaxis are idiopathic (non-IgE mediated).

Management

You should consult the current resuscitation guidelines. Protocols will guide the physician according to treatment, if CPR is needed, or if the allergic symptoms are worsening. Such clinical indicators include lip swelling, itch, wheeze, fainting, hypotension, tachycardia, cyanosis, abdominal pain or vomiting. If there are worsening allergic features, and the patient does not require CPR, the following aspects of the **initial** management plan are normally recommended.

- Summon assistance from colleague.
- Call 999 to transfer patient to Emergency Department.
- Maintain airway and administer oxygen via non-rebreathing mask at 15 L per minute.
- Administer intramuscular adrenaline at the correct dosage.
- Observe continually until transfer; monitor and record blood pressure, pulse and respiratory rates.
- If no clinical improvement in 5 minutes, repeat administration of intramuscular adrenaline at the correct dosage.

2. Common allergies

Allergies occur when a specific substance is inhaled and the body reacts to it in a hypersensitive way. Although many adult allergies stem from childhood allergies, for others, allergies may not occur until adulthood.

Symptoms

Allergy symptoms can vary from person to person. For pollens, moulds and pet dander, a typical response is allergic rhinitis, or hay fever, in which the symptoms include nasal congestion, itchy throat, watery eyes, sneezing and coughing. In more severe cases, asthma may appear.

Prevention

Preventing contact with allergens is crucial in treating allergies. At home, use high-efficiency particulate air (HEPA) filters on vacuums, air purifiers and air conditioners. These powerful filters have the ability to remove any micro-size allergens like pollens or pet dander which may be floating in your home. Also, hay fever sufferers are advised to check pollen and mould forecasts online to see when the counts in a sufferer's local area are high. When they are, an individual is advised to try to plan activities indoors and limit time outside.

Management

Many good over-the-counter and prescription medications can control and prevent symptoms. To control reactions, antihistamines and decongestants are widely used. It is important to take these at the first sign of any reaction as they can take up to 30 minutes before any relief is felt.

To prevent symptoms, oral corticosteroid and nasal inhalers are effective in dramatically reducing inflammation. This type of medication is meant for long-term use, so relief may not be felt for several weeks. For severe reactions such as asthma and anaphylaxis, it is imperative that special medications be carried at all times. Asthmatics should always have a fast-acting inhaler on hand, and those who risk anaphylaxis should always have an auto-inject medication with them.

Immunotherapy is still an area of much interest in this field.

3. Urticaria and angioedema

[*See* Chapter 2.]

R. Oncology and palliative care

1. Malignancy-associated hypercalcaemia (MAH)

Although primary hyperparathyroidism is the most common cause of hyper-calcaemia, accounting for more than 90% of cases, **malignancy-associated hypercalcaemia** (MAH) represents 65% of patients requiring admission to hospital for treatment.

Hypercalcaemia is defined as a corrected serum calcium (Ca^{2+}) concentration of more than 2.6 mmol/L. The majority of laboratories only measure total serum calcium; however, approximately 40% of plasma calcium is bound to albumin and is biologically inactive.

MAH affects approximately 1.5% of cancer patients humoral hypercalcaemia, which results from secretion of parathyroid hormone-related protein (PTHrP), accounts for approximately 80% of cases. PTHrP is a protein with close homology to parathyroid hormone (PTH). It binds to the PTH receptor, thus mimicking the physiological effects of PTH, including increased bone resorption, increased calcium reabsorption in the distal renal tubule and inhibition of phosphate transport mechanism in the proximal renal tubule. Osteolytic bone metastases account for approximately 20% of cases.

The clinical features of hypercalcaemia are often non-specific and include anorexia, fatigue, muscular weakness, nausea, abdominal pain, constipation, anxiety and confusion. Hence they are classically described as *'bones, stones, abdominal groans and psychic moans'.* Patients with skeletal metastases may have bony tenderness. Patients with severe hypercalcaemia can present with life-threatening complications such as acute pancreatitis, acute renal failure and coma.

Investigations

Baseline laboratory investigations include full blood count, electrolytes, renal and liver function tests, serum calcium, phosphate and magnesium concentration and PTH concentrations.

A plain chest radiograph should be performed as squamous cell carcinoma of the lung is the most common malignant cause of hypercalcaemia.

Currently PTHrP concentration is not routinely measured.

Management

The majority of patients with MAH can be managed on a medical ward and do not require oncology involvement.

Patients presenting with life-threatening complications require admission to a high-dependency unit. The patient's medication should be reviewed and contributing drugs (for example, thiazide diuretics, calcium supplements) should be discontinued. The patient's fluid intake and urinary output should be monitored strictly as patients with hypercalcaemia are often dehydrated because of inadequate fluid intake due to anorexia and nausea, which are compounded by nephrogenic diabetes insipidus resulting from raised serum calcium concentrations.

Initial management should therefore include fluid replacement with intravenous normal saline. The rate of fluid replacement is determined by the serum calcium concentration, the severity of dehydration and co-morbidity such as impaired cardiac function.

Intravenous saline therapy increases glomerular filtration rate, thus increasing the load of filtered calcium passing in to the renal tubular lumen. However, intravenous saline therapy alone is rarely adequate to correct anything more than mild hypercalcaemia.

Following rehydration, bisphosphonates are the recommended first-line medical treatment of hypercalcaemia. Currently the bisphosphonates recommended for treating MAH are zoledronic acid or pamidronate.

Biochemical response is usually observed within 2–4 days following treatment with a bisphosphonate and the nadir is reached within 7–10 days. Normocalcaemia is attained after the first dose in up to 90% of patients, and is usually maintained for up to 3 weeks following treatment.

Although the majority of patients respond to rehydration and bisphosphonates, a minority are resistant to treatment and such patients should be referred for a specialist endocrinology opinion.

2. Superior vena cava obstruction (SVCO)

Superior vena cava obstruction (SVCO) is most likely caused by bronchogenic carcinoma, especially small cell carcinoma (10% of small cell cancers present with SVCO) due to mediastinal lymphadenopathy. Other causes include:

- lymphoma
- aortic aneurysm
- mediastinal fibrosis and
- mediastinal goitre

Chemotherapy ± radiotherapy is the treatment of choice in small cell carcinoma. Radiotherapy may be the treatment of choice for non-small cell carcinoma. Median survival of lung cancer presenting with SVCO, even with treatment, is 5 months. Lymphoma has a better prognosis and will require specific chemotherapy ± radiotherapy.

Recurrent laryngeal nerve palsy usually occurs with malignant tumour but can occur with aneurysm of aortic arch. There may also be Horner's syndrome due to involvement of sympathetic chain. Compression of vital structures can result in stridor and dysphagia.

SVCO is associated with elevated non-pulsatile jugular venous pressure (JVP). Kussmaul's sign is the paradoxical rise in JVP on inspiration due to constrictive pericarditis or significant pericardial effusion.

The commonest symptoms are usually cough and chest pain due to the distortion of mediastinal anatomy. Physical signs are often absent or minimal, but classically there are facial and periorbital oedema, chemosis and distended veins.

3. Spinal cord compression

Please refer to CG75 2008 NICE clinical guideline metastatic cord compression.

Spinal cord compression is an oncological emergency and affects up to 5% of cancer patients. It is commoner in patients with lung, breast and prostate cancer.

Features

+ back pain: may be worse on lying down and coughing
+ neurological signs depend on the level of the lesion; tendon reflexes tend to be increased below the level of the lesion and absent at the level of the lesion

Management

+ high-dose oral dexamethasone
+ urgent oncological assessment for consideration of radiotherapy or surgery
+ urgent MRI neuroimaging is obligatory, prior to oncological/neurosurgical referral

Recent NICE guidelines suggest contacting the local metastatic spinal cord compression coordinator in this situation. This should hopefully prevent delays in treatment by ensuring the patient is admitted to the most appropriate place.

4. Examples of common cancers

Bladder cancer: risk factors

The following factors are associated with the development of **bladder cancer**:

+ smoking
+ occupational: aniline dyes used in printing and textile industry, rubber manufacture
+ schistosomiasis
+ drugs: cyclophosphamide (*see* Chapter 11)

Oesophageal cancer

Oesophageal cancer is most commonly due to a squamous carcinoma but the incidence of adenocarcinoma is rising rapidly. Adenocarcinoma is the most common type of cancer to develop in patients with a history of gastro-oesophageal reflux disease (GORD) or Barrett's oesophagus.

The majority of tumours are in the middle third of the oesophagus.

Risk factors

- smoking
- alcohol
- gastro-oesophageal reflux disease
- Barrett's oesophagus
- achalasia
- Plummer-Vinson syndrome
- *rare*: coeliac disease, scleroderma

Gastric cancer
Epidemiology

- overall incidence is decreasing, but incidence of tumours arising from the cardia is increasing
- peak age = 70–80 years
- more common in Japan, China, Finland and Columbia than the West
- more common in males, 2 : 1

Associations

- *H. pylori* infection
- blood group A: gastric cancer
- gastric adenomatous polyps
- pernicious anaemia
- smoking
- diet: salty, spicy, nitrates
- may be negatively associated with duodenal ulcer

Investigation

- diagnosis: endoscopy with biopsy
- staging: CT or endoscopic ultrasound – endoscopic ultrasound has recently been shown to be superior to CT

Thymoma
Thymomas are the most common tumour of the anterior mediastinum.

Associated with

+ myasthenia gravis (30%–40% of patients with thymoma)
+ red cell aplasia
+ dermatomyositis
+ *also* SLE, SIADH

Causes of death

+ compression of airway
+ cardiac tamponade

5. Paraneoplastic syndromes

Recent medical advances have improved the understanding, diagnosis and treatment of **paraneoplastic syndromes**.

These disorders arise from tumour secretion of hormones, peptides or cytokines or from immune cross-reactivity between malignant and normal tissues. Paraneoplastic syndromes may affect diverse organ systems, most notably the endocrine, neurologic, dermatological, rheumatological and indeed haematological systems.

The most commonly associated malignancies include small cell lung cancer, breast cancer, gynaecological tumours and haematological malignancies. In some instances, the timely diagnosis of these conditions may lead to detection of an otherwise clinically occult tumour at an early and highly treatable stage.

As paraneoplastic syndromes often cause considerable morbidity, effective treatment can improve a patient's well-being, enhance the delivery of cancer therapy and prolong survival.

Treatments include addressing the underlying malignancy, immunosuppression and correction of electrolyte and hormonal derangements (for endocrine paraneoplastic syndromes).

6. Bladder cancers associated with analgesia

There is limited, however intriguing evidence on the effects of other drugs on bladder cancer risk, particularly analgesics and anti-inflammatory drugs.

Phenacetin, an analgesic drug, was classified by the International Agency for Research on Cancer (IARC) in 1987 as being probably carcinogenic to humans, and analgesic mixtures containing phenacetin as being carcinogenic.

Two epidemiological studies of bladder cancer included in the IARC report indicated an excess risk of two- to over sixfold associated with use of phenacetin-containing drugs. One additional study found a fourfold increased risk of bladder cancer among phenacetin abusers. However, these were relatively small studies, and were not able to demonstrate dose-related effects.

7. Palliative care prescribing for pain

SIGN issued guidance on the control of pain in adults with cancer in 2008 (SIGN guideline 106).

Selected points

- The breakthrough dose of morphine is roughly a sixth the daily dose of morphine.
- All patients who receive opioids should be prescribed a laxative.
- Opioids should be used with caution in patients with chronic kidney disease. Alfentanil, buprenorphine and fentanyl are preferred.
- Metastatic bone pain may respond to NSAIDs, bisphosphonates or radiotherapy.

8. Tumour markers

Tumour markers may be divided into:

- monoclonal antibodies against carbohydrate or glycoprotein tumour antigens
- tumour antigens
- enzymes (alkaline phosphatase, neurone specific enolase)
- hormones (e.g. calcitonin, ADH)

It should be noted that tumour markers usually have a low specificity.

TABLE 5.3 Common tumour markers

Tumour marker	Association
CA 125	Ovarian cancer
CA 19-9	Upper GI, lower GI, pancreatic cancer
CA 15-3	Breast cancer

References

Muñoz M, García-Erce JA, Remacha AF. Disorders of iron metabolism. Part 1: molecular basis of iron homoeostasis. *J Clin Pathol*. 2011; **64**(4): 281–6.

National Institute for Health and Clinical Excellence. Metastatic cord compression. NICE guideline 75. London: NIHCE; 2008. www.nice.org.uk/Guidance/CG75/NiceGuidance/pdf/English

Smith A, Wisloff F, Samson D. Guidelines on the diagnosis and management of multiple myeloma. *Br J Haematol*. 2006; **132**(4): 410–51.

Scottish Intercollegiate Guidelines Network (SIGN). Control of pain in adults with cancer: guideline number 106. Edinburgh: SIGN; November 2008. Available at: www.sign.ac.uk/pdf/SIGN106.pdf (accessed 17 September 2011).

Working Group of the Resuscitation Council (UK). *Emergency Treatment of Anaphylactic Reactions: guidelines for healthcare providers*. London: Resuscitation Council (UK); 2008.

Chapter 6

Infectious diseases (and tropical medicine and sexually transmitted diseases)

The Foundation Programme and MRCP(UK) Part 1 syllabus (from the JRCPMTB) specify what is required in terms of competencies, skills and knowledge from junior physicians in core medical training in infectious diseases, tropical medicine and sexually transmitted diseases. You are advised to consult carefully this syllabus, which emphasises the importance of basic medical sciences as well as a competent level of applied clinical practice.

A. Introduction to pathology and infectious diseases

1. Mechanisms of transmission of pathogens

Micro-organisms that cause disease in humans and other species are known as pathogens. The transmission of pathogens to a human or other host can occur in a number of ways, depending upon the micro-organism.

A common route is via water. The ingestion of contaminated water introduces the microbes into the digestive system, potentially causing intestinal upsets. As well, an organism may be capable of entering the cells that line the digestive tract and gaining entry to the bloodstream. From there, an infection can become widely dispersed. A prominent example of a waterborne pathogen is *Vibrio cholerae*, the bacterium that causes cholera. The contamination of drinking water by this bacterium is still at epidemic proportions in some areas of the world.

Pathogens can also be transmitted via the air. Viruses and bacterial spores are light enough to be lifted on the breeze. These agents can subsequently be inhaled, where they cause lung infections. An example of such a virus is the Hanta virus.

Still other microbial pathogens are transmitted from one human to another via body fluids such as the blood. This route is utilised by a number of viruses, e.g. HIV, and the viruses that cause haemorrhagic fever (e.g. ebola) are transmitted in the blood.

Transmission of pathogens can occur directly as well as indirectly. An intermediate host that harbours the micro-organism can transfer the microbes to humans via a bite or by other contact. *Coxiella burnetti*, the bacterium that causes Q fever, is transmitted to humans from the handling of animals such as sheep.

Finally, some viruses are able to transmit infection over long periods of time by becoming latent in the host. More specifically, the genetic material of viruses such as the hepatitis viruses and the herpes virus can integrate and be carried for decades in the host genome before the symptoms of infections appear.

2. How epidemics happen

In epidemiology, an epidemic occurs when new cases of a certain disease, in a given human population, and during a given period, substantially exceed what is 'expected', based on recent experience (the number of new cases in the population during a specified period of time is called the 'incidence rate'). In recent usages, the disease is not required to be communicable; examples include cancer or heart disease.

Factors that have been proposed as explaining the rise of new epidemics include:

◆ alterations in agricultural practices and land usage

◆ changes in society and human demographics

◆ poor population health (e.g. malnutrition, high prevalence of HIV)

◆ hospitals and medical procedures

◆ evolution of the pathogen (e.g. increased virulence, drug resistance)

◆ contamination of water supplies and food sources

◆ international travel

◆ failure of public health programs

◆ international trade

◆ climate change

3. Knowledge of key terms in infectious diseases

The definition of a **carrier state** is an animal which harbours a disease organism in its body without manifest signs, thus acting as a carrier or distributor of infection. A carrier may be one with a latent infection and which appears healthy. Other types of carriers are the incubatory carrier, when the animal is not yet showing clinical signs, or a convalescent carrier when it has passed the clinical stage.

The **reservoir** for a disease is the site where the infectious agent survives. For example, humans are the reservoir for the measles virus because it does not infect other organisms. Animals often serve as reservoirs for diseases that infect humans. The major reservoir for *Yersinia pestis*, the bacteria that causes plague, is wild rodents. There are also non-living reservoirs. Soil is the reservoir for many pathogenic fungi as well as some pathogenic bacteria such as *Clostridium tetani*, which causes tetanus.

Transmission of infectious diseases may also involve a **vector**. Vectors may be mechanical or biological. A mechanical vector picks up an infectious agent on the outside of its body and transmits it in a passive manner.

4. Immunisations

Common misconceptions regarding immunisations include:

+ a family history of adverse reaction, or a previous history of pertussis, measles, rubella or mumps infection
+ prematurity or low birth weight
+ stable neurological conditions such as cerebral palsy or Down's syndrome
+ asthma, eczema, hay fever or snuffles
+ contact with an infectious disease, or treatment with antibiotics or topical steroids
+ pregnant mother or a mother who is breastfeeding
+ prolonged jaundice
+ patients on replacement corticosteroids

Oral polio vaccine should not be given to immunosuppressed children, their siblings or household contacts.

In children with HIV, there is little evidence that they themselves will have problems, but excretion may be prolonged, and this may give rise to an increased risk of infection of HIV-positive household contacts.

5. Pertussis immunisation

True contraindications to pertussis immunisation include:

+ acute illness – until recovered

+ previous reaction to pertussis:

  - **Local** – an extensive area of redness and swelling which becomes indurated, involving most of the anterolateral surface of the thigh or a major part of the circumference of the upper arm.

  - **General** – fever equal to or more than 39.5°C within 48 hours of vaccine, anaphylaxis, bronchospasm, laryngeal oedema, collapse, prolonged hyporesponsiveness, prolonged inconsolable or high-pitched screaming of more than 4 hours, convulsions or encephalopathy occurring within 72 hours.

A personal family history of allergy is not a contraindication, nor are stable neurological conditions such as cerebral palsy or spina bifida. In patients who have had a previous reaction, immunisations should be completed with DT vaccine, and a cellular vaccine considered.

B. Control of communicable diseases

1. Post-exposure prophylaxis

Hepatitis A

Human normal immunoglobulin (HNIG) or hepatitis A vaccine may be used depending on the clinical situation.

Hepatitis B

+ HBsAg-positive source: if the person exposed is a known responder to HBV vaccine then a booster dose should be given. If they are in the process of being vaccinated or are a non-responder they need to have hepatitis B immune globulin (HBIG) and the vaccine.

+ Unknown source: for known responders the green book advises considering a booster dose of HBV vaccine. For known non-responders HBIG + vaccine should be given whilst those in the process of being vaccinated should have an accelerated course of HBV vaccine.

Hepatitis C

+ monthly PCR – if seroconversion then interferon +/– ribavirin

HIV

◆ a combination of oral antiretrovirals (e.g. tenofovir, emtricitabine, lopinavir and ritonavir) as soon as possible (i.e. within 1–2 hours, but may be started up to 72 hours following exposure) for 4 weeks

◆ serological testing at 12 weeks following completion of post-exposure prophylaxis

◆ reduces risk of transmission by 80%

Varicella zoster

◆ VZIG for IgG-negative pregnant women/immunosuppressed

2. Antibiotics: mechanisms of action

The lists below summarise the site of action of the commonly used antibiotics.

Inhibit cell wall formation

◆ penicillins

◆ cephalosporins

Inhibit protein synthesis

◆ aminoglycosides (cause misreading of mRNA)

◆ chloramphenicol

◆ macrolides (e.g. erythromycin)

◆ tetracyclines

◆ fusidic acid

Inhibit DNA synthesis

◆ quinolones (e.g. ciprofloxacin)

◆ metronidazole

◆ sulphonamides

◆ trimethoprim

Inhibit RNA synthesis

◆ rifampicin

3. Antiviral drugs: mechanisms of action

Acyclovir

+ acyclovir is phosphorylated by thymidine kinase which in turn inhibits the viral DNA polymerase

Ribavirin

+ effective against a range of DNA and RNA viruses
+ interferes with the capping of viral mRNA

Interferons

+ inhibit synthesis of mRNA, translation of viral proteins, viral assembly and release

Amantadine

+ used to treat influenza
+ inhibits uncoating of virus in cell

4. Anti-retroviral agents used in HIV

Nucleoside analogue reverse transcriptase inhibitors (NRTI)

+ examples: zidovudine (AZT), didanosine, lamivudine, stavudine, zalcitabine

Protease inhibitors (PI)

+ inhibits a protease needed to make the virus able to survive outside the cell
+ examples: indinavir, nelfinavir, ritonavir, saquinavir

Non-nucleoside reverse transcriptase inhibitors (NNRTI)

+ examples: nevirapine, efavirenz

C. Specific infections/syndromes

1. Bacterial septicaemia, meningitis and encephalitis

Investigations for meningitis

- blood cultures
- blood PCR
- lumbar puncture
- full blood count and clotting to assess for disseminated intravascular coagulation

Meningitis and encephalitis

CSF analysis

TABLE 6.1 Typical CSF findings in meningitis

	Bacterial	Viral	Tuberculous
Appearance	Cloudy	Clear/cloudy	Fibrin web
Glucose	Low (<½ plasma)	Normal	Low (<½ plasma)
Protein	High (>1 g/L)	Normal/raised	High (>1 g/L)
White cells	10-5000 polymorphs/ mm³	15–1000 lymphocytes/mm³	10–1000 lymphocytes/mm³

The **Ziehl-Neelsen stain** is only 20% sensitive in the detection of tuberculous meningitis and therefore PCR is sometimes used (sensitivity = 75%).

Management

- third-generation cephalosporins must be started immediately on suspicion of bacterial meningitis
- add vancomycin where resistance to cephalosporins on a rise
- if penicillin allergic then give chloramphenicol + vancomycin +/– rifampicin
- anti-tuberculous treatment for up to 1 year
- role of steroids is contoversial
- supportive care

Management of contacts

- prophylaxis needs to be offered to household and close contacts of patients affected with meningococcal meningitis

- rifampicin or ciprofloxacin may be used
- the risk is highest in the first 7 days but persists for at least 4 weeks
- meningococcal vaccination should be offered when serotype results are available, for close contacts who have not previously been vaccinated

2. Pneumonia: community-acquired

Community-acquired pneumonia (CAP) may be caused by the following infectious agents:

- *Streptococcus pneumoniae* (accounts for around 80% of cases)
- *Haemophilus influenzae*
- *Staphylococcus aureus*
- atypical pneumonias (e.g. due to *Mycoplasma pneumoniae*)
- viruses

Klebsiella pneumoniae is classically seen in alcoholics.

Streptococcus pneumoniae (pneumococcus) is the most common cause of community-acquired pneumonia.

Characteristic features of pneumococcal pneumonia:

- rapid onset
- high fever
- pleuritic chest pain
- herpes labialis

Antibiotic choices

- home-treated uncomplicated CAP: first line – oral amoxicillin
- hospitalised uncomplicated CAP: if admitted for other clinical reasons or not previously treated in the community for this episode then oral amoxicillin, otherwise amoxicillin + macrolide

3. Therapy of tuberculosis

The standard therapy for treating active tuberculosis is as follows.

Initial phase – first 2 months (RIPE)

- rifampicin
- isoniazid
- pyrazinamide
- ethambutol (the 2006 NICE guidelines now recommend giving a 'fourth drug' such as ethambutol routinely; previously this was only added if drug-resistant tuberculosis was suspected)

Continuation phase – next 4 months

- rifampicin
- isoniazid

The treatment for latent tuberculosis is isoniazid alone for 6 months.

Patients with meningeal tuberculosis are treated for a prolonged period (at least 12 months) with the addition of steroids.

Directly observed therapy with a thrice weekly dosing regimen may be indicated in certain groups, including:

- homeless people with active tuberculosis
- patients who are likely to have poor concordance
- all prisoners with active or latent tuberculosis

Contact tracing

According to **NICE guideline 33**, once a patient has been diagnosed with active TB, inform colleagues so that need for contact tracing can be assessed. The clinician should not delay contact tracing until notification.

4. Pyrexia of unknown origin
Defined as a prolonged fever of >3 weeks which resists diagnosis after a week in hospital.

Neoplasia
+ lymphoma
+ hypernephroma
+ preleukaemia
+ atrial myxoma

Infections
+ abscess
+ TB

5. Soft-tissue infection and osteomyelitis
Acute epiglottitis is a rare but serious infection caused by *Haemophilus influenzae* type B. Prompt recognition and treatment is essential as airway obstruction may develop. Epiglottitis generally occurs in children between the ages of 2 and 6 years. The incidence of epiglottitis has decreased since the introduction of the Hib vaccine.

Features
+ rapid onset
+ unwell, toxic child
+ stridor
+ drooling of saliva

6. Streptococcal infection
Streptococci may be divided into alpha and beta haemolytic types.

Alpha-haemolytic streptococci
The most important alpha-haemolytic *Streptococcus* is *Streptococcus pneumoniae* (pneumococcus). Pneumococcus is a common cause of pneumonia, meningitis and otitis media. Another clinical example is *Streptococcus viridians.*

Beta-haemolytic streptococci

These can be subdivided into groups A and B.

Group A

✦ most important organism is *Streptococcus pyogenes*

✦ responsible for erysipelas, impetigo, cellulitis, type 2 necrotising fasciitis and pharyngitis/tonsillitis

✦ immunological reactions can cause rheumatic fever or post-streptococcal glomerulonephritis

✦ erythrogenic toxins cause scarlet fever

Group B

✦ *Streptococcus agalactiae* may lead to neonatal meningitis and septicaemia

Intra-abdominal sepsis: pyogenic liver abscess
Management

✦ drainage (needle aspiration or catheter) should always be performed

✦ amoxicillin + ciprofloxacin + metronidazole

✦ if penicillin allergic: ciprofloxacin + clindamycin

7. Food poisoning

Gastroenteritis may either occur whilst at home or whilst travelling abroad (travellers' diarrhoea). Travellers' diarrhoea may be defined as at least three loose to watery stools in 24 hours with or without one or more of abdominal cramps, fever, nausea, vomiting or blood in the stool. The most common cause is *Escherichia coli.*

Another pattern of illness is 'acute food poisoning'. This describes the sudden onset of nausea, vomiting and diarrhoea after the ingestion of a toxin. Acute food poisoning is typically caused by *Staphylococcus aureus, Bacillus cereus* or *Clostridium perfringens.* Stereotypical histories of infective gastroenteritis are provided as a brief overview in Table 6.2.

TABLE 6.2 Stereotypical histories in gastroenteritis

Escherichia coli	Common amongst travellers
	Watery stools
	Abdominal cramps and nausea
Giardiasis	Prolonged, non-bloody diarrhoea
Cholera	Profuse, watery diarrhoea
	Severe dehydration resulting in weight loss
	Not common amongst travellers
Shigella	Bloody diarrhoea
	Vomiting and abdominal pain
Staphylococcus aureus	Severe vomiting
	Short incubation period
Campylobacter	A flu-like prodrome is usually followed by crampy abdominal pains, fever and diarrhoea which may be bloody
	Complications include Guillain-Barré syndrome

Incubation period

+ 1–6 hrs: *Staphylococcus aureus, Bacillus cereus*
+ 12–48 hrs: *Salmonella, Escherichia coli*
+ 48–72 hrs: *Shigella, Campylobacter*
+ >7 days: giardiasis, amoebiasis

8. Giardiasis

Giardiasis is a major diarrhoeal disease found throughout the world. The flagellate protozoan *Giardia lamblia*, its causative agent, is the most commonly identified intestinal parasite in the United States and the most common protozoal intestinal parasite isolated worldwide. Giardiasis usually represents a zoonosis with cross-infectivity between animals and humans.

Presentation

A broad spectrum of clinical syndromes may occur. The vast majority of symptoms are GI in nature.

Gastrointestinal symptoms: a small number of persons develop abrupt onset of explosive, watery diarrhoea, abdominal cramps, foul flatus, vomiting, fever and malaise. These symptoms last 3–4 days before transition into the more common subacute syndrome. Most patients experience a more insidious onset of symptoms, which are recurrent or resistant.

Stools become malodorous, mushy and greasy. Watery diarrhoea may alternate with soft stools or even constipation. Stools do not contain blood or pus because dysenteric symptoms are not a feature of giardiasis.

Upper GI symptoms, often exacerbated by eating, accompany stool changes or may be present in the absence of soft stools. These include upper and midabdominal cramping, nausea, early satiety, bloating, sulphurous belching, substernal burning and acid indigestion.

Constitutional symptoms including anorexia, fatigue, malaise and weight loss are common.

Weight loss occurs in more than 50% of patients.

Treatment
Emergency care for giardiasis consists of restoration of volume status with oral hydration or intravenous crystalloid solution. If diagnosis is made in the ED, antimicrobial therapy should be instituted. A number of antibiotic regimens may be used.

D. Tropical infections

1. Falciparum malaria
Features of severe malaria
+ schizonts on a blood film
+ parasitaemia >2%
+ hypoglycaemia
+ temperature >39°C
+ severe anaemia
+ complications *as below*

Complications
+ cerebral malaria: seizures, coma
+ acute renal failure: blackwater fever, secondary to intravascular haemolysis, mechanism unknown
+ acute respiratory distress syndrome (ARDS)
+ hypoglycaemia

◆ disseminated intravascular coagulation (DIC)

Uncomplicated falciparum malaria

◆ strains resistant to chloroquine are prevalent in certain areas of Asia and Africa

◆ first choice is oral quinine for 5 days followed by sulfadoxine-pyrimethamine or doxycycline

◆ alternative regimes include atovaquone-proguanil or artemether-lumefantrine

Severe falciparum malaria

◆ a parasite count of more than 2% will usually need parenteral treatment irrespective of clinical state

◆ options include intravenous quinine or artemisinins

◆ if parasite count >10% then exchange transfusion should be considered

◆ shock may indicate coexistent bacterial septicaemia; malaria rarely causes haemodynamic collapse

2. Non-falciparum malaria

The most common cause of non-falciparum malaria is *Plasmodium vivax*, with *Plasmodium ovale* and *Plasmodium malariae* accounting for the other cases. *Plasmodium vivax* is often found in Central America and the Indian subcontinent whilst *Plasmodium ovale* typically comes from Africa.

Benign malarias have a hypnozoite stage and may therefore relapse following treatment.

Treatment

◆ non-falciparum malarias are almost always chloroquine sensitive

◆ primaquine should be used in *Plasmodium vivax* and *Plasmodium ovale* infection to destroy liver hypnozoites

3. Leishmaniasis

Leishmaniasis is a protozoal disease capable of causing a spectrum of clinical syndromes ranging from cutaneous ulcerations to systemic infections. With the exception of Australia, the Pacific Islands and Antarctica, the parasites have been identified throughout large portions of the world. The protozoa are transmitted to mammals via the bite of the female sandfly of the genera *Phlebotomus* in the Old World and *Lutzomyia* in the New World. Humans are generally considered incidental hosts. For most species of *Leishmania*, an animal reservoir is required for endemic conditions to persist.

Cutaneous leishmaniasis

Inoculation occurs after a sandfly bites an exposed part of the body (usually the legs, arms, neck or face). Incubation occurs over weeks to months followed by the appearance of an erythematous papule, which can evolve into a plaque or ulcer.

Diffuse cutaneous leishmaniasis

Infection is characterised by a primary lesion, which spreads to involve multiple areas of the skin. Plaques, ulcers and nodules may form over the entire body, resembling lepromatous leprosy. However, no neurological or systemic invasion is involved.

Mucocutaneous leishmaniasis

Mucocutaneous disease is most commonly caused by New World species infection by *Leishmania (Viannia) braziliensis*. It may lead to mucosal involvement in up to 10% of infections depending on the region in which it was acquired. Initial infection is characterised by a persistent cutaneous lesion that eventually heals, although as many as 30% of patients report no prior evidence of leishmaniasis. Several years later, oral and respiratory mucosal involvement occurs, causing inflammation and mutilation of the nose, mouth, oropharynx and trachea. Progressive disease is difficult to treat and often recurs.

Visceral leishmaniasis

Visceral disease, the most devastating and fatal form, is classically known as kala-azar or black fever. The syndrome is characterised by the pentad of fever, weight loss, hepatosplenomegaly, pancytopaenia and hypergammaglobulinaemia. Patients may report night sweats, weakness and anorexia. Melanocyte stimulation and xerosis can occur, causing characteristic skin hyperpigmentation.

The mainstay in treatment are the pentavalent antimony compounds first introduced in the 1930s. The two available preparations, sodium stibogluconate (pentostam) and meglumine antimonite, have similar efficacy.

4. Hookworms

Hookworms represent a widespread and clinically important human nematode infection. Hookworm infection is acquired through skin exposure to larvae in soil contaminated by human faeces.

Adults, especially agricultural workers, are at equal or higher risk of exposure than children. Most individuals who develop hookworm infection are from known endemic areas. Early symptoms of hookworm infection are proportional to the intensity of exposure.

Severe infection with either *Ancylostoma duodenale* or *Necator americanus* may produce pneumonitis ('*Loeffler-like syndrome*') that manifests as cough, fever and malaise. As worms mature in the jejunum, patients may experience diarrhoea, vague abdominal pain, colic and/or nausea.

These symptoms are more common with initial exposures than with subsequent exposures. Patients with severe iron deficiency anaemia may present with lassitude, headache, palpitations, dyspnoea and oedema. Albendazole or mebendazole is the drug of choice for hookworm infection.

5. Viral haemorrhagic fevers

Viral haemorrhagic fevers are a group of aetiologically diverse viral diseases unified by common underlying pathophysiology. These febrile diseases result from infection by viruses from four viral families: Arenaviridae, Bunyaviridae, Filoviridae, and Flaviviridae.

The viruses in the four families are all RNA viruses. Survival and perpetuation of the viruses is dependent on an animal host known as a natural reservoir; humans are not the natural reservoir. With the exception of a vaccine for yellow fever and ribavirin, which is used as a drug treatment for some arenaviral infections, no cures or drug treatments for viral haemorrhagic fever exist. Only supportive treatment is possible.

Not all viruses in these families cause viral haemorrhagic fever. Viral haemorrhagic fevers share certain clinical manifestations, regardless of the virus that causes the disease. Common clinical manifestations of viral haemorrhagic fever are increased capillary permeability, leucopenia and thrombocytopaenia. Viral haemorrhagic fever is manifested by sudden onset, fever, headache, generalised myalgia, backache, petechiae and conjunctivitis.

The severity of symptoms varies.

Common symptoms include the following:

- myalgia
- fever
- prostration
- vomiting
- headache
- petechial haemorrhages
- hypotension
- flushing of the head and the chest
- oedema
- malaise
- diarrhoea

Severe viral haemorrhagic fever tends to evolve to shock and generalised mucous membrane haemorrhage. Viral haemorrhagic fever is often accompanied by neurologic, hematopoietic or pulmonary involvement.

Intensive supportive care is necessary for most cases of viral haemorrhagic fever. General supportive care principles apply to the treatment of haemo-dynamic, haematologic, pulmonary and neurological manifestations of viral haemorrhagic fever. Supportive care entails maintaining the patient's oxygen status and blood pressure and balancing fluid and electrolyte levels.

6. Schistosomiasis

Schistosomiasis (also known as *bilharzia*) is a human disease syndrome caused by infection from one of several species of parasitic trematodes of the genus *Schistosoma*. Schistosomiasis is a major source of morbidity and mortality for developing countries in Africa, South America, the Caribbean, the Middle East and Asia.

Patients with acute schistosomiasis (Katayama fever) present several weeks after contact with infested water. Obtaining a careful travel history, including drinking water sources and recreational activities, is important. In A&E, the physician confirms the diagnosis, begins antibiotic therapy and stabilises patients with acute complications of schistosomiasis.

Symptoms are likely secondary to immune complex formation. Following egg deposition in tissues, the illness resembles serum sickness.

Features

◆ fever

◆ headache

◆ malaise

◆ athralgias/myalgias

◆ cough

◆ bloody diarrhoea

◆ right upper quadrant pain

◆ rash

Patients with symptomatic chronic schistosomiasis may present months to years after primary exposure. Many patients have few or mild symptoms. Individuals with symptoms may present with non-specific complaints reflecting their level of infection, the primary location of egg production for the schistosomal species involved (e.g. mesenteric, bladder wall), the extent of hepatosplenic involvement, the extent of cardiopulmonary involvement and the presence of ectopic sites (e.g. CNS).

Management

◆ single oral dose of praziquantel

7. Viral hepatitis
Hepatitis is a general term that refers to inflammation of the liver. This condition may result from various infectious and non-infectious aetiologies.

Infectious aetiologies include viral, bacterial, fungal and parasitic organisms. In the United States, viral hepatitis is most commonly caused by hepatitis A virus (HAV), hepatitis B virus (HBV) and hepatitis C virus (HCV). These three viruses can all result in an acute disease process with symptoms of nausea, abdominal pain, fatigue, malaise and jaundice. Additionally, HBV and HCV can also lead to chronic infection.

Patients who are chronically infected may go on to develop cirrhosis and hepatocellular carcinoma. Furthermore, chronic hepatitis carriers remain infectious and may transmit the disease for many years.

Clinical presentation of infectious hepatitis varies from person to person as well as with the aetiology of infection. Some patients may present as entirely asymptomatic or only mildly symptomatic. Others may present with rapid onset of fulminant hepatic failure. The classic presentation of infectious hepatitis involves four phases.

Phase 1 – Viral replication
Patients are asymptomatic during this phase. Laboratory studies demonstrate serologic and enzyme markers of hepatitis.

Phase 2 – Prodromal phase
Patients experience anorexia, nausea, vomiting, alterations in taste, arthralgias, malaise, fatigue, urticaria and pruritus.

Phase 3 – Icteric phase
Patients may note dark urine, followed by pale-coloured stools. In addition to the predominant gastrointestinal symptoms and malaise, patients become icteric and may develop right upper quadrant pain with hepatomegaly.

Phase 4 – Convalescent phase
Symptoms and icterus resolve. Liver enzymes return to normal. No specific treatment is usually indicated other than supportive care including intravenous rehydration. A liver abscess, however, requires intravenous antibiotic therapy directed toward the most likely pathogens and consultation for possible surgical or percutaneous drainage.

Hepatitis B serology
Interpreting hepatitis B serology is a dying art form which still occurs at regular intervals in medical exams (including the MRCP(UK) PACES exam).

It is important to remember a few key 'background' facts:

◈ Surface antigen (HBsAg) is the first marker to appear and causes the production of anti-HBs antibody.

◈ HBsAg normally implies acute disease (present for 1–6 months).

◈ If HBsAg is present for >6 months then this implies chronic disease (i.e. infective).

◈ Anti-HBs implies immunity (either exposure or immunisation). It is negative in chronic disease.

◈ Anti-HBc implies previous (or current) infection. IgM anti-HBc appears during acute or recent hepatitis B infection and is present for about 6 months.

◆ HbeAg results from breakdown of core antigen from infected liver cells and is therefore a marker of infectivity.

Example results

◆ previous immunisation: anti-HBs positive, all others negative

◆ previous hepatitis B (>6 months ago), not a carrier: anti-HBc positive, HBsAg negative

◆ previous hepatitis B, now a carrier: anti-HBc positive, HBsAg positive

8. Scabies

Scabies is quite a common condition caused by infestation with the mite *Sarcoptes scabiei*.

Transmission is by skin-to-skin contact.

It tends to occur in young adults or institutionalised patients.

Clinical presentation can take several weeks, as it takes time to become sensitised to the mites. **Treatment** is through malathion, benzyl benzoate or permethrin.

It is common to treat all contacts, i.e. members of the family, other ward members. Treatment failure is common.

9. Glandular fever syndrome and its differentiation from HIV seroconversion illness

HIV seroconversion is symptomatic in 60%–80% of patients and typically presents as a glandular fever-type illness. Increased symptomatic severity is associated with poorer long-term prognosis. It typically occurs 3–12 weeks after infection.

Features

◆ sore throat

◆ lymphadenopathy

◆ malaise, myalgia, arthralgia

◆ diarrhoea

◆ maculopapular rash

◆ mouth ulcers

◆ rarely, meningoencephalitis

Diagnosis

- antibodies to HIV may not be present
- HIV PCR and p24 antigen tests can confirm diagnosis

10. Staphylococcal toxic shock syndrome

Staphylococcal toxic shock syndrome describes a severe systemic reaction to staphylococcal exotoxins. It came to prominence in the early 1980s following a series of cases related to infected tampons.

Centers for Disease Control and Prevention diagnostic criteria

- fever: temperature >38.9°C
- hypotension: systolic blood pressure <90 mmHg
- diffuse erythematous rash
- desquamation of rash, especially of the palms and soles
- involvement of three or more organ systems, e.g. gastrointestinal (diarrhoea and vomiting), mucous membrane erythema, renal failure, hepatitis, thrombocytopaenia, CNS involvement (e.g. confusion)

11. Measles

- RNA paramyxovirus
- spread by droplets
- infective from prodrome until 5 days after rash starts
- incubation period = 10–14 days

Features

- prodrome: irritable, conjunctivitis, fever
- Koplik spots (before rash): white spots ('grain of salt') on buccal mucosa
- rash: starts behind ears then to whole body, discrete maculopapular rash becoming blotchy and confluent

Complications

- encephalitis: typically occurs 1–2 weeks following the onset of the illness
- subacute sclerosing panencephalitis: very rare, may present 5–10 years following the illness
- febrile convulsions
- pneumonia, tracheitis

+ keratoconjunctivitis, corneal ulceration

+ diarrhoea

+ increased incidence of appendicitis

+ myocarditis

Management of contacts

+ if a child not immunised against measles comes into contact with measles then MMR should be offered (vaccine-induced measles antibody develops more rapidly than that following natural infection)

+ this should be given within 72 hours

12. *Legionella*

Legionnaire's disease is caused by the intracellular bacterium *Legionella pneumophila*. It typically colonises water tanks and hence questions may hint at hotel air-conditioning systems or foreign holidays. Person-to-person transmission is not seen.

Features

+ flu-like symptoms such as headache and myalgia

+ dry cough

+ confusion

+ abdominal pain

+ lymphopenia

+ hyponatraemia

+ deranged LFTs

Diagnosis

+ urinary antigen, IgM for *Legionella* (acute and convalescent only)

+ blood film nay show a normal WCC/leucopenia

Management

+ treat with erythromycin

+ consider adding rifampicin

13. Herpes simplex virus

There are two strains of the herpes simplex virus (HSV) in humans: HSV-1 and HSV-2. Whilst it was previously thought HSV-1 accounted for oral lesions (cold sores) and HSV-2 for genital herpes, it is now known there is considerable overlap.

Features

◆ primary infection: may present with a severe gingivostomatitis

◆ cold sores

◆ painful genital ulceration

14. Chickenpox

Chickenpox is caused by primary infection with varicella zoster virus. Shingles is the reactivation of the dormant virus in dorsal root ganglion. Chickenpox is highly infectious.

◆ spread via the respiratory route

◆ can be caught from someone with shingles

◆ infectivity = 4 days before rash, until 5 days after the rash first appeared

◆ incubation period = 10–21 days

Clinical features (tend to be more severe in older children/adults)

◆ fever initially

◆ itchy, rash starting on head/trunk before spreading. Initially macular then papular then vesicular

◆ systemic upset is usually mild

Management is supportive

◆ keep cool, trim nails

◆ calamine lotion

◆ school exclusion: current HPA advice is 5 days from start of skin eruption

◆ immunocompromised patients and newborns with peripartum exposure should receive varicella zoster immunoglobulin (VZIG). If chickenpox develops then IV acyclovir should be considered

Complications

A common complication is secondary bacterial infection of the lesions. Rare complications include:

+ pneumonia

+ encephalitis (cerebellar involvement may be seen)

+ disseminated haemorrhagic chickenpox

+ arthritis, nephritis and pancreatitis may very rarely be seen

Chickenpox exposure in pregnancy

Chickenpox is caused by primary infection with varicella zoster virus. Shingles is the reactivation of the dormant virus in dorsal root ganglion. In pregnancy there is a risk to both the mother and the foetus, a syndrome now termed foetal varicella syndrome.

Foetal varicella syndrome (FVS)

+ risk of FVS following maternal varicella exposure is around 1% if occurs before 20 weeks' gestation

+ studies have shown a very small number of cases occurring between 20 and 28 weeks' gestation and none following 28 weeks

+ features of FVS include skin scarring, eye defects (microphthalmia), limb hypoplasia, microcephaly and learning disabilities

Management of chickenpox exposure

+ If there is any doubt about the mother previously having chickenpox maternal blood should be checked for varicella antibodies.

+ If the pregnant woman is not immune to varicella she should be given varicella zoster immunoglobulin (VZIG) as soon as possible. RCOG and *Green Book* guidelines suggest VZIG is effective up to 10 days post-exposure.

+ Consensus guidelines suggest oral acyclovir should be given if pregnant women with chickenpox present within 24 hours of onset of the rash

15. Epstein-Barr virus: associated malignancies

Examples are:

- Burkitt's lymphoma
- Hodgkin's lymphoma
- nasopharyngeal carcinoma
- hairy leucoplakia
- HIV-associated central nervous system lymphomas

16. Splenectomy

Following a **splenectomy**, patients are particularly at risk from pneumococcus, *Haemophilus*, meningococcus and *Capnocytophaga canimorsus* infections, usually from dog bites.

Vaccination

- if elective, should be done 2 weeks prior to operation
- pneumococcal, Hib, meningitis A and C, and annual influenza vaccination

Antibiotic prophylaxis

- Penicillin V: unfortunately, clear guidelines do not exist of how long antibiotic prophylaxis should be continued. It is generally accepted, though, that penicillin should be continued for at least 2 years and at least until the patient is 16 years of age, although the majority of patients are usually put on antibiotic prophylaxis for life.

17. Leptospirosis

Leptospirosis is distributed worldwide (sparing the polar regions) but is most common in the tropics. Humans and a wide range of animals can develop *Leptospira* infection. However, humans are rarely chronic carriers and are therefore considered accidental hosts. Leptospirosis is transmitted via direct contact with the body fluid of an acutely infected animal or by exposure to soil or fresh water contaminated with the urine of an animal that is a chronic carrier.

Human leptospirosis is often acquired via contact with fresh water contaminated by rat, or urine as part of occupational contact with these animals. The disease is also acquired during adventure travel or vacations that involve water sports or hiking, or even as a consequence of flooding.

Expert consensus is that leptospirosis occurs as two recognisable clinical syndromes.

Anicteric leptospirosis is a self-limited disease similar to a mild flu-like illness.

Icteric leptospirosis, also known as *Weil's disease*, is a severe illness characterised by multiorgan involvement or even failure.

Leptospirosis is treated primarily with antimicrobial therapy.

In uncomplicated infections that do not require hospitalisation, oral doxycycline has been shown to decrease duration of fever and most symptoms.

Hospitalised patients should be treated with intravenous penicillin G therapy, which is the treatment of choice.

Severe cases of leptospirosis can affect any organ system and can lead to multiorgan failure.

In addition to antimicrobials, therapy is supportive.

18. *Borrelia*

Lyme disease is a systemic infection caused by the spirochete *Borrelia burgdorferi*. The bacterium is inoculated into the skin by a tick bite. The tick is almost always of the genus *Ixodes*.

Systemic manifestations

◈ Fever is generally low grade.

◈ Fatigue is common.

◈ Myalgias and arthralgias occur early.

◈ Flu-like illness (undifferentiated febrile illness) may occur.

Cutaneous symptoms

◈ The classic rash erythema migrans (EM) is present in about 75% of patients. About 20% of patients with Lyme disease have multiple lesions (from haematogenous dissemination).

Neurological symptoms

◈ Headache can occur in early infection as a non-specific finding and can herald CNS penetration and lymphocytic meningitis.

◈ Patients notice facial weakness, which is similar to a typical Bell's palsy and which can be the presenting symptom of Lyme disease.

◈ Late Lyme disease can cause paresthesias or pain due to peripheral neuropathy and personality, cognitive, and sleep disturbances from chronic encephalopathy.

Other involvement

◈ palpitations

◈ Lyme pericarditis, myocarditis and myopericarditis

◈ red, sore and itchy eyes from conjunctivitis

◈ nausea and vomiting

Emergency care of patients with Lyme disease depends on the presenting complaint. In general, Lyme disease is not fatal, and the emergency physician may be able to consult specialists and refer the patient to a primary care physician. However, it makes sense to start antimicrobial therapy in the ED, or with a prescription to be filled upon leaving the ED.

Early disseminated disease findings such as isolated facial palsy or secondary skin lesions (not meningitis) or disease with first-degree heart block (not a high-degree heart block) may be treated with oral antibiotics for 21–30 days. Early disseminated disease with meningitis or a high-degree heart block may be treated with intravenous ceftriaxone for 2–4 weeks.

19. Cholera

Cholera is caused by *Vibrio cholerae* – a Gram-negative bacterium.

Features

◈ profuse *'rice water'* diarrhoea

◈ dehydration

◈ hypoglycaemia

Management

◈ oral rehydration therapy

◈ antibiotics: doxycycline, ciprofloxacin

20. Zoonoses

Zoonotic diseases are diseases caused by infectious agents that can be transmitted between (or are shared by) animals and humans.

Cat scratch disease

Cat scratch disease is generally caused by the Gram-negative rod *Bartonella henselae*.

Features

- fever
- history of a cat scratch
- regional lymphadenopathy
- headache, malaise

Orf

Orf is generally a condition found in sheep and goats, although it can be transmitted to humans. It is caused by the parapox virus.

In animals

- 'scabby' lesions around the mouth and nose

In humans

- generally affects the hands and arms
- initially small, raised, red-blue papules
- later may increase in size to 2–3 cm and become flat-topped and haemorrhagic

E. Sexually transmitted diseases

1. HIV/AIDS infections

Toxoplasmosis

Toxoplasma gondii is a protozoa which infects the body via the GI tract, lung or broken skin. Its oocysts release trophozoites which migrate widely around the body including to the eye, brain and muscle. The usual animal reservoir is the cat, although other animals such as rats carry the disease.

Most infections are asymptomatic. Symptomatic patients usually have a self-limiting infection, often having clinical features resembling infectious mononucleosis (fever, malaise, lymphadenopathy). Other less common manifestations include meningo-encephalitis and myocarditis.

Investigation

◆ antibody test

◆ Sabin-Feldman dye test

Treatment is usually reserved for those with severe infections or patients who are immunosuppressed.

◆ pyrimethamine plus sulphadiazine for at least 6 weeks

Congenital toxoplasmosis is due to transplacental spread from the mother. It causes a variety of effects to the unborn child, including microcephaly, hydrocephalus, cerebral calcification and choroidoretinitis.

Pneumocystis carinii pneumonia

Whilst the organism *Pneumocystis carinii* is now referred to as *Pneumocystis jirovecii*, the term *Pneumocystis carinii* pneumonia (PCP) is still in common use.

◆ *Pneumocystis jirovecii* is a unicellular eukaryote, generally classified as a fungus but some authorities consider it a protozoa.

◆ PCP is the most common opportunistic infection in AIDS.

◆ All patients with a CD4 count <200/mm^3 should receive PCP prophylaxis.

Features

◆ dyspnoea

◆ dry cough

◆ fever

◆ very few chest signs

Extrapulmonary manifestations are rare (1%–2% of cases); they include:

+ hepatosplenomegaly
+ lymphadenopathy
+ choroid lesions

Investigation

+ CXR: typically shows bilateral interstitial pulmonary infiltrates but can present with other X-ray findings, e.g. lobar consolidation; may be normal
+ exercise-induced desaturation
+ sputum often fails to show PCP, bronchoalveolar lavage (BAL) often needed to demonstrate PCP (silver stain)

Management

+ co-trimoxazole
+ IV pentamidine in severe cases
+ steroids if hypoxic (if pO_2 <9.3 kPa then steroids reduce risk of respiratory failure by 50% and death by a third)

Pregnancy

With the increased incidence of HIV infection amongst the heterosexual population there are an increasing number of HIV-positive women giving birth in the UK. In London the incidence may be as high as 0.4% of pregnant women. The aim of treating HIV-positive women during pregnancy is to minimise harm to both the mother and foetus, and to reduce the chance of vertical transmission.

Factors which reduce vertical transmission (from 25%–30% to 2%)

+ maternal antiretroviral therapy
+ mode of delivery (caesarean section)
+ neonatal antiretroviral therapy
+ infant feeding (bottle feeding)

Screening

+ NICE guidelines recommend offering HIV screening to all pregnant women.

Antiretroviral therapy

◈ All pregnant women should be offered antiretroviral therapy regardless of whether they were taking it previously.

◈ If women are not currently taking antiretroviral therapy it is usually commenced between 28 and 32 weeks of gestation and should be continued intrapartum.

Mode of delivery

◈ elective caesarean section

◈ a zidovudine infusion should be started 4 hours before beginning the caesarean section

Neonatal antiretroviral therapy

◈ Zidovudine is usually administered orally to the neonate for 4–6 weeks.

Infant feeding

◈ In the UK all women should be advised not to breast feed.

Diarrhoea

Diarrhoea is common in patients with HIV. This may be due to the effects of the virus itself (HIV enteritis) or opportunistic infections.

Possible causes

◈ *Cryptosporidium* + other protozoa (most common)

◈ *Cytomegalovirus*

◈ *Mycobacterium avium-intracellulare*

◈ *Giardia*

Cryptosporidium is the most common infective cause of diarrhoea in HIV patients. It is an intracellular protozoa and has an incubation period of 7 days.

Presentation is very variable, ranging from mild to severe diarrhoea.

A modified Ziehl-Neelsen stain (acid-fast stain) of the stool may reveal the characteristic red cysts of *Cryptosporidium*. Treatment is difficult, with the mainstay of management being supportive therapy.

Mycobacterium avium-intracellulare is an atypical mycobacteria seen when the CD4 count is below 50.

Typical features include fever, sweats, abdominal pain and diarrhoea. There may be hepatomegaly and deranged LFTs. Diagnosis is made by blood cultures and bone marrow examination. Management is with rifabutin, ethambutol and clarithromycin.

Kaposi's sarcoma

Caused by HHV-8 (human herpes virus 8).

+ presents as purple papules or plaques on the skin or mucosa (e.g. gastrointestinal and respiratory tract)
+ skin lesions may later ulcerate
+ respiratory involvement may cause massive haemoptysis and pleural effusion
+ radiotherapy + resection

2. Gonorrhoea

Gonorrhoea is caused by the Gram-negative diplococcus *Neisseria gonorrhoeae*. Acute infection can occur on any mucous membrane surface, typically genitourinary but also rectum and pharynx. The incubation period of gonorrhoea is 2–5 days.

Features

+ males: urethral discharge, dysuria
+ females: cervicitis, e.g. leading to vaginal discharge
+ rectal and pharyngeal infection is usually asymptomatic

Local complications that may develop include urethral strictures, epididymitis and salpingitis (hence may lead to infertility). Disseminated infection may occur.

Management

+ Ciprofloxacin is a treatment of choice.
+ However, there is increased resistance to ciprofloxacin and therefore cephalosporins are now used.
+ Other options now include cefixime or ceftriaxone.

Disseminated gonococcal infection (DGI) – including gonococcal arthritis – may also occur, with gonococcal infection being the most common cause of septic arthritis in young adults. The pathophysiology of DGI is not fully understood but is thought to be due to haematogenous spread from mucosal infection (e.g. asymptomatic genital infection). Initially there may be a classic triad of symptoms: tenosynovitis, migratory polyarthritis and dermatitis. Later complications include septic arthritis, endocarditis and perihepatitis (Fitz-Hugh-Curtis syndrome).

Key features

◆ tenosynovitis

◆ migratory polyarthritis

◆ dermatitis (lesions can be maculopapular or vesicular)

3. Chlamydia

Chlamydia is the most prevalent sexually transmitted infection in the UK and is caused by *Chlamydia trachomatis*, an obligate intracellular pathogen. The incubation period is around 7–21 days, although it should be remembered a large percentage of cases are asymptomatic.

Features

◆ asymptomatic in around 70% of women and 50% of males

◆ women: cervicitis (discharge, bleeding), dysuria

◆ men: urethral discharge, dysuria

Potential complications

◆ epididymitis

◆ pelvic inflammatory disease

◆ endometritis

◆ increased incidence of ectopic pregnancies

◆ infertility

◆ reactive arthritis

◆ perihepatitis (*Fitz-Hugh-Curtis* syndrome)

Investigation

◆ Traditional cell culture is no longer widely used.

✦ Nuclear acid amplification tests (NAATs) are now rapidly emerging as the investigation of choice.

✦ Urine (first void urine sample), vulvovaginal swab or cervical swab may be tested using the NAAT technique.

Management

✦ doxycycline (7-day course) or azithromycin (single dose)

✦ if pregnant then erythromycin or amoxicillin may be used

✦ contacts of confirmed *Chlamydia* cases should be offered treatment prior to the results of their investigations being known (treat then test)

4. Genital ulcers

Painful: herpes – chancroid

> **Painless:** syphilis – lymphogranuloma venereum + granuloma inguinale
>
> **Lymphogranuloma venereum** usually involves three stages:

1. small painless pustule which later forms an ulcer
2. painful inguinal lymphadenopathy
3. proctocolitis

Genital herpes is most often caused by the herpes simplex virus (HSV) type 2 (cold sores are usually due to HSV type 1). Primary attacks are often severe and associated with fever whilst subsequent attacks are generally less severe and localised to one site.

Syphilis is a sexually transmitted infection caused by the spirochaete *Treponema pallidum*. Infection is characterised by primary, secondary and tertiary stages. A painless ulcer (*chancre*) is seen in the primary stage. The incubation period = 9–90 days.

Chancroid is a tropical disease caused by *Haemophilus ducreyi*. It causes painful genital ulcers associated with inguinal lymph node enlargement.

Lymphogranuloma venereum is caused by *Chlamydia trachomatis*. Typically infection comprises three stages:

✦ stage 1: small painless pustule which later forms an ulcer

✦ stage 2: painful inguinal lymphadenopathy

✦ stage 3: proctocolitis

Other causes of genital ulcers

◆ Behçet's disease

◆ carcinoma

◆ granuloma inguinale: *Klebsiella granulomatis*

5. Spirochaetosis

Syphilis

Syphilis is a venereal disease caused by infection with the spirochaete *Treponema pallidum*. Untreated syphilis progresses through four stages: primary, secondary, latent and tertiary.

Primary syphilis

Primary syphilis manifests mainly on the glans penis in males and on the vulva or cervix in females. Regional nontender lymphadenopathy follows invasion. Lesions (chancres) are usually solitary, raised, firm papules that can be several centimeters in diameter.

The chancre erodes to create an ulcerative crater within the papule, with slightly elevated edges around the central ulcer.

Secondary syphilis

Secondary syphilis manifests in various ways. It usually includes a localised or diffuse mucocutaneous rash and generalised nontender lymphadenopathy.

Constitutional symptoms of secondary syphilis include malaise, sore throat, headache, fever, anorexia and meningismus (rarely).

Other less common manifestations include GI involvement, hepatitis, nephropathy, proctitis, arthritis and optic neuritis.

Latent syphilis

Syphilis primarily spreads during the first year after infection. Affected patients may recall symptoms of primary and secondary syphilis. They are asymptomatic during the latent phase, and the disease is detected only by serologic tests.

Tertiary syphilis

Late syphilis is slowly progressive and may affect any organ. The disease is generally not thought to be infectious at this stage.

Clinical and serological conversions are the endpoints of medical treatment for syphilis. Penicillin is the treatment of choice for treating syphilis. Surgical care is reserved for treating the complications of tertiary syphilis (e.g. aortic valve replacement).

Investigation

Treponema pallidum is a very sensitive organism and cannot be grown on artificial media. The diagnosis is therefore usually based on clinical features, serology and microscopic examination of infected tissue.

Serological tests can be divided into:

- cardiolipin tests (not treponeme specific)
- treponemal specific antibody tests

Cardiolipin tests

- syphilis infection leads to the production of non-specific antibodies that react to cardiolipin
- examples include VDRL (Venereal Disease Research Laboratory) and RPR (rapid plasma reagin)
- insensitive in late syphilis
- becomes negative after treatment

Treponemal specific antibody tests

- example: TPHA (*Treponema pallidum* haemagglutination test)
- remains positive after treatment

Causes of false positive cardiolipin tests

- pregnancy
- SLE, anti-phospholipid syndrome
- TB
- leprosy
- malaria
- HIV

Chapter 7

Neurology

The Foundation Programme and MRCP(UK) Part 1 syllabus (from the JRCPMTB) specify what is required in terms of competencies, skills and knowledge from junior physicians in core medical training in neurology. You are advised to consult carefully this syllabus, which emphasises the importance of basic medical sciences as well as a competent level of applied clinical practice.

A. Neurogenetics

You are expected to have knowledge of recent advances in the understanding of the genetic basis for various neurological disorders.

1. Myotonic dystrophy

Myotonic dystrophy (also called *dystrophia myotonica*) is an inherited myopathy with features developing at around 20–30 years old. It affects skeletal, cardiac and smooth muscle. These are trinucleotide repeats transcribed in RNA, but which are not translated into protein. There are two main types of myotonic dystrophy, DM1 and DM2.

Genetics

◈ autosomal dominant

◈ a trinucleotide repeat disorder

◈ DM1 is caused by a CTG repeat at the end of the *DMPK* (dystrophia myotonica protein kinase) gene on chromosome 19

◈ DM2 is caused by a repeat expansion of the *ZNF9* gene on chromosome 3

The key differences are listed in Table 7.1.

TABLE 7.1 Types of myotonic dystrophy (DM)

DM1	DM2
• *DMPK* gene on chromosome 19q13.3	• *ZNF9* gene on chromosome 3q21
• distal weakness more prominent	• proximal weakness more prominent
	• severe congenital form not seen

General features

✦ myotonic facies (long, 'haggard' appearance)

✦ frontal balding

✦ bilateral ptosis

✦ cataracts

✦ dysarthria

Other features

✦ myotonia (tonic spasm of muscle)

✦ weakness of arms and legs (distal initially)

✦ mild mental impairment

✦ diabetes mellitus

✦ testicular atrophy

✦ cardiac involvement: heart block, cardiomyopathy

✦ dysphagia

2. Genetic aspects of Alzheimer's disease

Most cases are sporadic.

✦ Five per cent are inherited as an autosomal dominant trait.

Mutations in the amyloid precursor protein (chromosome 21), presenilin 1 (chromosome 14) and presenilin 2 (chromosome 1) genes are thought to cause the inherited form.

Apoprotein E allele E4 – encodes a cholesterol transport protein

An area of growing interest has been genetic testing for Alzheimer's disease. Until recently, clinical gene testing only included apolipoprotein E genotyping and testing for presenilin 1 mutations.

In 2008, testing in the US expanded to include the presenilin 2 and amyloid precursor protein genes. Despite these advances, genetic testing is currently not

appropriate for most individuals diagnosed with AD, and has limited utility for predictive purposes.

B. Cell biology

Questions in this area will relate to advances in the cellular mechanisms of certain neurological disease processes which have provided better understanding of disease mechanisms and which might, in the future, lead to more rational therapy.

1. The genesis of tissue damage in stroke and the role of certain excitatory neurotransmitters

Knowledge of the molecular mechanisms that underlie neurone death following stroke is important to allow the development of effective neuroprotective strategies.

Neurological research focuses on information derived from animal models of ischaemic injury. The two principal models for human stroke are induced in rodents either by global or focal ischaemia.

In both cases, blood flow disruptions limit the delivery of oxygen and glucose to neurones, causing ATP reduction and energy depletion, initiating excitotoxic mechanisms that are deleterious for neurones. These include activation of glutamate receptors and release of excess glutamate in the extracellular space, inducing neurone depolarisation and dramatic increase of intracellular calcium that in turn activates multiple intracellular death pathways.

The notion that excitotoxicity leads only to neurone necrosis has largely been abandoned now, as ultrastructural and biochemical analysis have shown signs of apoptotic and autophagic cell death in ischaemic neurones, and this has been further confirmed in neurones subjected to in vitro ischaemia models.

2. The role of the dopaminergic system in various extrapyramidal disorders

It is our understanding of the degeneration of the nigrostriatal dopaminergic system that is the rationale for using dopamine as an enhancer in Parkinson's disease. Currently accepted practice in the management of patients with Parkinson's disease (PD) is to delay treatment until the onset of disabling symptoms and then to introduce a dopamine receptor agonist. If the patient is elderly, levodopa is sometimes used as an initial treatment.

Dopamine receptor agonists

✦ e.g. bromocriptine, ropinirole, cabergoline, apomorphine

✦ Ergot-derived dopamine receptor agonists (bromocriptine, cabergoline, pergolide) have been associated with pulmonary, retroperitoneal and cardiac fibrosis. The **Committee on Safety of Medicines** advise that an ESR, creatinine and chest X-ray should be obtained prior to treatment and patients should be closely monitored.

Levodopa

✦ usually combined with a decarboxylase inhibitor (e.g. carbidopa or benserazide) to prevent peripheral metabolism of levodopa to dopamine

✦ reduced effectiveness with time (usually by 2 years)

✦ unwanted effects: dyskinesia, 'on-off' effect

✦ no use in neuroleptic induced Parkinsonism

L-dopa and dopamine agonists are the treatment of choice for bradykinesia and rigidity.

Monoamine oxidase-B (MAO-B) inhibitors

✦ e.g. selegiline

✦ inhibits the breakdown of dopamine secreted by the dopaminergic neurons

Amantadine

✦ mechanism is not fully understood, probably increases dopamine release and inhibits its uptake at dopaminergic synapses

Catechol-O-methyl transferase (COMT) inhibitors

✦ e.g. entacapone

✦ COMT is an enzyme involved in the breakdown of dopamine, and hence may be used as an adjunct to levodopa therapy

✦ used in established PD

Antimuscarinics

✦ block cholinergic receptors

✦ now used more to treat drug-induced Parkinsonism rather than idiopathic Parkinson's disease

◆ help tremor and rigidity

◆ e.g. procyclidine, benzotropine, trihexyphenidyl (benzhexol)

Note carefully that anticholinergic treatment (for example, benzhexol) is the treatment of choice of tremor, predominantly Parkinson's disease.

Oculogyric crisis

Oculogyric crisis is an acute dystonic reaction of the face/eyes and is usually a consequence of typical neuroleptic drugs such as haloperidol and chlorpromazine but is unusual with newer agents such as olanzapine anad clozapine.

The condition is often precipitated by reintroduction of the agent.

The condition should be treated with procyclidine (usually IV or IM) or benztropine.

Chronic treatment beyond a couple of days is not required.

C. Neuropharmacology

You are expected to have some knowledge of new drug developments in neurology, as well as the established drug therapies.

1. Dementia: Alzheimer's disease

Hypotheses implicating defects within both neurotransmitter systems in Alzheimer's disease are well recognised now in the literature, following the seminal paper by Bartus *et al.* (1982) implicating dysfunction of the cholinergic system.

This knowledge coupled with ongoing discoveries about the multiple pathophysiologic pathways involved in development and progression of AD has given rise to several plausible therapeutic targets. Therapies addressing some of these targets (i.e. acetylcholine, glutamate) have already shown clinical efficacy in treating AD while other targets continue to be investigated.

2. Atypical antipsychotics

Atypical antipsychotics should now be used first-line in patients with schizophrenia, according to 2005 NICE guidelines.

'Schizophrenia – atypical antipsychotics' NICE technology appraisal 43 (June 2002). NICE recommended the use of atypical (newer) oral antipsychotic drugs for a person who has been newly diagnosed with schizophrenia and for people who are currently taking typical (older) antipsychotic drugs that are controlling their symptoms of schizophrenia but are causing side effects. The main advantage of the atypical agents is a significant reduction in extrapyramidal side effects.

Adverse effects of atypical antipsychotics

◈ weight gain

◈ olanzapine and risperidone are associated with an increased risk of stroke in elderly patients

◈ clozapine is associated with agranulocytosis (see below)

Examples of atypical antipsychotics

◈ clozapine

◈ olanzapine

◈ risperidone

◈ quetiapine

◈ amisulpride

Clozapine

Clozapine, one of the first atypical agents to be developed, carries a significant risk of agranulocytosis, and full blood count monitoring is therefore essential during treatment. For this reason clozapine should only be used in patients resistant to other antipsychotic medication.

Adverse effects of clozapine

◈ agranulocytosis (1%), neutropaenia (3%)

◈ reduced seizure threshold – can induce seizures in up to 3% of patients

3. Antioxidants

Riluzole is a sodium channel blocker that inhibits the release of glutamate and has several other potentially neuroprotective effects: it had a modest effect in prolonging survival in motor neurone disease.

There have been, thus far, no well-powered trials of antioxidant compounds in motor neurone disease: a small scale trial using *N*-acetylcysteine found a non-significant improvement in survival in patients whose disease symptoms started in the limb muscles.

D. Localisation of function

1. Ulnar nerve

Overview

◆ arises from medial cord of brachial plexus (C8, T1)

Motor to

◆ medial two lumbricals

◆ adductor pollicis

◆ interossei

◆ hypothenar muscles: abductor digiti minimi, flexor digiti minimi

◆ flexor carpi ulnaris

Sensory to medial 1½ fingers (palmar and dorsal aspects)

Patterns of damage
Damage at wrist

◆ 'claw hand'

◆ wasting and paralysis of intrinsic hand muscles (except lateral two lumbricals)

◆ wasting and paralysis of hypothenar muscles

◆ sensory loss to the medial 1½ fingers (palmar and dorsal aspects)

Damage at elbow

◆ as above

◆ radial deviation of wrist

2. Acoustic neuroma (acoustic neurinoma)

Acoustic neuromas account for approximately 5% of intracranial tumours and 90% of cerebellopontine angle.

Features can be predicted by the affected cranial nerves:

◈ cranial nerve VIII: hearing loss, vertigo, tinnitus

◈ cranial nerve V: absent corneal reflex

◈ cranial nerve VII: facial palsy

Bilateral acoustic neuromas are seen in neurofibromatosis type 2.

MRI of the cerebellopontine angle is the investigation of choice.

Basic features

◈ caused by compression of lateral cutaneous nerve of thigh

◈ typically burning sensation over antero-lateral aspect of thigh

3. Intracranial venous thrombosis

Overview

◈ can cause cerebral infarction, much lesson common than arterial causes

◈ 50% of patients have isolated sagittal sinus thromboses; the remainder have coexistent lateral sinus thromboses and cavernous sinus thromboses

Features

◈ headache (may be sudden onset)

◈ nausea and vomiting

◈ papilloedema

Sagittal sinus thrombosis

◈ may present with seizures and hemiplegia

◈ parasagittal biparietal or bifrontal haemorrhagic infarctions are sometimes seen

Cavernous sinus thrombosis

◈ other causes of cavernous sinus syndrome: local infection (e.g. sinusitis), neoplasia, trauma

◈ ophthalmoplegia due to IIIrd, IVth and VIth cranial nerve damage

- trigeminal nerve involvement may lead to hyperaesthesia of upper face and eye pain
- central retinal vein thrombosis
- swollen eyelids

Lateral sinus thrombosis
- VIth and VIIth cranial nerve palsies

4. Pituitary apoplexy
Definition: sudden enlargement of pituitary tumour secondary to haemorrhage or infarction.

Neurological features
- sudden onset headache similar to that seen in subarachnoid haemorrhage
- vomiting
- neck stiffness
- visual field defects: classically bitemporal superior quadrantic defect
- extraocular nerve palsies
- features of pituitary insufficiency, e.g. hypotension secondary to hypoadrenalism

Please note that pituitary failure in the context of adrenal insufficiency is discussed as an important endocrine emergency in Chapter 3.

E. Common and important neurological syndromes
1. Dementia
Dementia is a clinical state characterised by loss of function in multiple cognitive domains beyond what might be expected from normal ageing. Particularly affected areas may be memory, attention, language and solving.

The most common form of dementia, **Alzheimer's disease**, accounts for 50%–75% of all cases of dementia. The cluster of conditions commonly referred to as 'Alzheimer's disease' should strictly speaking be referred to as a clinical syndrome. Another 20%–30% is due to blood vessel disease (post-stroke dementia). The remaining cases result from a variety of less common disorders.

Given the relatively insidious onset of an individual's memory loss, accompanied by visuospatial dysfunction, unremarkable cardiovascular examination and relatively normal CT head, Alzheimer's dementia could be the most likely diagnosis in a scenario in the MRCP(UK) Part 1 examination.

Short-term memory impairment is the commonest clinical presentation of Alzheimer's disease. Usually patients are fully orientated in time, person and place. Long-term memory is usually intact. The best way to test short-term memory is to ask the patient to recall new information in the next few minutes.

The pathogenesis of AD is complex and not yet fully understood. A number of factors, including amyloid plaques, NFTs and inflammatory processes, are likely to contribute to development of the disease. Acetylcholine and glutamate are intimately involved in learning and memory.

Management
The key points, relevant to medial care, are as follows (from CG42 NICE guidelines on dementia):

◆ Memory assessment services (which may be provided by a memory assessment clinic or by community mental health teams) should be the single point of referral for all people with a possible diagnosis of dementia.

◆ Structural imaging should be used in the assessment of people with suspected dementia to exclude other cerebral pathologies and to help establish the subtype diagnosis. Magnetic resonance imaging (MRI) is the preferred modality to assist with early diagnosis and detect subcortical vascular changes, although computed tomography (CT) scanning could be used. Specialist advice should be taken when interpreting scans in people with learning disabilities.

◆ People with dementia who develop non-cognitive symptoms that cause them significant distress or who develop behaviour that challenges should be offered an assessment at an early opportunity to establish the likely factors that may generate, aggravate or improve such behaviour.

Diffuse Lewy body disease
This is the third-commonest cause of dementia (after Alzheimer's disease and vascular dementia).

It presents with:

◆ cognitive impairment

◆ visual hallucinations

◆ Parkinsonism

A common manifestation of the disease is severe neuroleptic treatment intolerance which can be fatal.

2. Cortical lesions

Lesions of the frontal lobe include difficulties with task sequencing and executive skills, expressive aphasia (receptive aphasias a temporal lobe lesion), primitive reflexes, perseveration (repeatedly asking the same question or performing the same task), anosmia and changes in personality.

Lesions of the parietal lobe include apraxias, neglect, astereognosis (unable to recognise an object by feeling it) and visual field defects (typically homonymous inferior quadrantanopia). They may also cause alcalculia (inability to perform mental arithmetic).

Lesions of the temporal lobe cause visual field defects (typically homonymous superior quadrantanopia), Wernicke's (receptive) aphasia, auditory agnosia and memory impairment.

Occipital lobe lesions include cortical blindness (blindness due to damage to the visual cortex and may present as *Anton's syndrome*, where there is blindness but the patient is unaware or denies blindness), homonymous hemianopia and visual agnosia (seeing but not percieving objects – it is different to neglect since in agnosia the objects are seen and followed but cannot be named).

3. Chronic subdural haematoma

Overview

- most commonly secondary to trauma, e.g. old person/alcohol-influenced falling over
- initial injury may be minor and is often forgotten
- caused by bleeding from damaged bridging veins between cortex and venous sinuses

Features

- headache
- classically fluctuating conscious level
- raised intracranial pressure

Treatment

- needs neurosurgical review

4. Epilepsy

Generalised – no focal features, consciousness lost immediately:

+ grand mal (tonic-clonic)
+ petit mal (absence seizures)
+ partial seizures progressing to generalised seizures
+ atonic
+ infantile spasms

Partial – focal features depending on location:

+ simple (no disturbance of consciousness or awareness)
+ complex (consciousness is disturbed)
+ temporal lobe $\Rightarrow$ aura, déjà vu, jamais vu motor $\Rightarrow$ Jacksonian 'march'
+ simple partial followed by impaired consciousness, or consciousness impaired at onset

Unclassified aversive seizures are a form of simple partial seizure, consisting of head turning and conjugate eye movements.

Forms

+ **Rasmussen's encephalitis** is a subacute inflammatory encephalitis, and is one cause of *epilepsia partialis continua*.
+ **Rolandic epilepsy** is a benign partial epilepsy associated with centro-temporal spikes. There is an excellent prognosis.
+ **Complex partial seizures** often contain automatisms which may be elementary (including lip smacking, chewing, swallowing or salivation), or automatic behaviour (semi-purposive uncoordinated or unplanned gestures, including picking and pulling at clothing).

Management

Most neurologists now start anti-epileptics following a second epileptic seizure. NICE guidelines suggest starting anti-epileptics after the first seizure if any of the following are present:

+ The patient has a neurological deficit.
+ Brain imaging shows a structural abnormality.
+ The EEG shows unequivocal epileptic activity.

⬥ The patient or their family or carers consider the risk of having a further seizure unacceptable.

Sodium valproate is considered the first-line treatment for patients with generalised seizures, with carbamazepine used for partial seizures.

Adverse effects of anticonvulsants

⬥ gastrointestinal: nausea and increased appetite and weight gain

⬥ alopecia: regrowth may be curly

⬥ ataxia

⬥ tremor

⬥ hepatitis

⬥ pancreatitis

⬥ teratogenic

Overview of management strategies

Absences, generalised tonic-clonic seizures and myoclonus are features of primary generalised epilepsy. The treatment of choice includes sodium valproate, lamotrigine and topiramate. Clonazepam is useful in myoclonus, ethosuximide in isolated absences and gabapentin in partial seizures.

Tonic-clonic seizures

⬥ sodium valproate

⬥ *second-line*: lamotrigine, carbamazepine

Absence seizures (petit mal)

⬥ sodium valproate or ethosuximide

⬥ sodium valproate is particularly effective if co-existent tonic-clonic seizures in primary generalised epilepsy

Myoclonic seizures

⬥ sodium valproate

⬥ *second-line*: clonazepam, lamotrigine

Partial seizures

⬥ carbamazepine

⬥ *second-line*: lamotrigine, sodium valproate

5. Multiple sclerosis (MS)

Diagnosis

Since the early 1980s, the *'Poser criteria'* were used to classify **multiple sclerosis**. This relied upon evidence of at least two relapses typical of multiple sclerosis and evidence of involvement of white matter in more than one site in the central nervous system – the concept of *'lesions scattered in time and space'*.

Attacks or exacerbations of multiple sclerosis are characterised by new symptoms that reflect CNS involvement. These symptoms are typically separated in time (e.g. by months or years) and in anatomical location (e.g. weakness of one or more limbs, optic neuritis, sensory symptoms). Recognising that physical and cognitive disability progression in MS may occur in the absence of clinical exacerbations is important. Although most patients have a wide range of symptoms from lesions in different areas of the brain and spinal cord, others may present with predominantly visual, cognitive or cerebellar symptoms.

A new system of classification, the *'McDonald criteria'*, incorporates clinical and laboratory elements, allowing an earlier confirmation of the diagnosis and thus enabling earlier decisions about starting disease-modifying therapies. Therefore, in summary, multiple sclerosis is now a clinical diagnosis on the basis of two episodes involving two or more areas of the central nervous system over time, but the McDonald criteria incorporate magnetic resonance imaging to demonstrate multiple areas of involvement and also involvement over time with the appearance of new enhancing lesions.

Progression

About 85% of patients with multiple sclerosis present with the relapsing-remitting form, comprising episodic relapses and remissions that may be partial or complete.

A first attack is categorised as a *'clinically isolated syndrome'*. After many years most of these patients will enter a phase of progression with or without attacks, called secondary 'progressive multiple sclerosis'.

About 15% of patients present without relapses but show a slowly progressive pattern called primary progressive multiple sclerosis. A few of them may later relapse, called progressive-relapsing multiple sclerosis. Fifteen per cent of patients with relapsing-remitting multiple sclerosis likewise have a mild course with minimal disability after 15 years, called benign multiple sclerosis.

Classification of multiple sclerosis is important as all the disease-modifying drugs have shown benefit only in the relapsing-remitting type and no benefit in the primary progressive form.

Management
Acute attacks

Unless an attack is mild, such as minor sensory symptoms, the treatment is intravenous methylprednisolone daily for 3 days. Protocols vary, but this is the most widely used.

Patients are usually not admitted to hospital for this therapy unless severe problems justify other approaches.

Large doses of oral steroids may achieve comparable results, but further studies are required.

Contemporary aspects

Management in multiple sclerosis is focused at reducing the frequency and duration of relapses. There is no cure. High-dose steroids (e.g. IV methylprednisolone) may be given for 3–5 days to shorten the length of an acute relapse. Baclofen is helpful in controlling spasticity. Hallucinations are occasionally seen on the withdrawal of baclofen.

Beta-interferon has been shown to reduce the relapse rate by up to 30%. Certain criteria have to be met before it is used:

◆ relapsing-remitting disease + 2 relapses in past 2 years + able to walk 100 m unaided

◆ secondary progressive disease + 2 relapses in past 2 years + able to walk 10 m (aided or unaided)

Beta-interferon reduces number of relapses and MRI changes, however does not reduce overall disability.

Other drugs used in the management of multiple sclerosis include:

◆ Glatiramer acetate: immunomodulating drug.

◆ Natalizumab: a recombinant monoclonal antibody that antagonises alpha4beta1 integrin found on the surface of leucocytes, thus inhibiting migration of leucocytes across the endothelium into parenchymal tissue.

◆ Symptom control.

◆ Spasticity: baclofen and gabapentin are first-line. Other options include diazepam, dantrolene and tizanidine.

◆ Botulinum toxin is the treatment of choice for focal dystonia (such as torticollis and hemifacial spasm) and focal dystonia. The primary action of the toxin is to block acetylcholine release at the neuromuscular junction and so to produce muscle weakness. Occasionally systemic absorption of the toxin can affect distal muscles causing symptoms such as diplopia and dysphagia.

 For a review of the most up-to-date (at the time of publication) guidance on multiple sclerosis in the UK, please refer to **NICE CG8**.

6. Guillain-Barré syndrome

Guillain-Barré syndrome is a peripheral neuropathy that causes acute neuromuscular failure. Misdiagnosis is common and can be fatal because of the high frequency of respiratory failure, which contributes to the 10% mortality seen in prospective studies. Around 75% of patients have a history of preceding infection, usually of the respiratory and GI tract.

Clinical features

All types of Guillain-Barré syndrome present with acute neuropathy, defined as progressive onset of limb weakness that reaches its worst within 4 weeks.

Limb weakness is usually global – both proximal and distal – unlike that of back axonopathy, such as neuropathy associated with drug toxins or alcohol, which is usually distal.

Sensory loss is variable in acute inflammatory demyelinating polyradiculoneuropathy. Typically there are sensory symptoms but few sensory signs.

Reflexes are usually lost early in the illness, although acute motor axonal neuropathy can be associated with retained reflexes or even brisk reflexes. Autonomic signs such as tachycardia, hypertension, or lack of sinus arrhythmia are common.

The respiratory system is affected in a third of cases, but this may not be associated with clear dyspnoea, which makes it more difficult to assess. It is essential to measure vital capacity in such cases to anticipate declining respiratory effort.

BOX 7.1   A note on the vital capacity

A falling vital capacity is a more useful warning sign of incipient respiratory arrest than blood gases or oxygen saturation, which often remain normal until breathing stops altogether.

The cranial nerves are often affected, with facial weakness and bulbar palsy the most common problems, followed by an eye movement disorder.

Diagnosis

♦ Nerve conduction studies are the most useful confirmatory test and are abnormal in 85% of patients, even early on in the disease. Typically these show signs of conduction block, prolonged distal latencies, delayed F waves. Motor conduction velocities are usually normal initially but may slow later.

♦ An increase in cerebrospinal fluid protein, which is helpful diagnostically but is not specific to Guillain-Barré syndrome, has long been recognised.

♦ Finally, it may be helpful to measure antiganglioside antibodies, as well as antibodies to *Campylobacter jejuni*.

Management

A Cochrane review has shown that plasma exchange is better than supportive measures.

Intravenous immunoglobulin has now become the standard treatment for the syndrome because it can be given rapidly and has fewer side effects than plasma exchange. The standard regimen of 0.4 g/kg body weight each day for five consecutive days is well tolerated, but side effects include dermatitis and much more rarely renal impairment and hyperviscosity effects, including strokes.

Unusually for a disease that is thought to have an immunological aetiology, steroids are ineffective.

Miller-Fisher syndrome

Miller-Fisher syndrome is a variant/spectrum of Guillain-Barré syndrome (GBS).

GBS is associated with *Campylobacter jejuni* infection, which can trigger this syndrome.

The Miller-Fisher syndrome is classically described as a triad of:

♦ external ophthalmoplegia

♦ ataxia

♦ areflexia

7. Peripheral neuropathy

Alcohol abuse and diabetes are the commonest causes of **peripheral neuropathy** in the UK.

Vitamin B$_{12}$ deficiency causes neuropathy that affects only the dorsal column (joint position, light touch and vibration).

Lead neuropathy is purely motor affecting mainly the upper limbs.

Chronic inflammatory demyelinating polyradiculopathy causes mainly motor impairment (distal and proximal).

8. Neuralgic amyotrophy

Neuralgic amyotrophy is a brachial plexopathy (usually upper brachial plexus) usually preceded by an infective picture.

A typical history might be a 30-year-old male presenting with a week-long history of right arm weakness. It might be, originally, that the problem began with severe pain in the neck which radiated into the right shoulder, which was followed by weakness.

Examination might reveal winging of the right scapula with weakness of right shoulder abduction and elbow extension. There could be some sensory loss over the lateral aspect of the right shoulder and right triceps reflex was absent.

It usually presents with severe pain for days to weeks followed by weakness and sensory loss over the corresponding territory of the brachial plexus (more commonly C5–C7).

It is a self-limiting condition but recovery may be slow (years).

9. Polymyositis and respiratory failure

Acid maltase deficiency typically presents with insidious onset of proximal myopathy and early respiratory muscle weakness.

Respiratory failure in inflammatory myopathies (polymyositis, dermatomyositis, inclusion body myositis) and limb girdle muscular dystrophy are relatively rare. Muscle biopsy shows vacuolation in muscle fibres.

10. Headache
Headaches are chronic or acute.

Chronic headaches
Cluster headaches
Cluster headaches are more common in men (5 : 1) and smokers.

Features

- constant, intense, and boring pain typically occurs once or twice a day, each episode lasting 15 minutes to 2 hours
- paroxysmal, with clusters typically lasting 4–12 weeks
- intense unilateral pain around one eye (recurrent attacks 'always' affect same side)
- patient is restless during an attack
- 80%–90% have attacks at the same time each day
- alcohol is often a trigger
- accompanied by redness, lacrimation, lid swelling
- nasal stuffiness or congestion
- miosis and ptosis (in a minority)
- more common in men (M : F, 10 : 1)
- usually present nocturnally (early morning)
- examination between the attacks should be normal

Management

- acute: 100% oxygen, subcutaneous sumatriptan, nasal lidocaine
- prophylaxis: verapamil, lithium, sodium valproate, prednisolone
- consider specialist referral

Migraine
A typical history might be a 25-year-old woman who presents with 2 hours of a unilateral temporal headache increasing in severity. The pain is of a throbbing character and is exacerbated by light. There are no abnormal signs on examination. Migraine is the commonest cause of headache in young patients. Photophobia, unilateral presentation and normal examination will be consistent with migraine.

Tension headaches

Tension headaches are one of the most common forms of headaches. They may occur at any age, but are most common in adults and adolescents.

If a headache occurs two or more times a week for several months or longer, the condition is considered chronic. Chronic daily headaches can result from the under- or overtreatment of a primary headache (*'analgesia-overuse headache'*). Tension headaches can occur when the patient also has a migraine.

Tension headaches occur when neck and scalp muscles become tense or contract. The muscle contractions can be a response to stress, depression, a head injury or anxiety. Any activity that causes the head to be held in one position for a long time without moving can cause a headache.

Other triggers of tension headaches include:

- alcohol
- caffeine (too much or withdrawal)
- colds and the flu
- dental problems such as jaw clenching or teeth grinding
- eye strain
- excessive smoking
- fatigue
- nasal congestion
- overexertion
- sinus infection

Symptoms

The headache pain may be described as:

- dull, pressure-like (not throbbing)
- a tight band or vice on the head
- 'all over' (i.e. not just in one point or one side)
- worse in the scalp, temples or back of the neck, and possibly in the shoulders

The pain may occur as an isolated event, constantly or daily. Pain may last for 30 minutes to 7 days. It may be triggered by or get worse with stress, fatigue, noise or glare.

Investigations

A headache that is mild to moderate, not accompanied by other symptoms, and responds to home treatment within a few hours may not need further examination or testing, especially if it has occurred in the past. A tension headache reveals no abnormal findings on a neurological exam. However, tender points (trigger points) in the muscles are often seen in the neck and shoulder areas.

Management

- headache diary
- cold or hot showers
- changing sleep habits
- (*the role of pharmacological interventions is currently being actively researched*)

Paroxysmal hemicranias

Paroxysmal hemicrania is characterised by multiple, brief, intense, daily focal head pain attacks. The pain is unilateral and always affects the same side. The pain is usually most severe in the auriculotemporal area, the forehead and above or behind the ear. It may spread to involve the ipsilateral shoulder, arm and neck. The pain is described as excruciating, throbbing, boring or pulsating. Between attacks, the patient may have tenderness in the symptomatic area.

Paroxysmal hemicrania usually begins in early adulthood. As in adults, the differential diagnosis with cluster headache can be troublesome. The attack profile of paroxysmal hemicrania is highly characteristic. The frequency of attacks varies enormously within any 24-hour period. Attacks usually last between 2 and 25 minutes and occasionally as long as 60 minutes.

Ipsilateral lacrimation is reported to occur in about 80% of attacks. When the lacrimation is bilateral, it is predominantly on the side of the pain. Photophobia may accompany some attacks, and increased forehead sweating, especially on the symptomatic side, is observed in a few patients.

There is much interest in the best management of these headaches, with indomethacin being suggested currently.

The acute new headache
Subarachnoid haemorrhage (SAH)

The cardinal symptom of a **subarachnoid haemorrhage** (SAH) is headache, present in 85%–100% (those without a headache are usually unconscious, and therefore not able to give a history).

Approximately 85% of SAHs are secondary to a ruptured intracranial saccular aneurysm.

The presence of nausea, vomiting, neck stiffness, transient loss of consciousness, or focal neurological symptoms are supportive of the diagnosis of SAH. However, absence of these symptoms cannot be taken as reassurance that the patient has not had an SAH, as a proportion will present with headache as the only symptom.

The prognosis of SAH is poor: about 25% of patients will die within 24 hours of their ictus (that is, either before they reach the ED, or very shortly thereafter), a further 25% will die within hospital and of the survivors, up to 50% will be disabled.

Those who survive their aneurysmal SAH but do not have the aneurysm secured (either by clipping or endovascular treatment) have a 3% per year risk of re-bleeding.

Vascular causes other than SAH

Intraventricular or primary intracerebral haemorrhage, and ischaemic stroke, may present with headache. By definition, however, there will be other focal symptoms to alert the neurologist.

Some patients will be comatose early (usually those with haemorrhagic stroke, particularly in the posterior fossa), and urgent CT is required for the diagnosis.

Dissection of the carotid or vertebrobasilar arteries may present with predominantly head, neck or facial pain. Dissection of the internal carotid artery causes ipsilateral facial, dental or cervical pain; neurological features may be minimal or absent initially, but an ipsilateral Horner's syndrome should be looked for. More obvious features are ipsilateral monocular blindness or contralateral motor or sensory symptoms. Vertebrobasilar dissection may cause ipsilateral pain in the back of the neck and/or occiput, and may lead to brainstem symptoms. The neurological symptoms in arterial dissection may fluctuate considerably. Dissection may also be a rare cause of SAH.

Intracranial venous thrombosis presents in a diverse manner, ranging from intracranial hypertension to rapid onset coma and death.

A proportion will present with acute onset headache indistinguishable from SAH, the diagnosis only becoming clear with further investigations, such as CT angiography.

Meningo-encephalitis

Although **meningeal infection** usually presents in a subacute manner, patients may either present comatose (that is, with no history available from them), or occasionally with true sudden onset headache indistinguishable from SAH.

Untreated bacterial meningitis has a poor prognosis, and immediate treatment with antibiotics is essential. The presence of a high fever (>38°C), features of septic shock or a purpuric rash should be sought.

Benign headache syndromes

Physical exertion (including sexual activity) may precede SAH or benign syndromes such as thunderclap, benign exertional or coital headache, but it is rarely possible to differentiate between these on clinical grounds alone.

Thunderclap headache is a diagnosis of exclusion, **and is only acceptable once SAH and other serious intracranial causes have been excluded.**

11. Neurofibromatosis

There are two types of **neurofibromatosis**, NF1 and NF2. Both are inherited in an autosomal dominant fashion.

NF1 is also known as von Recklinghausen's syndrome. It is caused by a gene mutation on chromosome 17 which encodes neurofibromin and affects around one in 4000.

NF2 is caused by gene mutation on chromosome 22 and affects around one in 100 000.

Features

TABLE 7.2

NF1	NF2
Café au lait spots (= 6–15 mm in diameter)	Bilateral acoustic neuromas
Axillary/groin freckles	
Peripheral neurofibromas	
Iris: Lisch nodules in >90%	
Scoliosis	

12. Paraneoplastic syndromes affecting nervous systems

Lambert-Eaton myasthenic syndrome

◆ associated with small cell lung cancer (also breast and ovarian)

◆ antibody directed against pre-synaptic voltage gated calcium channel in the peripheral nervous system

◆ can also occur independently as autoimmune disorder

Anti-Hu

◆ associated with small cell lung carcinoma and neuroblastomas

◆ sensory neuropathy – may be painful

◆ cerebellar syndrome

◆ encephalomyelitis

Anti-Yo

◆ associated with ovarian and breast cancer

◆ cerebellar syndrome

Anti-GAD antibody

◆ associated with breast, colorectal and small cell lung carcinoma

◆ stiff person syndrome

Anti-Ri

◆ associated with breast and small cell lung carcinoma

◆ ocular opsoclonus-myoclonus

13. Parkinson's disease

Presentation

The cardinal symptoms of **Parkinson's disease** are shaking, stiffness, and slowness and poverty of movement.

The condition leads to physical signs, including tremor at rest, rigidity on passive movement, slowness of movement (bradykinesia) and poverty of movement (hypokinesia). These features are unilateral at onset, but become bilateral as the condition progresses. Later, postural instability and falls, orthostatic hypotension and dementia can develop.

The motor features of Parkinson's disease can be controlled reasonably well in most patients with the measures outlined above. It is the non-motor features of the disorder, such as anxiety and depression, which now present the greatest management challenge in the earliest stages.

Diagnosis

The diagnosis of Parkinson's disease remains clinical in most cases. Most experts use the **UK Parkinson's Disease Society Brain Bank diagnostic criteria.**

The **NICE guidelines** recommend that people with suspected Parkinson's disease should be referred quickly and untreated to a specialist with expertise in differential diagnosis. They recommend that all patients with suspected Parkinson's disease should be reviewed regularly and the diagnosis reviewed if atypical features develop.

It is difficult for experts to differentiate essential tremor from Parkinson's disease when asymmetric postural and action tremor of the upper limbs appears at rest. In this situation, single photon emission computed tomography (SPECT) is useful and is supported by NICE. Uptake is normal in controls and in patients with essential tremor, neuroleptic induced Parkinsonism and psychogenic Parkinsonism, but is reduced in those with Parkinson's disease, Parkinson's disease dementias and Parkinsonian syndromes.

Pharmacological treatment

[This is described in section 4 of this chapter.]

Surgery

Improved understanding of the neural mechanism of Parkinson's disease showed that the subthalamic nucleus is overactive. This led to the development of bilateral subthalamic stimulation surgery to switch off this nucleus.

Role of the multidisciplinary team

Clarke (2007) helpfully reviewed the importance of the multidisciplinary team in a recent review article amongst other aspects.

14. Essential tremor

Essential tremor (previously called 'benign essential tremor') is an autosomal dominant condition which usually affects both upper limbs.

Features

◆ postural tremor: worse if arms outstretched

◆ improved by alcohol and rest

◆ most common cause of titubation (head tremor)

Management

◆ propranolol is first-line

◆ primidone is sometimes used

15. Multiple system atrophy

Shy-Drager syndrome is a type of multiple system atrophy.

Features

◆ Parkinsonism

◆ autonomic disturbance (atonic bladder, postural hypotension)

◆ cerebellar signs

16. Motor neurone disease

Motor neurone disease is relatively uncommon, with an annual incidence of two in 100 000 and prevalence of five to seven per 100 000.

Medical care

Multidisciplinary motor neurone disease clinics improve care, reduce the frequency and length of inpatient stays, and improve survival.

The team may include a neurologist, physiotherapist, occupational therapist, specialist nurse, social worker, dietitian, speech and language therapist, respiratory nurse, and respiratory and palliative care doctors.

A medication with promise is riluzole, described in section 3 of this chapter.

The greatest advance in recent years in treating motor neurone disease has been the discovery of the beneficial effects of non-invasive ventilation, in which the patient uses a mask ventilator system (usually bilateral positive airway pressure) overnight during sleep. The machines are small and portable, and various face masks are available.

Presentation

Motor neurone disease is largely a sporadic disease of middle and elderly life presenting in the sixth and seventh decades, although the disease can present in much younger patients. A younger presentation is more often seen in familial motor neurone disease, which accounts for approximately 5% of cases.

The classic form of the disease is also referred to as amyotrophic lateral sclerosis and presents with a mixture of upper and lower motor neurone features, such as wasted fasciculating biceps with a brisk or easily obtained biceps deep tendon reflex. The rarer variants of the disease can have a pure upper motor neurone presentation, primary lateral sclerosis, or a pure lower motor neurone presentation, progressive muscular atrophy.

Classic motor neurone disease tends to be focal in onset, with a particular group of muscles affected first. Of the three recognised patterns – limb, bulbar and respiratory onset – limb onset is by far the commonest. In the upper limbs early symptoms are most commonly due to asymmetrical distal weakness, causing patients to drop objects or have difficulty manipulating objects with one hand, such as turning keys, writing and opening bottles. Wasting of the intrinsic small muscles of the hand is common, particularly flattening of the thenar eminence and the first dorsal interosseous muscle, and often patients or relatives will have noticed this. In the lower limbs early symptoms include foot drop, a sensation of heaviness of one or both legs, or a tendency to trip. Patients may also notice difficulty in rising from low chairs and climbing stairs or excessive fatigue when walking.

Bulbar onset motor neurone disease occurs in about 20% of those affected. The first sign is usually slurring of the speech, caused by impaired tongue movement, which may be accompanied by obvious wasting and fasciculation of the tongue. Dysphagia tends to occur later, when speech difficulties have become significant. Bulbar symptoms in motor neurone disease, as with other causes of pseudobulbar palsy, are often associated with emotional lability, manifesting as inappropriate laughing or crying.

The least common pattern of onset is when the respiratory muscles are affected first. Patients can present with dyspnoea and orthopnoea or more subtly with the clinical features resulting from hypoventilation overnight, including frequent waking, unrefreshing sleep, hypersomnolence and early morning headaches.

Diagnosis

A diagnosis of motor neurone disease relies on interpretation of the clinical symptoms and signs and use of investigations to exclude other causes.

A person who presents with a painless, progressive loss of function in a weak, wasted limb or with one of the presentations described above would benefit from a neurological opinion. The lack of a definitive test can cause problems, particularly if patients are seen very early after onset of symptoms, when the signs may be limited. In these cases waiting and observation of the condition over weeks and months are needed. Other tests such as a muscle biopsy may be useful in excluding diagnoses.

As with other disorders with such a grave prognosis, alternative cause for the patient's symptoms and signs must be excluded. Several conditions can mimic motor neurone disease, such as benign cramp fasciculation syndrome, cervical radiculomyelopathy, multifocal motor neuropathy with conduction block and inclusion body myositis.

17. Idiopathic intracranial hypertension

Idiopathic intracranial hypertension (also known as pseudotumour cerebri and formerly benign intracranial hypertension) is a condition classically seen in young, overweight females.

Features
- headache
- blurred vision
- papilloedema (usually present)
- enlarged blind spot
- sixth nerve palsy may be present

Risk factors
- obesity
- female sex
- pregnancy
- drugs: oral contraceptive pill, steroids, tetracycline, vitamin A

Management
- weight loss
- diuretics, e.g. acetazolamide
- repeated lumbar puncture
- surgery: optic nerve sheath decompression and fenestration may be

needed to prevent damage to the optic nerve (a lumboperitoneal or ventriculoperitoneal shunt may also be performed to reduce intracranial pressure)

The best long-term management is weight reduction, which can improve the patient's symptoms.

Changing the combined oral contraceptive pill to a more oestrogen-based one can worsen the symptoms.

Lumbar puncture and acetazolamide can help improve the symptoms, but should not be considered as long-term management.

18. Herpes simplex encephalitis

Herpes simplex (HSV) encephalitis is a common topic in the MRCP(UK). The virus characteristically affects the temporal lobes – questions may give the result of imaging or describe temporal lobe signs, e.g. aphasia.

Features

◆ fever, headache, peculiar behaviour/psychiatric symptoms such as hallucinations, seizures, vomiting
◆ focal features, e.g. dysphasia, aphasia
◆ peripheral lesions (e.g. cold sores) have no relation to presence of HSV encephalitis
◆ there are usually no skin manifestations of herpes simplex infections

Pathophysiology

◆ HSV-1 responsible for 95% of cases in adults
◆ typically affects temporal and inferior frontal lobes

Investigation

◆ CSF: lymphocytosis, elevated protein (virus rarely isolated)
◆ PCR for HSV
◆ CT: medial temporal and inferior frontal changes (e.g. petechial haemorrhages) – normal in one-third of patients
◆ MRI is better (and often brings up the characteristic 'cortical ribboning effect')
◆ EEG pattern: lateralised periodic discharges at 2 Hz

Treatment

◆ intravenous acyclovir

The prognosis is dependent on whether acyclovir is commenced early. If treatment is started promptly the mortality is 10%–20%. Left untreated the mortality approaches 80%.

19. Normal pressure hydrocephalus

Normal pressure hydrocephalus is a reversible cause of dementia seen in elderly patients. It is thought to be secondary to reduced CSF absorption at the arachnoid villi. These changes may be secondary to head injury, subarachnoid haemorrhage or meningitis.

A classical triad of features is seen:

◆ urinary incontinence

◆ dementia and bradyphrenia

◆ gait abnormality (may be similar to Parkinson's disease)

Imaging

◆ hydrocephalus with an enlarged fourth ventricle

Management

◆ ventriculoperitoneal shunting

20. Restless legs syndrome

Restless legs syndrome (RLS) is a syndrome of spontaneous, continuous lower limb movements that may be associated with paraesthesia. It is extremely common, affecting between 2%–10% of the general population. Males and females are equally affected and a family history may be present.

Clinical features

Although no specific tests exist for the diagnosis it is based on the **International Restless Legs Syndrome Study Group four basic criteria for diagnosing RLS**:

1. a desire to move the limbs, often associated with paraesthesias or dysesthesias
2. symptoms that are worse or present only during rest and are partially or temporarily relieved by activity
3. motor restlessness
4. nocturnal worsening of symptoms

Causes and associations

✦ there is a positive family history in 50% of patients with idiopathic RLS

✦ iron deficiency anaemia

✦ uraemia

✦ diabetes mellitus

✦ pregnancy

The diagnosis is clinical although bloods to exclude iron deficiency anaemia may be appropriate.

Management

✦ simple measures: walking, stretching, massaging affected limbs

✦ treat any iron deficiency

✦ dopamine agonists are first-line treatment (e.g. pramipexole, ropinirole)

✦ benzodiazepines

✦ gabapentin

21. Risk factors for stroke

A **stroke** happens when the blood supply to the brain is disrupted. This can be by a blood clot blocking an artery in your brain (ischaemic stroke) or a blood vessel bursting in your brain (haemorrhagic stroke).

Risk factors for stroke include:

✦ smoking

✦ high blood pressure

✦ high cholesterol

✦ being overweight or obese

✦ diabetes

✦ a family history of stroke/heart disease

✦ abnormal heart beat (arrhythmia)

✦ conditions that increase your bleeding tendency (e.g. haemophilia)

✦ regular, heavy drinking

✦ using illegal drugs, such as cocaine

A stroke can also happen after an injury to an artery in your neck. This is called cervical artery dissection.

Management of stroke

Antiplatelet therapy plays a major role in the secondary prevention of ischaemic stroke. The antiplatelet agents that are most used in the clinic include aspirin, dipyridamole and clopidogrel. These agents inhibit platelet activation through different mechanisms of action.

Aspirin is the first-line drug in the secondary prevention of stroke – a combination of aspirin with dipyridamole produces a synergistic antithrombotic effect. Clopidogrel is slightly more effective than aspirin at reducing the risk of ischaemic events. Trials comparing the combination of aspirin and clopidogrel versus aspirin are underway. Intravenous antiplatelet therapy with glycoprotein IIb/IIIa receptor inhibitors for acute stroke and as an adjunct to carotid artery stenting appears promising. However, oral GPIIb/IIIa receptor inhibitors appear hazardous.

A recent meta-analysis of 21 trials that enrolled 18 270 patients with prior ischaemic stroke and transient ischaemic attack (TIA) demonstrated that antiplatelet agents reduced the relative risk of vascular events by 17% as compared with controls (Antithrombotic Trialists' Collaboration, 2002).

22. Transient ischaemic attack

NICE issued updated guidelines relating to stroke and transient ischaemic attack (TIA) in 2008. They advocated the use of the ABCD2 prognostic score for risk stratifying patients who have had a suspected TIA (*see* Table 7.3):

TABLE 7.3

	Criteria	Points
A	Age = 60 years	1
B	Blood pressure = 140/90 mmHg	1
C	Clinical features	
	• unilateral weakness	2
	• speech disturbance, no weakness	1
D	Duration of symptoms	
	• >60 minutes	2
	• 10–59 minutes	1
	Patient has diabetes	1

This gives a total score ranging from 0 to 7. People who have had a suspected TIA who are at a higher risk of stroke (that is, with an ABCD2 score of 4 or above) should have:

+ aspirin (300 mg daily) started immediately
+ specialist assessment and investigation within 24 hours of onset of symptoms
+ measures for secondary prevention introduced as soon as the diagnosis is confirmed, including discussion of individual risk factors

If the ABCD2 risk score is 3 or below:

+ specialist assessment within 1 week of symptom onset, including decision on brain imaging
+ if vascular territory or pathology is uncertain, refer for brain imaging

People with crescendo TIAs (two or more episodes in a week) should be treated as being at high risk of stroke, even though they may have an ABCD2 score of 3 or below.

NICE also published a technology appraisal in 2005 on the use of clopidogrel and dipyridamole.

Recent recommendations from NICE include:

+ Low-dose aspirin combined with modified-release dipyridamole is recommended as first-line treatment. After two years treatment should revert to low-dose aspirin alone.
+ If aspirin cannot be taken, treat with clopidogrel alone.

With regard to carotid artery endarterectomy:

+ Recommend if patient has suffered stroke or TIA in the carotid territory and is not severely disabled.

Endarterectomy should only be considered if carotid stenosis >70% according to European Carotid Surgery Trialists' Collaborative Group (ECST) criteria or >50% according to North American Symptomatic Carotid Endarterectomy Trial (NASCET) criteria.

23. Stroke: highlighted points from the guidelines on management

Selected points relating to the management of acute stroke include:

◆ Blood glucose, hydration, oxygen saturation and temperature should be maintained within normal limits.

◆ Blood pressure should not be lowered in the acute phase unless there are complications, e.g. hypertensive encephalopathy.

◆ Aspirin 300 mg orally or rectally should be given as soon as possible if a haemorrhagic stroke has been excluded.

◆ With regard to atrial fibrillation, the RCP state: 'anticoagulants should not be started until brain imaging has excluded haemorrhage, and usually not until 14 days have passed from the onset of an ischaemic stroke'.

◆ If the cholesterol is >3.5 mmol/L patients should be commenced on a statin.

Thrombolysis

Thrombolysis should only be given if:

◆ it is administered within 3–4½ hours (alteplase is currently recommended by NICE) of onset of stroke symptoms (unless as part of a clinical trial)

◆ haemorrhage has been definitively excluded (i.e. imaging has been performed)

F. Investigative methods

1. A brief note on nerve conduction studies

Nerve conduction studies (NCSs) are useful in determining between axonal and demyelinating pathology.

Axonal

◆ normal conduction velocity

◆ reduced amplitude

Demyelinating

◆ reduced conduction velocity

◆ normal amplitude

References

Antithrombotic Trialists' Collaboration. Collaborative meta-analysis of randomised trials of antiplatelet therapy for prevention of death, myocardial infarction, and stroke in high risk patients. *BMJ*. 2002; **324**(7329): 71–86.

Bartus RT, Dean RL, Beer B, *et al*. The cholinergic hypothesis of geriatric memory dysfunction. *Science*. 1982; **217**(4558): 408–14.

Clarke CE. Parkinson's disease. *BMJ*. 2007; **335**(7617): 441–5.

National Institute for Health and Clinical Excellence. Parkinson's Disease: Diagnosis and Management in Primary and Secondary Care: NICE guideline 35. London: NIHCE; 2006. http://guidance.nice.org.uk/CG35

National Institute for Health and Clinical Excellence. Diagnosis and Initial Management of Acute Stroke and Transient Ischaemic Attack. NICE guideline 68. London: NIHCE; 2008. www.nice.org.uk/Guidance/CG68/NiceGuidance/pdf/English

National Institute for Health and Clinical Excellence. Clopidogrel and Dipyridamole for the Prevention of Atherosclerotic Events. NICE guideline 90. London: NIHCE; 2005. http://guidance.nice.org.uk/TA90

National Institute for Health and Clinical Excellence. Multiple Sclerosis. NICE guideline 8. London: NIHCE; 2003. http://guidance.nice.org.uk/CG8

The International Restless Legs Syndrome Study Group. Validation of the international restless legs syndrome study group rating scale for restless legs syndrome. *Sleep Med* 2003; **4**(2):121–32.

Chapter 8

Ophthalmology

The Foundation Programme and MRCP(UK) Part 1 syllabus (from the JRCPMTB) specify what is required in terms of competencies, skills and knowledge from junior physicians in core medical training in ophthalmology. You are advised to consult carefully this syllabus, which emphasises the importance of basic medical sciences as well as a competent level of applied clinical practice.

A. Ophthalmic emergencies

1. Acute angle-closure glaucoma

Acute angle-closure glaucoma is an ocular emergency and receives distinction due to its acute presentation, need for immediate treatment and well-established anatomic pathology. Rapid diagnosis, immediate intervention and referral can have profound effects on patient outcome and morbidity.

History: (for example), red eye of an acute, painful, dull nature, with photophobia and reduced vision in a hypermetropic person is highly indicative of acute angle-closure glaucoma.

The pupil in this condition is usually mid-dilated oval shaped.

Any sharp ocular pain is more suggestive of corneal/ocular surface pathologies, and hence herpetic keratitis is the most likely diagnosis.

The patient should be brought to the hospital in an expeditious manner to have intraocular pressure (IOP) reduced. The treatment of acute angle-closure glaucoma (AACG) consists of IOP reduction, suppression of inflammation, and the reversal of angle closure. Once diagnosed, the initial intervention includes acetazolamide, a topical beta-blocker, and a topical steroid.

2. Posterior communicating artery aneurysm (PCOM)

History: (for example), a history of anisocoria, with headaches and diplopia should ring alarm bells, in that a life-threatening posterior communicating artery aneurysm/berry aneurysm needs to be excluded urgently.

A **posterior communicating artery (PCOM) aneurysm** may have no symptoms at all. Preceding rupture of an aneurysm, patients may report severe headache, stiff neck, nausea, vomiting and vision impairment. In some cases, the patient may lose consciousness. Aneurysm rupture results in bleeding into the brain or the lining of the brain with sudden onset of symptoms.

Oculomotor nerve palsy is a notable sign specific to PCOM aneurysm. The oculomotor nerve provides the nerve supply to the muscles that lift the eyelid and move the eye up, down and inward. Additionally, the nerves that constrict the pupil in bright light travel with the oculomotor nerve.

If a patient has an oculomotor palsy, he will have a droopy upper eyelid, double vision, a deviated eye that moves improperly and, possibly, a large unresponsive pupil. Patients experiencing these symptoms should undergo immediate brain imaging to search for a PCOM aneurysm.

3. Eye movements

Ocular motility abnormalities include:

Nuclear and fascicular nerve palsies: VIth nerve palsies are the most common, followed by IIIrd nerve palsies, which may be partial. IVth nerve palsies are rare.

Internuclear ophthalmoplegia: Internuclear tracts connect the ocular motor nuclei within the brainstem and coordinate eye movements. When affected by multiple sclerosis, there is limitation or slowing of adduction associated with abducting nystagmus in the fellow eye. A wall-eyed bilateral internuclear ophthalmoplegia (WEBINO) is also possible. This is a failure to adduct both eyes, but preservation of up and down gaze suggests a demyelinating process, and failure of ocular adduction in such cases should prompt the diagnosis of internuclear ophthalmoplegia.

Supranuclear vertical gaze palsies, e.g. Parinaud's syndrome. Parinaud's syndrome is a cluster of abnormalities of eye movement and pupil dysfunction, characterised by: paralysis of up gaze, the pseudo-Argyll Robertson pupil, accommodation paresis, mid-dilated pupils, nystagmus, eyelid retraction (Collier's sign), and conjugate down gaze in the primary position: *'setting-sun sign'.*

Nystagmus

This may result from cerebellar involvement, or demyelination within the gaze-holding brainstem centres.

B. The lens

1. Subluxation of the lens

Ectopia lentis/subluxation of the lens is associated with:

+ Ehlers-Danlos syndrome
+ Marfan's syndrome
+ Weill-Marchesani syndrome (short stature, skeletal abnormalities and ectopia lentis)
+ Refsum's disease
+ homocystinuria

2. Cataracts

Cataracts are an important general medical topic. The lens is made mostly of water and protein. Specific proteins within the lens are responsible for maintaining its clarity. Over many years, the structures of these lens proteins are altered, ultimately leading to a gradual clouding of the lens. Rarely, cataracts can present at birth or in early childhood as a result of hereditary enzyme defects, and severe trauma to the eye, eye surgery or intraocular inflammation can also cause cataracts to occur earlier in life. Other factors that may lead to development of cataracts at an earlier age include excessive ultraviolet-light exposure, diabetes, smoking or the use of certain medications, such as oral, topical or inhaled steroids. Other medications that are more weakly associated with cataracts include the long-term use of statins and phenothiazines.

3. Osmotic changes in a newly diagnosed diabetic eye

History: (for example), six-week history of blurring of vision, who on presentation reveals a high fasting plasma glucose. Such a patient could be a newly diagnosed diabetic as we are told they were previously fit and well.

Therefore the most probable explanation for blurred vision is osmotic change.

C. Retinal disorders

1. Retinitis pigmentosa

Retinitis pigmentosa (RP) has a prevalence of about one in 4000; an estimated 2 million people are affected worldwide. The condition is most often inherited by an autosomal dominant, autosomal recessive or X-linked mode of transmission.

Mutations in over 45 causative genes account for 50%–60% of cases; the most common genes involved are the rhodopsin gene, the Usher IIA gene and the RPGR gene. These genes may be subclassified based on the known or presumed function of encoded proteins.

2. Angioid retinal streaks

Angioid retinal streaks are seen on fundoscopy as irregular dark red streaks radiating from the optic nerve head. The elastic layer of Bruch's membrane is characteristically thickened and calcified.

Causes

+ pseudoxanthoma elasticum (this makes a nice PACES case!)
+ Ehler-Danlos syndrome
+ Paget's disease
+ sickle cell anaemia
+ acromegaly

Pseudoxanthoma elasticum with angioid streaks is also known as Grönblad-Strandberg syndrome.

3. Kearns-Sayre syndrome

History: of night blindness and gradual deterioration of the patient's peripheral visual fields bilaterally.

Kearns-Sayre syndrome is a mitochondrial inherited disease, and as such is only passed on by mothers to offspring. Red ragged fibres found in mitochondrial cytopathy are found in Kearns-Sayre syndrome; mitochondrial myopathy, lactic acidosis and stroke-like episodes (MELAS); and Leber's optic atrophy.

It is a slowly progressive neuromuscular disorder associated with progressive external ophthalmoplegia and heart conduction defect.

Ocular manifestations include ptosis and peripheral retinal bony spiculed appearances. Ocular examination can reveal bony spiculed lesions in the peripheral retina of both eyes with attenuated retinal blood vessels.

4. CMV retinitis

History: for example, an acute onset of reduced vision in the left eye.

Cytomegalovirus (CMV) retinitis is very often secondary to human immunodeficiency virus (HIV).

Fundoscopy of the affected eye reveals an extensive 'brushfire-like' lesion in the major superior temporal arcade with a large patch of white fluffy lesion mixed with extensive retinal haemorrhages.

Affected patients usually report night deficiency and difficulty with adaptation in adolescence, loss of mid-peripheral and then far peripheral visual field in young adulthood, development of tunnel vision in middle life and eventual loss of central vision after age 60.

Clinical findings

These typically include elevated final dark adaptation thresholds, attenuated retinal vessels, intraretinal bone spicule pigmentation around the midperiphery in most cases and reduced and delayed full-field electroretinograms (ERGs).

The ERGs show more loss of rod function than cone function or comparable loss of rod and cone function. The majority develop central posterior subcapsular cataracts and some have cystoid macular oedema.

Many develop waxy pallor of the optic discs in the advanced stage. About 20% of cases have associated hearing loss designated as Usher syndrome. Histologic studies of autopsy eyes have shown that loss of vision is due to degeneration of rod and cone photoreceptors across the retina.

Treatment options

While monitoring the natural course of RP, a risk factor analysis revealed that patients self-treating with a separate capsule of vitamin A showed less progression by ERG testing than those taking only a multivitamin or no vitamin supplements.

During the vitamin A and E trial, a subset of patients with higher red blood cell (RBC) docosahexaenoic acid (DHA) levels were found to have a significantly slower rate of progression of retinitis pigmentosa than a subset with lower RBC DHA levels. This prompted a second randomised controlled trial which showed, in fact, that DHA supplementation 1200 mg/day did **not**, on average, slow the course of this condition over 4 years.

5. Optic atrophy

Optic atrophy is seen as pale, well-demarcated disc on fundoscopy. It is usually bilateral and causes a gradual loss of vision. Causes may be acquired or congenital.

Acquired causes

◆ multiple sclerosis

◆ papilloedema (longstanding)

◆ raised intraocular pressure (e.g. glaucoma, tumour)

◆ retinal damage (e.g. choroiditis, retinitis pigmentosa)

◆ ischaemia

◆ toxins: tobacco amblyopia, quinine, methanol, arsenic, lead

◆ nutritional: vitamin B_1, B_2, B_6 and B_{12} deficiency

Congenital causes

◆ Friedreich's ataxia

◆ mitochondrial disorders, e.g. Leber's optic atrophy

DIDMOAD – the association of cranial Diabetes Insipidus, Diabetes Mellitus, Optic Atrophy and Deafness (also known as Wolfram's syndrome).

6. Macular degeneration

Macular degeneration is the most common cause of blindness in the UK. Degeneration of the central retina (macula) is the key feature with changes usually bilateral. Two forms of macular degeneration are seen:

◆ Dry macular degeneration: characterised by drusen – yellow round spots in Bruch's membrane.

◆ Wet (exudative, neovascular) macular degeneration: characterised by choroidal neovascularisation. Leakage of serous fluid and blood can subsequently result in a rapid loss of vision. Carries worst prognosis.

Risk factors

◆ age: most patients are over 60 years of age

◆ family history

◆ smoking

◆ more common in Caucasians

◆ female sex

Features

◈ reduced visual acuity: 'blurred', 'distorted' vision, central vision is affected first

◈ central scotomas

◈ fundoscopy: drusen, pigmentary changes

General management

◈ stopping smoking

◈ high does of beta-carotene, vitamins C and E, and zinc may help to slow down visual loss for patients with established macular degeneration; should be avoided in smokers due to an increased risk of lung cancer

Dry macular degeneration

◈ no medical treatments currently

Wet macular degeneration

◈ photocoagulation

◈ photodynamic therapy

◈ anti-vascular endothelial growth factor (anti-VEGF) treatments: intravitreal ranibizumab

D. General medical disorders

1. Temporal arteritis

Temporal arteritis is large vessel vasculitis which overlaps with polymyalgia rheumatica (PMR). Histology shows changes which characteristically *'skip'* certain sections of affected artery whilst damaging others.

Features

◈ typically patient >60 years old

◈ usually rapid onset (e.g. <1 month)

◈ headache (found in 85%)

◈ jaw claudication (65%)

◈ possibly visual disturbance

◈ tender, palpable temporal artery

♦ features of polymyalgia rheumatica (PMR): aching, morning stiffness in proximal limb muscles (not weakness)

♦ also lethargy, depression, low-grade fever, anorexia, night sweats

Investigations

♦ ESR >50 mm/hr (note ESR <30 in 10% of patients)

♦ temporal artery biopsy: skip lesions may be present

♦ note CK and EMG normal

♦ reduced CD8 + T cells

♦ normochronic/normocytic anaemia

♦ raised alkaline phosphatase (ALP) and raised C-reactive protein (CRP)

Treatment

High-dose prednisolone should produce a dramatic response. If not, the diagnosis should be reconsidered.

2. Homocystinuria

Homocystinuria is a rare autosomal recessive disease caused by deficiency of cystathione beta-synthetase. This results in an accumulation of homocysteine which is then oxidised to homocystine.

Features

♦ often patients have fine, fair hair

♦ musculoskeletal: may be similar to Marfan's syndrome – arachnodactyly, etc.

♦ neurological patients may have learning difficulties, seizures

♦ ocular: downwards dislocation of lens

♦ increased risk of arterial and venous thromboembolism

♦ also malar flush, *livedo reticularis*

Diagnosis is made by the cyanide-nitroprusside test, which is also positive in cystinuria.

Treatment is vitamin B_6 supplements.

3. Marfan's syndrome

Marfan's syndrome is an autosomal dominant connective tissue disorder. It is caused by a defect in the fibrillin-1 gene on chromosome 15.

Features

◆ tall stature with arm span > height ratio >1.05

◆ high-arched palate

◆ arachnodactyly

◆ *pectus excavatum*

◆ *pes planus*

◆ scoliosis of >20 degrees

◆ heart: dilation of the aortic sinuses (seen in 90%) which may lead to aortic regurgitation, mitral valve prolapse (75%), aortic dissection

◆ lungs: repeated pneumothoraces

◆ eyes: upwards lens dislocation (superotemporal ectopia lentis), blue sclera (the upward dislocation is in contrast to the downward dislocation in homocystinuria)

4. Rheumatoid arthritis: ocular manifestations

Ocular manifestations of **rheumatoid arthritis** are common, with 25% of patients having eye problems.

Ocular manifestations

◆ keratoconjunctivitis sicca (*most common*)

◆ episcleritis (erythema)

◆ scleritis (erythema and pain)

◆ corneal ulceration

◆ keratitis

Iatrogenic

◆ steroid-induced cataracts

◆ chloroquine retinopathy

E. The pupil

1. Pathway of pupillary light reflex

◆ afferent: retina > optic nerve > lateral geniculate body > midbrain

◆ efferent: Edinger-Westphal nucleus (midbrain) > oculomotor nerve

2. Causes of a small pupil

These include:

◆ Horner's syndrome

◆ old age

◆ pontine haemorrhage

◆ Argyll Robertson pupil

◆ drugs and poisons (e.g. opiates, organophosphates)

3. Causes of a large pupil

These include:

◆ Holmes-Adie (myotonic) pupil

◆ third nerve palsy

◆ drugs and poisons (atropine, cobalt, ethylene glycol)

Drug causes of mydriasis

◆ topical mydriatics: tropicamide, atropine

◆ sympathomimetic drugs: amphetamines

◆ anticholinergic drugs: tricyclic antidepressants

4. Adie's tonic pupil

An **Adie's tonic pupil** is charateristically seen in young women, and may occur after an episode of zoster infection.

At the beginning of the condition the pupil is large, but over time becomes small and poorly reactive. Slit-lamp examination may reveal small worm-like contractions of the iris, but the usual diagnostic test is to use weak pilocarpine eye drops, which induce vigorous pupil contraction on the affected side, but only weak contraction of the pupil on the unaffected side.

In adults, this tends to be a benign condition and is simply observed, however infants are usually referred because of an association with familial dystonias.

5. Relative afferent pupillary defect

The **relative afferent pupillary defect** is also known as the *Marcus Gunn pupil*. A relative afferent pupillary defect is found by the 'swinging light test'. It is caused by a lesion anterior to the optic chiasm, i.e. optic nerve or retina.

Causes

◆ retina: detachment

◆ optic nerve: optic neuritis, e.g. multiple sclerosis

6. Herpetic keratitis

Patients with **herpetic keratitis** may complain of the following with a history of a day or two:

◆ pain

◆ photophobia

◆ blurred vision

◆ tearing

◆ redness

A history of prior episodes in patients with recurrent disease may exist. Since most cases of HSV epithelial keratitis resolve spontaneously within 3 weeks, the rationale for treatment is to minimise stromal damage and scarring. Gentle epithelial debridement may be performed to remove infectious virus and viral antigens that may induce stromal keratitis.

Reference

Wood-Gush HG. Retinitis pigmentosa research: a review. *J R Soc Med.* 1989; **82**(6): 355–8.

Chapter 9

Clinical pharmacology (and toxicology and therapeutics)

The Foundation Programme and MRCP(UK) Part 1 syllabus (from the JRCPMTB) specify what is required in terms of competencies, skills and knowledge from junior physicians in core medical training in clinical pharmacology. You are advised to consult carefully this syllabus, which emphasises the importance of basic medical sciences as well as a competent level of applied clinical practice.

A. An outline of medications requiring therapeutic monitoring

Emphasis will be given to the areas of clinical practice and therapeutics where the narrow therapeutic range of particular pharmacokinetic properties of the drug make this approach important.

1. Lithium

◆ range = 0.4–1.0 mmol/L

◆ take 12 hours post-dose

Lithium is a mood-stabilising drug used most commonly prophylactically in bipolar disorder but also as an adjunct in refractory depression. It has a very narrow therapeutic range (0.4–1.0 mmol/L) and a long plasma half-life, being excreted primarily by the kidneys.

Mechanism of action – not fully understood, two theories:

◆ interferes with inositol triphosphate formation

◆ interferes with cAMP formation

Adverse effects

- nausea/vomiting, diarrhoea
- fine tremor
- polyuria
- thyroid enlargement, may lead to hypothyroidism
- ECG: T wave flattening/inversion
- weight gain

Toxicity

Lithium toxicity generally occurs following concentrations >1.5 mmol/L.

Toxicity may be precipitated by dehydration, renal failure, diuretics (especially bendroflumethiazide) or ACE inhibitors.

Features

- coarse tremor (a fine tremor is seen in therapeutic levels)
- acute confusion
- seizure
- coma

Management

- Mild–moderate toxicity may respond to volume resuscitation with normal saline.
- Haemodialysis may be needed in severe toxicity.
- Sodium bicarbonate is sometimes used but there is limited evidence to support this. By increasing the alkalinity of the urine it promotes lithium excretion.

2. Cyclosporin

- trough levels immediately before dose

3. Digoxin

- at least 6 hours post-dose

4. Phenytoin

◆ trough levels immediately before dose

Side effects

Phenytoin is associated with a large number of adverse effects. These may be divided into acute, chronic, idiosyncratic and teratogenic.

Acute

◆ initially: vertigo, diplopia, nystagmus, slurred speech, ataxia
◆ later: confusion, seizures

Chronic

◆ *common*: gingival hyperplasia, hirsutism, coarsening of facial features
◆ megaloblastic anaemia (secondary to altered folate metabolism)
◆ peripheral neuropathy
◆ enhanced vitamin D metabolism causing osteomalacia
◆ lymphadenopathy
◆ dyskinesia

Idiosyncratic

◆ fever
◆ rashes, including severe reactions such as toxic epidermal necrolysis
◆ hepatitis
◆ Dupuytren's contracture
◆ aplastic anaemia
◆ drug-induced lupus

Teratogenic

◆ associated with cleft palate and congenital heart disease

B. Adverse drug reactions

You should have an understanding of the epidemiology of adverse drug reactions and know how to recognise and avoid them.

You must also be aware of important adverse effects of commonly used drugs and have an understanding of the importance of adverse drug reaction reporting schemes.

1. Drugs causing visual disturbance

Cataracts

+ steroids

Corneal opacities

+ amiodarone
+ indomethacin

Optic neuritis

+ ethambutol
+ amiodarone
+ metronidazole

Retinopathy

+ chloroquine, quinine

Sildenafil can cause both blue discolouration and non-arteritic anterior ischaemic neuropathy.

2. Drugs causing photosensitivity

+ thiazides
+ tetracyclines, sulphonamides, ciprofloxacin
+ amiodarone
+ NSAIDs, e.g. piroxicam
+ psoralens
+ sulphonylureas

3. Gingival hyperplasia

Drug causes of gingival hyperplasia:

+ phenytoin

+ cyclosporin

+ calcium channel blockers (especially nifedipine)

Other causes of gingival hyperplasia include:

+ acute myeloid leukaemia (myelomonocytic and monocytic types)

4. Side effects of sildenafil

Sildenafil (Viagra®) is a phosphodiesterase type V inhibitor used in the treatment of impotence.

Contraindications

+ patients taking nitrates and related drugs ('nitrate derivatives') such as nicorandil

+ hypotension

+ recent stroke or myocardial infarction

+ non-arteritic anterior ischaemic optic neuropathy

Adverse effects

+ visual disturbances, e.g. blue discolouration, non-arteritic anterior ischaemic neuropathy

+ nasal congestion

+ influenza-like symptoms

+ dry mouth

+ flushing

+ gastrointestinal side effects

5. Side effects of sulphonylureas

Sulphonylureas are oral hypoglycaemic drugs used in the management of type 2 diabetes mellitus.

They work by increasing pancreatic insulin secretion and hence are only effective if functional B cells are present.

Common adverse effects

◆ hypoglycaemic episodes (more common with long-acting preparations such as chlorpropamide)

◆ increased appetite and weight gain

Rarer adverse effects

◆ syndrome of inappropriate ADH secretion

◆ bone marrow suppression

◆ liver damage (cholestatic jaundice and hepatitis)

◆ photosensitivity

◆ (peripheral neuropathy)

Sulphonylureas should be avoided in breastfeeding and pregnancy.

6. Sodium valproate

Sodium valproate is used in the management of epilepsy and is first-line therapy for generalised seizures. It works by increasing GABA activity.

Adverse effects

◆ gastrointestinal: nausea, diarrhoea

◆ increased appetite and weight gain

◆ alopecia: regrowth may be curly

◆ ataxia

◆ tremor

◆ hepatitis

◆ thrombocytopaenia

◆ pancreatitis

◆ teratogenic

7. Combined oral contraceptive pill: contraindications

The decision of whether to start a woman on the combined oral contraceptive pill is now guided by the UK Medical Eligibility Criteria (UKMEC). This categorises the potential cautions and contraindications according to a four-point scale, as detailed below:

- UKMEC 1: unrestricted use
- UKMEC 2: advantages generally outweigh the disadvantages
- UKMEC 3: disadvantages generally outweigh the advantages
- UKMEC 4: represents an unacceptable health risk

Examples of UKMEC 3 conditions include:

- more than 35 years old and smoking less than 15 cigarettes/day
- BMI 35–9 kg/m^2
- migraine without aura and more than 35 years old
- family history of thromboembolic disease in first-degree relatives <45 years
- controlled hypertension
- multiple risk factors for cardiovascular disease
- history of gall bladder disease, cholestasis or cirrhosis
- breast cancer in remission for 5 years
- immobility, e.g. wheelchair use
- breastfeeding 6 weeks – 6 months post-partum

Examples of UKMEC 4 conditions include:

- more than 35 years old and smoking more than 15 cigarettes/day
- BMI >40 kg/m^2
- migraine with aura
- history of thromboembolic disease or thombogenic mutation
- history of stroke or ischaemic heart disease
- uncontrolled hypertension
- breast cancer
- active hepatitis, decompensated liver disease or liver tumours
- major surgery with prolonged immobilisation

Diabetes mellitus with complications or diagnosed >20 years ago is classified as UKMEC 3 or 4 depending on severity.

8. Isotretinoin
Adverse effects

- teratogenicity – females *must* be taking contraception
- mood changes
- dry eyes and lips
- raised triglycerides, glucose and/or transaminases
- haematological changes
- hair thinning
- nose bleeds

[*See also* Chapter 2.]

9. Cyclosporin
[*See* Chapters 9 and 11.]

10. Cytotoxic agents
[*See* Chapter 5.]

11. Hormone replacement therapy: adverse effects
Hormone replacement therapy (HRT) involves the use of a small dose of oestrogen (combined with a progestogen in women with a uterus) to help alleviate menopausal symptoms.

Side effects
- nausea
- breast tenderness
- fluid retention and weight gain

Potential complications
- increased risk of breast (and ovarian) cancer: increased by the addition of a progestogen
- increased risk of endometrial cancer: reduced by the addition of a

progestogen but not eliminated completely; the BNF states that the additional risk is eliminated if a progestogen is given continuously

◆ increased risk of venous thromboembolism: increased by the addition of a progestogen

◆ increased risk of coronary heart disease if started more than 10 years after the menopause

Breast cancer

◆ In the **Women's Health Initiative (WHI) study** there was a relative risk of 1.26 at 5 years of developing breast cancer.

◆ The increased risk relates to duration of use.

◆ Breast cancer incidence is higher in women using combined preparations compared to oestrogen-only preparations.

◆ The risk of breast cancer begins to decline when HRT is stopped, and by 5 years it reaches the same level as in women who have never taken HRT.

12. Finasteride

Finasteride is an inhibitor of 5-α-reductase, an enzyme which metabolises testosterone into dihydrotestosterone.

Indications

◆ benign prostatic hyperplasia

◆ male pattern baldness

Adverse effects

◆ impotence

◆ decreased libido

◆ ejaculation disorders

◆ gynaecomastia and breast tenderness

Finasteride causes decreased levels of serum prostate specific antigen.

C. Therapeutics for specific patient groups

You should understand the principles of therapeutics as they apply in special groups.

1. Pregnancy and breastfeeding

The major breastfeeding contraindications tested in exams relate to drugs (see below). Other contraindications of note include:

◆ galactosaemia

◆ viral infections – this is controversial with respect to HIV in the developing world; this is because there is such an increased infant mortality and morbidity associated with bottle-feeding that some doctors think the benefits outweigh the risk of HIV transmission

Drug contraindications (always check the BNF)

The following drugs can be given to mothers who are breastfeeding:

◆ antibiotics: penicillins, cephalosporins, trimethoprim

◆ endocrine: glucocorticoids (avoid high doses), levothyroxine

◆ epilepsy: sodium valproate, carbamazepine

◆ asthma: salbutamol, theophyllines

◆ psychiatric drugs: tricyclic antidepressants, antipsychotics

◆ hypertension: beta-blockers, hydralazine, methyldopa

◆ anticoagulants: warfarin, heparin

◆ digoxin

The following drugs should be avoided:

◆ antibiotics: ciprofloxacin, tetracycline, chloramphenicol, sulphonamides

◆ psychiatric drugs: lithium, benzodiazepines

◆ aspirin

◆ carbimazole

◆ sulphonylureas

◆ cytotoxic drugs

◆ amiodarone

2. Epilepsy: pregnancy and breastfeeding

The risks of uncontrolled epilepsy during pregnancy generally outweigh the risks of medication to the foetus. All women thinking about becoming pregnant should be advised to take folic acid 5 mg per day well before pregnancy to minimise the risk of neural tube defects – always check the BNF.

Other important points

◆ aim for monotherapy
◆ there is no indication to monitor anti-epileptic drug levels
◆ sodium valproate: associated with neural tube defects
◆ phenytoin: associated with cleft palate

Breastfeeding is generally considered safe for mothers taking anti-epileptics, with the possible exception of the barbiturates.

It is advised that pregnant women taking phenytoin are given vitamin K in the last month of pregnancy to prevent clotting disorders in the newborn.

A note on folic acid metabolism

Drugs which inhibit dihydrofolate reductase are:

◆ methotrexate
◆ pyrimethamine
◆ trimethoprim

Drugs which interfere with absorption/storage of folate are:

◆ phenytoin
◆ primidone
◆ oral contraceptives

3. General prescribing in pregnancy

Very few drugs are known to be completely safe in pregnancy. The list below largely comprises those known to be harmful – always check the BNF. Some countries have developed a grading system.

Antibiotics

◆ tetracyclines
◆ aminoglycosides

+ sulphonamides and trimethoprim
+ quinolones: the BNF advises to avoid due to arthropathy in some animal studies

Other drugs

+ ACE inhibitors, $AT_{2,1}$ receptor antagonists
+ statins
+ warfarin
+ sulphonylureas
+ retinoids (including topical)
+ cytotoxic agents

The majority of anti-epileptics including valproate, carbamazepine and phenytoin are known to be potentially harmful. The decision to stop such treatments however is difficult as uncontrolled epilepsy is also a risk.

4. Effects of renal or liver impairment in old age or pregnancy
Patients with renal disease

Nephrotoxic agents can exacerbate renal damage and other drugs, especially those that are water soluble and therefore eliminated largely by the kidneys, may accumulate in patients with a low glomerular filtration rate, leading to toxic effects. Drugs that may accumulate and cause toxicity in patients with severe renal failure include:

+ digoxin: cardiac arrhythmias, heart block
+ erythromycin: encephalopathy
+ lithium: cardiac arrythmias and seizures
+ penicillins and cephalosporins: lead to encephalopathy

Nephrotoxic drugs may lead to an acute deterioration of renal function in patients with chronic renal failure and can severely exacerbate renal failure in acute renal failure. If treatment is considered essential (e.g. gentamicin) then levels should be carefully monitored – always check the BNF. Examples of nephrotoxic drugs include:

+ aminoglycosides
+ amphotericin

✦ NSAIDs

✦ cisplatin

BOX 9.1   A note on the side effects of cisplatin

These commonly include:

- marrow toxicity
- ototoxicity
- peripheral neuropathy
- nephrotoxicity
- alopecia
- changes in taste

Patients with hepatic disease

Chronic liver disease is more predictably associated with impaired metabolism of drugs than acute liver dysfunction. However, in cases of severe acute liver failure, the capacity to metabolise the drug may be significantly impaired.

In the chronic state, cirrhosis of any aetiology, viral hepatitis and hepatoma can decrease drug metabolism. In moderate to severe liver dysfunction, rates of drug metabolism may be reduced by as much as 50%. The mechanism is thought to be due to spatial separation of blood from the hepatocyte by fibrosis along the hepatic sinusoids.

The use of certain drugs in patients with cirrhosis occasionally increases the risk of hepatic decompensation. An example of this is the increased risk of hepatic encephalopathy in some patients who receive pegylated interferon alpha-2α in combination with ribavirin for the treatment of chronic active hepatitis related to the hepatitis C virus. In addition, co-infection with hepatitis B or C virus, even in the absence of cirrhosis, increases the risk of hepatotoxicity from antiretroviral therapy in patients with coexistent HIV infection.

In the presence of chronic liver disease, there is potential for changing the systemic availability of high extraction drugs, thereby affecting plasma concentrations.

A potential consequence of liver disease is the development of portosystemic shunts that may carry a drug absorbed from the gut through the mesenteric veins directly into the systemic circulation. As such, oral treatment with high hepatic clearance drugs such as morphine or propranolol can lead to high plasma concentrations and an increased risk of adverse effects.

Liver damage can also affect drugs with low hepatic clearance. For instance, the effect of warfarin, which has a low extraction ratio, is increased due to the reduced production of vitamin K-dependent clotting factors.

The pharmacokinetic interaction between alcohol and drugs is more complex. An acute ingestion of alcohol may inhibit a drug's metabolism by competing with the drug for the same set of metabolising enzymes. Conversely, hepatic enzyme induction may occur with chronic excessive alcohol ingestion via CYP2E1 resulting in increased clearance of certain drugs (for example, phenytoin, benzodiazepines). After these enzymes have been induced, they remain so in the absence of alcohol for several weeks after cessation of drinking. In addition, some enzymes induced by chronic alcohol consumption transform some drugs (for example, paracetamol) into toxic compounds that can damage the liver.

In the presence of cholestatic jaundice, drugs and their active metabolites that are dependent on biliary excretion for clearance will have impaired elimination. Further impairment will occur if the compound is excreted as a glucuronide and is subject to enterohepatic circulation.

> **The bottom line: always check the BNF.**

D. Clinical toxicology

You should understand the principles of management of patients who have been poisoned with drugs or other toxic substances. This should include assessment, recognition of common symptom patterns, principles of removal of toxic substances (e.g. activated charcoal if substances ingested within the previous 2 hours) and their antidotes where these approaches may be appropriate.

1. Paracetamol overdose

Metabolic pathways

The liver normally conjugates paracetamol with glucuronic acid/sulphate. During an overdose the conjugation system becomes saturated, leading to oxidation by P450 mixed function oxidases. This explains why there is a lower threshold for treating patients who take P450-inducing medications, e.g. phenytoin or rifampicin. This produces a toxic metabolite (*N*-acetyl-*p*-benzoquinone imine).

Normally glutathione acts as a defence mechanism by conjugating with the toxin forming the non-toxic mercapturic acid. If glutathione stores run out, the toxin forms covalent bonds with cell proteins, denaturing them and leading to cell death. This occurs not only in hepatocytes but also in the renal tubules.

N-acetylcysteine is used in the management of paracetamol overdose as it is a precursor of glutathione and hence can increase hepatic glutathione production.

Management

KING'S COLLEGE HOSPITAL CRITERIA FOR LIVER TRANSPLANTATION (PARACETAMOL LIVER FAILURE)

Arterial pH <7.3, 24 hours after ingestion or all of the following:

- prothrombin time >100 seconds
- creatinine >300 µmol/L
- grade III or IV encephalopathy

---

2. Salicylate overdose

A key concept for the exam is to understand that salicylate overdose leads to a mixed respiratory alkalosis and metabolic acidosis. Early stimulation of the respiratory centre leads to a respiratory alkalosis, whilst later the direct acid effects of salicylates (combined with acute renal failure) may lead to an acidosis. In children metabolic acidosis tends to predominate.

Features

- hyperventilation (centrally stimulates respiration)
- tinnitus
- lethargy
- sweating, pyrexia
- nausea/vomiting
- hyperglycaemia and hypoglycaemia
- seizures (evidence of neurotoxicity)
- coma

Treatment

- general (ABC, charcoal)
- urinary alkalinisation is now rarely used – it is contraindicated in cerebral

and pulmonary oedema, with most units now proceeding straight to haemodialysis in cases of severe poisoning

◆ haemodialysis

Indications for haemodialysis in salicylate overdose

◆ serum concentration >700 mg/L

◆ metabolic acidosis resistant to treatment

◆ acute renal failure

◆ pulmonary oedema

◆ seizures

◆ coma

3. Ethylene glycol overdose

Ethylene glycol is a type of alcohol used as a coolant or antifreeze.

  Features of toxicity are divided into three stages:

◆ stage 1: symptoms similar to alcohol intoxication: confusion, slurred speech, dizziness

◆ stage 2: metabolic acidosis with high anion gap and high osmolar gap; also tachycardia, hypertension

◆ stage 3: acute renal failure

Management has evolved:

◆ ethanol had been used for many years

◆ works by competing with ethylene glycol for an isoform of the enzyme alcohol dehydrogenase

◆ this limits the formation of toxic metabolites (e.g. glycoaldehyde and glycolic acid) which are responsible for the haemodynamic/metabolic features of poisoning

◆ fomepizole, an inhibitor of alcohol dehydrogenase, is now used first-line in preference to ethanol

◆ haemodialysis also has a role in refractory cases

4. Tricyclic antidepressant overdose

Overdose of tricyclic antidepressants is a common presentation to A&E departments.

Early features relate to anticholinergic properties: dry mouth, dilated pupils, agitation, sinus tachycardia, blurred vision.

Features of severe poisoning include:

+ arrhythmias
+ seizures
+ metabolic acidosis
+ coma

ECG changes

+ sinus tachycardia
+ widening of QRS
+ prolongation of QT interval

Widening of QRS >100 ms is associated with an increased risk of seizures whilst QRS >160 ms is associated with ventricular arrhythmias.

Management

+ IV bicarbonate may reduce the risk of seizures and arrhythmias in severe toxicity.
+ Arrhythmias: class 1a (e.g. quinidine) and class Ic antiarrhythmics (e.g. flecainide) are contraindicated as they prolong depolarisation. Class III drugs such as amiodarone should also be avoided as they prolong the QT interval. Response to lignocaine is variable and it should be emphasised that correction of acidosis is the first line in management of tricyclic induced arrhythmias.
+ Dialysis is ineffective in removing tricyclic antidepressants.

5. Lithium poisoning

Lithium is a mood-stabilising drug, used most commonly prophylactically in bipolar affective disorder, but also as an adjunct in refractory depression. It has a very narrow therapeutic range (0.4–1.0 mmol/L), and a long plasma half-life, being excreted primarily by the kidneys.

Mechanism of action

Not fully understood, two theories:

◆ interferes with inositol triphosphate formation

◆ interferes with cAMP formation

Adverse effects

◆ nausea/vomiting, diarrhoea

◆ fine tremor, muscle twitching, seizures

◆ polyuria

◆ thyroid enlargement, may lead to hypothyroidism

◆ ECG: T wave flattening/inversion

◆ weight gain

◆ slurred speech

◆ movement disorders

◆ kidney failure

◆ psychosis

Lithium toxicity generally occurs following concentrations >1.5 mmol/L. Toxicity may be precipitated by dehydration, renal failure, diuretics (especially bendroflumethiazide) or ACE inhibitors.

Common features of toxicity

◆ coarse tremor (a fine tremor can be seen at therapeutic levels)

◆ acute confusion

◆ seizure

◆ coma

Management

◆ mild–moderate toxicity may respond to volume resuscitation with normal saline

◆ haemodialysis may be needed in severe toxicity

◆ sodium bicarbonate is sometimes used but there is limited evidence to support this; increasing the alkalinity of the urine promotes lithium excretion

6. Iron poisoning

Iron overload may develop chronically as well, especially in patients requiring multiple transfusions of red blood cells. This condition develops in patients with sickle cell disease, thalassaemia and myelodysplastic syndromes.

Possible symptoms

◆ iron ingestions with GI symptoms such as vomiting and diarrhoea

◆ haemorrhagic gastroenteritis, even in the absence of ingestion

◆ hyperglycaemia with metabolic acidosis during or following episodes of abdominal pain and gastroenteritis

◆ hypotension and shock

◆ drowsiness, convulsions, coma

Principles of acute medicine care

◆ Assume that symptomatic patients are hypovolemic. Administer vigorous isotonic crystalloid therapy (e.g. 0.9 isotonic NaCl solution) in 20 ml/kg boluses to attain and maintain haemodynamic stability.

◆ Gastric lavage with a large-bore orogastric tube or administration of *ipecac* syrup may remove iron from the stomach. However, ipecac is not used routinely for iron removal because it can mask clinical signs of iron toxicity (vomiting). Due to local caustic effect of iron, poisoned patients routinely are vomiting on their own, performing self-decontamination even without ipecac.

◆ Ideally, these treatments should be performed 1–2 hours post-ingestion or even later if evidence of iron products in the stomach are observed on a radiograph. Each modality has its disadvantages.

◆ Iron has a gelatinous texture and may be difficult to remove by lavage.

◆ Perform whole-bowel irrigation in patients with a radiopacity on KUB until the radiopacity clears.

◆ Activated charcoal does not bind iron but should be utilised if co-ingestants are suspected.

◆ Oxygen should be supplemented.

7. Digoxin poisoning

Digoxin is a cardiac glycoside, now used mainly in the management of atrial fibrillation.

Mechanism of action

◆ decreases conduction through the atrioventricular node which slows the ventricular rate in atrial fibrillation and flutter

◆ increases the force of cardiac muscle contraction due to inhibition of the Na^+/K^+ ATPase pump

Features

◆ generally unwell, lethargy, nausea and vomiting, confusion, yellow-green vision

◆ arrhythmias (e.g. AV block, bradycardia)

Precipitating factors

◆ classically: hypokalaemia

◆ myocardial ischaemia

◆ hypomagnesaemia, hypercalcaemia, hypernatraemia, acidosis

◆ hypoalbuminaemia

◆ hypothermia

◆ hypothyroidism

◆ drugs: amiodarone, quinidine, verapamil, spironolactone (compete for secretion in distal convoluted tubule, therefore reduce excretion)

Management

◆ correct electrolyte disturbances

◆ bicarbonate for acidosis

◆ atropine for bradyarrhythmias

◆ digibind

◆ haemodialysis for acidosis with hyperkalaemia

8. Lead poisoning

Lead can be absorbed through the skin and by inhalation. It is associated with iron deficiency and a microcytic anaemia.

The most common gastrointestinal symptoms are abdominal colic and constipation.

Lead poisoning also causes a peripheral neuropathy due to demyelination.

9. Differences between overdose treatments

Haemodialysis involves blood from the patient being pumped through an array of semi-permeable membranes in contact with dialysylate, which flows countercurrent to the blood. It is considered in severe poisoning from:

◆ lithium

◆ salicylates

◆ phenobarbital

◆ methanol

◆ ethylene glycol

Haemofiltration involves heparinised blood passing through devices containing absorbant particles, such as activated charcoal, to which the drugs are adsorbed. It is recommended for the treatment of severe poisoning for:

◆ medium- and short-acting barbiturates

◆ chloral hydrate

◆ theophylline

10. Intoxication due to drugs of abuse

Cocaine

Cocaine use may cause a wide variety of adverse effects.

Cardiovascular effects

- myocardial infarction
- both tachycardia and bradycardia may occur
- hypertension
- QRS widening and QT prolongation
- aortic dissection

Neurological effects

- seizures
- hypertonia
- hyperreflexia

Psychiatric effects

- agitation
- psychosis
- hallucinations

Others

- hyperthermia
- metabolic acidosis
- rhabdomyolysis
- retroperitoneal fibrosis
- pulmonary hypertension
- flash pulmonary oedema

Emergency treatment

- benzodiazepines
- physical cooling and paracetamol (for hyperpyrexia)

Ecstasy poisoning

Ecstasy (MDMA, 3,4-Methylenedioxymethamphetamine) use became popular in the 1990s during the emergence of dance music culture.

Clinical features

- neurological: agitation, anxiety, confusion, ataxia
- cardiovascular: tachycardia, hypertension
- water intoxication
- hyperthermia
- rhabdomyolysis

Management

- supportive
- dantrolene may be used for hyperthermia if simple measures fail

11. Carbon monoxide poisoning

Carbon monoxide has high affinity for haemoglobin and myoglobin resulting in a left shift of the oxygen dissociation curve and tissue hypoxia. There are approximately 50 deaths per year from accidental carbon monoxide poisoning in the UK.

Questions may hint at badly maintained housing, e.g. student houses, caravans, elderly flats.

Features of carbon monoxide toxicity

- headache: 90% of cases
- nausea and vomiting: 50%
- vertigo: 50%
- confusion: 30%
- subjective weakness: 20%
- (in cases of severe toxicity): 'pink' skin and mucosae, hyperpyrexia, arrhythmias, extrapyramidal features, coma, death

Typical carboxyhaemoglobin levels

- <3% non-smokers
- <10% smokers
- 10%–30% symptomatic: headache, vomiting
- >30% severe toxicity

Management

♦ 100% oxygen

♦ hyperbaric oxygen

Indications for hyperbaric oxygen as stated in the 2008 Department of Health publication *Recognising Carbon Monoxide Poisoning*:

♦ loss of consciousness at any point

♦ neurological signs other than headache

♦ myocardial ischaemia or arrhythmia

♦ pregnancy

12. Organophosphate insecticide poisoning

One of the effects of organophosphate poisoning is **inhibition of acetylcholinesterase.**

Features can be predicted by the accumulation of acetylcholine (mnemonic = SLUDGE):

♦ **S**alivation

♦ **L**acrimation

♦ **U**rination

♦ **D**efaecation

♦ **G**astric motility

♦ **E**mesis

♦ also cardiovascular: hypotension, bradycardia

♦ also neurological: small pupils, muscle fasciculation

Management

♦ atropine

♦ the role of pralidoxime is still unclear – meta-analyses to date have failed to show any clear benefit

13. Beta-blocker overdose

Features

+ bradycardia
+ hypotension
+ heart failure
+ syncope
+ weakness
+ drowsiness
+ confusion
+ convulsions

Management

+ if bradycardic then atropine
+ ionotropes may be required to maintain blood pressure
+ in resistant cases glucagon may be used

Haemodialysis is not effective in beta-blocker overdose.

Mechanism

+ Chronic alcohol consumption enhances GABA-mediated inhibition in the CNS (similar to benzodiazepines) and inhibits NMDA-type glutamate receptors.
+ Alcohol withdrawal is thought to lead to a different neuropharmacological scenario (decreased inhibitory GABA and increased NMDA glutamate transmission).

Features

+ symptoms start at 6–12 hours
+ peak incidence of seizures at 36 hours
+ peak incidence of delirium tremens at 72 hours

Management

+ benzodiazepines (chlordiazepoxide)
+ vitamin B supplementation for treatment or prophylaxis against Wernicke's encephalopathy (intravenously for 3 days followed by oral)

◆ carbamazepine also effective in treatment of alcohol withdrawal

◆ phenytoin is said not to be as effective in the treatment of alcohol withdrawal seizures

E. Drug interactions

Outline of importance of drug interactions and role of CYP450 isoenzymes.

1. Drug metabolism usually involves two types of biochemical reactions: phase I and phase II reactions

◆ **phase I reactions:** oxidation, reduction, hydrolysis. Mainly performed by the P450 enzymes but some drugs are metabolised by specific enzymes, for example alcohol dehydrogenase and xanthine oxidase. Products of phase I reactions are typically more active and potentially toxic.

◆ **phase II reactions:** conjugation. Products are typically inactive and excreted in urine or bile. Glucuronyl, acetyl, methyl, sulphate and other groups are typically involved.

The majority of phase I and phase II reactions take place in the liver.

First-pass metabolism

This is a phenomenon where the concentration of a drug is greatly reduced before it reaches the systemic circulation due to hepatic metabolism. As a consequence much larger doses are needed orally than if given by other routes. This effect is seen in many drugs, including:

◆ aspirin

◆ isosorbide dinitrate

◆ glyceryl trinitrate

◆ lignocaine

◆ propranolol

◆ verapamil

Carbamazepine

It is well recognised that carbamazepine is a P450 enzyme inducer but it is less well appreciated that it causes auto-induction, and so would require increase in dose to maintain the same therapeutic concentration.

Zero-order kinetics

Zero-order kinetics describes metabolism which is independent of the concentration of the reactant. This is due to metabolic pathways becoming saturated, resulting in a constant amount of drug being eliminated per unit time. This explains why people may fail a breathalyser test in the morning if they have been drinking the night before.

Drugs exhibiting zero-order kinetics (mnemonic: SHEP)

+ Salicylates

+ Heparin

+ Ethanol

+ Phenytoin

2. Acetylator status

Fifty per cent of the UK population are deficient in hepatic N-acetyltransferase.
  Drugs affected by acetylator status (mnemonic: **D-HIPS**):

+ Dapsone

+ Hydralazine

+ Isoniazid

+ Procainamide

+ Sulfasalazine

3. Interactions

Induction usually requires prolonged exposure to the inducing drug, as opposed to P450 inhibitors where effects are often seen rapidly.

Inducers of the P450 system include:

+ anti-epileptics: phenytoin, carbamazepine

+ barbiturates: phenobarbitone

+ rifampicin

+ St John's Wort

+ chronic alcohol intake

+ griseofulvin

+ smoking (affects CYP1A2, reason why smokers require more aminophylline)

Inhibitors of the P450 system include:

* antibiotics: ciprofloxacin, erythromycin
* isoniazid
* cimetidine
* omeprazole
* amiodarone
* allopurinol
* imidazoles: ketoconazole, fluconazole
* SSRIs: fluoxetine, sertraline
* ritonavir
* sodium valproate
* acute alcohol intake

A note on griseofulvin

> For an account of griseofulvin and Stevens-Johnson syndrome, read *Am J Emerg Med* 1984; 2: 129–135. Many other drugs are implicated in causing Stevens-Johnson syndrome.

Griseofulvin is active against trichophytons (*tinea*) and other dermatophytes. Treatment with griseofulvin is often needed for a long period, sometimes years, depending on the rate of nail growth. It is metabolised in the liver (note also, it is an enzyme inducer). Only 0.1%–0.2% is excreted in urine.

Chapter 10

Psychiatry

The Foundation Programme and MRCP(UK) Part 1 syllabus (from the JRCPMTB) specify what is required in terms of competencies, skills and knowledge from junior physicians in core medical training in psychiatry. You are advised to consult carefully this syllabus, which emphasises the importance of basic medical sciences as well as a competent level of applied clinical practice.

A. Affective disorders

1. Unipolar depression

Unipolar depression is marked by persistent low mood, loss of interest and enjoyment in usually pleasurable activities (anhedonia), reduced energy, fatigue and fatiguability, and diminished activity. Concentration, attention, self-esteem and self-confidence are often reduced, and the patient may have ideas of guilt and unworthiness, bleak and pessimistic views of the future, ideas or plans or acts of self-harm or suicide, poor sleep and poor appetite. Diurnal variation of mood is common (often worst in the morning), as is early morning waking, psychomotor retardation or agitation, loss of appetite and weight, and loss of libido.

ICD-10 criteria for diagnosis

Diagnostic criteria for depression ICD-10 uses an agreed list of 10 depressive symptoms.

Key symptoms

At least one of these, most days, most of the time for at least two weeks: persistent sadness or low mood; loss of interests or pleasure; fatigue or low energy.

If any of above present, ask about associated symptoms:
1. disturbed sleep
2. poor concentration or indecisiveness

3. low self-confidence
4. poor or increased appetite
5. suicidal thoughts or acts
6. agitation or slowing of movements
7. guilt or self-blame

The 10 symptoms then define the degree of depression, and management is based on the particular degree:

+ **not depressed** (fewer than four symptoms)

+ **mild depression** (four symptoms)

+ **moderate depression** (five to six symptoms)

+ **severe depression** (seven or more symptoms, with or without psychotic symptoms)

Symptoms should be present for a month or more and every symptom should be present for most of every day.

Treatment
Selective serotonin reuptake inhibitors
Selective serotonin reuptake inhibitors (SSRIs) are considered first-line for the majority of patients with depression. Citalopram and fluoxetine are currently the preferred SSRIs. Citalopram is useful for elderly patients as it is associated with lower risks of drug interactions. Sertraline is useful post-myocardial infarction as there is more evidence for its safe use in this situation than other antidepressants.

Patients sometimes fail to respond to SSRIs, and are as such advised to switch to another group of antidepressant; especially, a newer agent like mirtazapine is a feasible approach. For example, mirtazapine is a newer antidepressant that exhibits both noradrenergic and serotonergic activity and was found to be an effective treatment for a substantial proportion of patients for whom a selective serotonin reuptake inhibitor (SSRI) was ineffective and/or poorly tolerated.

Adverse effects of SSRIs

+ gastrointestinal symptoms are the most common side effects

+ patients should be counselled to be vigilant for increased anxiety and agitation

Following the initiation of antidepressant therapy, patients should normally be reviewed by a doctor after 2 weeks.

If patients make a good response to antidepressant therapy, they should continue on treatment for at least 6 months after remission as this reduces the risk of relapse.

When stopping an SSRI, the dose should be gradually reduced over a 4-week period to avoid the well-known *'serotonin discontinuation syndrome'.*

BOX 10.1   A note on treatment with electroconvulsive therapy

Side effects of ECT can occur. For example, ECT may result in seizures, cerebral ischaemia and cardiac arrhythmias.

Over the course of ECT, it may be more difficult for patients to remember newly learned information, though this difficulty disappears over the days and weeks following completion of the ECT course.

Some patients also report a partial loss of memory for events that occurred during the days, weeks and months preceding ECT. While most of these memories typically return over a period of days to months following ECT, some patients report longer-lasting problems with recall of these memories.

Other individuals report improved memory ability following ECT, because of its ability to remove the amnesia sometimes associated with severe depression.

Cardiac arrhythmia may be stimulated by the electrical shock of ECT.

Musculoskeletal injury has been reported after ECT, but with adequate anaesthetisation, this is rare.

---

2. Factors associated with risk of suicide following an episode of deliberate self-harm

+ efforts to avoid discovery
+ planning
+ leaving a written note
+ final acts such as sorting out finances
+ violent method

These are in addition to standard risk factors for suicide:

+ male sex
+ increased age

◆ unemployment or social isolation

◆ divorced or widowed

◆ history of mental illness (depression, schizophrenia)

◆ history of deliberate self-harm

◆ alcohol or drug misuse

3. Risk of a future suicide attempt

About one-third of people who attempt suicide will repeat the attempt within 1 year, and about 10% of those who threaten or attempt suicide eventually do kill themselves.

There are certain characteristics that have been found in those who are more likely to repeat an attempted suicide.

These characteristics include:

◆ age of 45 or more

◆ being male

◆ a previous attempt which resulted in hospital admission

◆ problems with drugs or alcohol

◆ a personality disorder

◆ living alone (especially if separated, divorced or widowed)

◆ previous history of psychiatric treatment

◆ criminal record

◆ unemployment

◆ lower social class

Relational pathology, for example an ongoing difficulty with female's relationship with her boyfriend, is also a recognised factor for repeat suicide attempts.

4. Anxiety
Characteristics of anxiety (after Lewis)
1. an emotional state with the subjectively experienced quality of fear
2. an unpleasant emotion which may be accompanied by a feeling of impending death
3. a feeling directed towards the future, perceiving a threat of some kind
4. there may be no recognisable threat or one which, by reasonable standards, is out of proportion to the emotion it seemingly provokes
5. there may be subjective bodily discomfort and manifest bodily disturbance

Biological markers of anxiety
Cardiac function

Electrodermal response

Peripheral blood flow
+ more vasodilatation
+ decreased renal and splanchnic flow

Neurotransmitter abnormalities
+ increased circulating adrenaline
+ increased circulating noradrenaline
+ increased platelet MAO
+ increased central NA and 5-HT activity

Physiological responses
Paraesthesia is often experienced with hyperventilation associated with anxiety disorders and is often in hands, feet and periorally.

Behaviour therapies
Systematic desensitisation
+ gradual exposure to phobic stimulus along hierarchy of increasing intensity until patient habituates and avoidance response is extinguished

Flooding (implosion)
+ supervised maximum exposure to feared stimulus until anxiety reduction, or exhaustion

✦ effective for phobias where free-floating anxiety is prominent

Modelling

✦ observation of therapist engaging in non-avoidance behaviour with the feared stimulus

✦ a combination of flooding, associated modelling, and moderate doses of diazepam given four hours before sessions may be particularly effective in agoraphobia

5. Phobic anxiety disorders

Mowrer's two-step conditioning (1971) aims to explain fear, and phobias:

✦ pairing of stimulus with fear (classical conditioning)

✦ reinforcing avoidance by anxiety reduction (operant conditioning)

6. Bipolar illness (mania)

In **bipolar illness**, there is usually more than one episode of depression and of mania, or multiple episodes of mania. Other features are:

1. commonly has a seasonal pattern
2. hypersomnia is more common
3. more common in males
4. family history of mania
5. earlier, more acute onset more episodes

Features

✦ depression tends to present first, with onset of mania after the age of 30

✦ manic episodes usually begin abruptly and last from 2 weeks to 5 months (median = 3–4 months)

✦ more than 50% of episodes last less than 1 month with treatment

✦ depressive episodes tend to last longer (median = 6 months)

B. Psychotic disorders

1. Schizophrenia and related syndromes

Schneider's first-rank symptoms include delusions of being controlled by an external force; the belief that thoughts are being inserted into or withdrawn from one's conscious mind; the belief that one's thoughts are being broadcast to other people; and hearing hallucinatory voices that comment on one's thoughts or actions or that have a conversation with other hallucinated voices.

Auditory hallucinations of a specific type

+ two or more voices discussing the patient in the third person
+ thought echo
+ voices commenting on the patient's behaviour

Thought disorder/thought alienation

+ thought insertion
+ thought withdrawal
+ thought broadcasting

Passivity phenomena

+ bodily sensations being controlled by external influence
+ actions/impulses/feelings – experiences which are imposed on the individual or influenced by others

Delusions

+ bizarre delusions
+ paranoid delusions

Other features of schizophrenia

+ impaired insight
+ incongruity/blunting of affect (inappropriate emotion for circumstances)
+ decreased speech
+ neologisms (made-up words)
+ catatonia
+ negative symptoms: incongruity/blunting of affect, anhedonia (inability to derive pleasure), alogia (poverty of speech), avolition (poor motivation)

Epidemiology
Risk of developing schizophrenia

+ monozygotic twin has schizophrenia = 50%

+ parent has schizophrenia = 10%–15%

+ sibling has schizophrenia = 10%

+ no relatives with schizophrenia = 1%

Prognostic factors
Factors associated with poor prognosis

+ strong family history

+ gradual onset

+ low IQ

+ premorbid history of social withdrawal

+ lack of obvious precipitant

Treatment
See section on neuropharmacology above. The pharmacological management has been heavily influenced by the dopamine hypothesis of schizophrenia, and vice versa.

C. Obsessive compulsive behaviour

1. OCD
Characteristics of compulsive acts (DSM III-R)

+ the act has to be a purposeful one

+ it has to be performed in accordance with a certain set of rules

+ the act is not an end in itself, but is designed to bring about another state of affairs (e.g. averting disaster)

+ there has to be a disconnection between the act itself and the state of affairs it is likely to engender: a magical quality between what the patient is doing and what he is trying to achieve or prevent must be present

Clinical features
Obsessions tend to increase anxiety in a sufferer of OCD, whilst carrying out a **compulsive** ritual tends to decrease anxiety.

Types of obsessions

+ obsessional thoughts/ideas
+ obsessional images
+ obsessive ruminations
+ obsessional doubts
+ obsessional convictions
+ compulsive rituals
+ obsessional slowness

Phenomenology

+ obsessive doubts
+ fears of contamination
+ bodily fears
+ insistence on symmetry
+ aggressive thoughts
+ checking compulsions
+ washing
+ counting

Epidemiology

Lifetime prevalence (ECA study) = 1.9%–3.1%

Aetiology
Biological

+ dysregulation of serotonin function

Genetic

+ MZ : DZ = 50%–80% : 25%
+ 35% of first-degree relatives also have OCD

Psychosocial, e.g. personality

+ 15%–35% of OCD patients have been noted to have previous anankastic personality traits
+ some personality traits which are said to characterise OCD sufferers are:

- abnormally high expectations of unpleasant outcomes
- failure to live up to perfectionist ideals should be punished
- magical rituals can prevent catastrophes
- erroneous perception of threat
- deficiency in ability to link concepts and integrate them
- give single events undue emphasis
- *'islands of certainty amid confusion'*

Treatment

- psychological: NB cognitive behavioural therapy and supportive therapy may be useful
- pharmacotherapy, e.g. clomipramine and SSRIs
- psychosurgery

Prognosis

better with:

- mild symptoms
- predominance of phobic ruminative ideas, absence of compulsions
- short duration of symptoms
- no childhood symptoms or abnormal personality traits

worse if:

- symptoms involving the need for symmetry and exactness
- male sex
- early onset
- family history of OCD
- presence of hopelessness, hallucinations or delusions

Associations

- depression (30%)
- schizophrenia (3%)
- Sydenham's chorea
- Tourette's syndrome
- anorexia nervosa

D. Stress reactions

1. Features of grief

Normal grief has three phases:

1. stunned (shock) phase (few hours to 2 weeks)
2. mourning (pining) phase (lasts for several weeks)
3. acceptance and adjustment

- initial shock and disbelief – 'a feeling of numbness'
- increasing awareness of the loss is associated with painful emotions of sadness and anger
- anger may be denied
- irritability

- somatic distress:
  - sleep disturbance
  - tearfulness
  - loss of appetite
  - weight loss
  - loss of libido
  - anhedonia
  - early morning wakening
- identification phenomena – in which the mannerisms and characteristics of the deceased person may be taken on
- preoccupation with deceased
- transient hallucinatory phenomena
- also may involve:
  - projection
  - wish fulfilment
  - denial
  - introjection
  - identity diffusion

2. Post-traumatic stress disorder

It is worth looking at the 2005 NICE PTSD guidelines (CG26). These guidelines are subject to regular review and revision.

Post-traumatic stress disorder (PTSD) can develop in people of any age following a traumatic event, for example a major disaster or childhood sexual abuse. It encompasses what became known as *'shell shock'* following the First World War. One of the DSM-IV diagnostic criteria is that symptoms have been present for more than 1 month.

Features

- re-experiencing: flashbacks, nightmares, repetitive and distressing intrusive images
- avoidance: avoiding people, situations or circumstances resembling or associated with the event
- hyperarousal: hypervigilance for threat, exaggerated startle response, sleep problems, irritability and difficulty concentrating
- emotional numbing: lack of ability to experience feelings, feeling detached from other people
- depression
- ?memory loss – due to the excitotoxic effect of the stress hormone cortisol on the hippocampus
- drug or alcohol misuse
- anger
- unexplained physical symptoms

Management

- Following a traumatic event, single-session interventions (often referred to as debriefing) are not recommended.
- *'Watchful waiting'* may be used for mild symptoms lasting less than 4 weeks.
- Trauma-focused cognitive behavioural therapy (CBT) or eye movement desensitisation and reprocessing (EMDR) therapy may be used in more severe cases.
- Drug treatments for PTSD should not be used as a routine first-line treatment for adults. If drug treatment is used then paroxetine or mirtazapine is recommended.

E. Acute confusional state

Introduction

The **acute confusional state** is a neuropsychiatric syndrome. Patients have difficulty sustaining attention, problems in orientation and short-term memory, poor insight and impaired judgement. Key elements here are fluctuating levels of consciousness. Impaired attention can be assessed with bedside tests that require sustained attention to a task that has not been memorised, such as reciting the days of the week or months of the year backwards, counting backwards from 20 or doing serial subtraction.

In addition in **delirium**, there are disorders of perception (hallucination, illusion, delusion).

Importantly, confusion and delirium are reversible.

DSM-IV-TR diagnostic criteria for delirium

- Disturbance of consciousness (i.e. reduced clarity of awareness of the environment) occurs, with reduced ability to focus, sustain or shift attention.

- Change in cognition (e.g. memory deficit, disorientation, language disturbance, perceptual disturbance) occurs that is not better accounted for by a pre-existing, established or evolving dementia.

- The disturbance develops over a short period (usually hours to days) and tends to fluctuate during the course of the day.

Evidence from the history, physical examination or laboratory findings is present that indicates the disturbance is caused by a direct physiological consequence of a general medical condition, an intoxicating substance, medication use or more than one cause.

Causes

'HIDEMAP'

- **H** = hypoxia (CCF, respiratory failure, ARF) or head trouble (head injury, SOL (SDH?, brain abscess?); meningitis or encephalitis

- **I** = infection (UTI, chest, wound, line, post-op, neutropenic sepsis, especially if immunosuppressed)

- **D** = drugs

- **E** = endocrine

- **M** = metabolic

+ **A** = alcohol or anaemia
+ **P**(s) = psychosis, post-ictal, post-op (e.g. post-fracture of the neck of the femur

Risk factors

+ dementia (i.e. worsening confusion)
+ alcohol or recreational drugs
+ recent surgery

Signs

+ record mental test score (partly as baseline)
+ needle tracks
+ signs of head injury or alcohol
+ constipation (in the case of confusion in the elderly)

Possible blood tests

+ blood tests (FBC although isolated anaemia is unlikely to cause delirium, U&Es, LFTs, ESR, CRP)
+ serum alcohol/toxicology screen
+ possibly serology (e.g. HIV test), if indicated

Possible other investigations

+ urinalysis
+ urine toxicology screen
+ CXR
+ AXR
+ CT + LP if not contraindicated
+ (*very rarely*) EEG

F. Eating disorders

1. Anorexia nervosa

Anorexia nervosa is an eating disorder characterised by refusal to maintain a healthy body weight and an obsessive fear of gaining weight. It is associated with the abnormal perception of body image. Patients generally feel well despite the protestations of others who think that they look awful. They exercise avidly and until the very late stages of the disease hold down full-time jobs.

Anorexia nervosa is associated with a number of characteristic clinical signs and physiological abnormalities which are summarised below.

Features

+ loss of axillary and pubic hair
+ bradycardia
+ hypotension
+ enlarged salivary glands

Physiological abnormalities

+ hypokalaemia
+ low FSH, LH, oestrogens and testosterone
+ raised cortisol and growth hormone
+ impaired glucose tolerance
+ hypercholesterolaemia
+ hypercarotinaemia
+ basal levels of TSH may be depressed in anorexia, though T_4 and T_3 may be normal
+ plasma testosterone levels are normal in females with anorexia
+ ferritin levels are low in a state of malnutrition

Cortisol levels may be increased but are typically within the 'normal range'. They may however fail to suppress with dexamethasone.

2. Bulimia nervosa

Bulimia nervosa is a type of eating disorder characterised by restraining of food intake for a period of time followed by an over-intake or bingeing period that results in feelings of guilt and low self-esteem. The median age of onset is 18 years. Sufferers attempt to overcome these feelings in a number of ways.

The most common form is defensive vomiting, sometimes called purging; fasting, the use of laxatives, enemas and diuretics, and over-exercising are also common. Bulimia nervosa is substantially more likely to occur in women than men.

Management

◆ Referral for specialist care is appropriate in all cases.

◆ Cognitive behaviour therapy (CBT) is currently considered first-line treatment.

◆ Interpersonal psychotherapy is also used but takes much longer than CBT.

◆ Pharmacological treatments have a limited role: a trial of high-dose fluoxetine is currently licensed for bulimia, but long-term data is felt by some to be lacking.

G. Unexplained symptoms

The term *'functional'* refers to an illness that is without a structural defect. Organic brain syndromes are physical conditions, including structural brain disease and metabolic disturbances causing mental dysfunction. Functional psychiatric illness rather than an organic brain disorder is suggested by a family history of psychiatric illness.

There are a wide variety of psychiatric terms for patients who have symptoms for which no organic cause can be found.

1. Somatisation disorder

◆ characterised by multiple, recurrent and changing symptoms for which no physical cause can be found

◆ patient refuses to accept reassurance or negative test results

Somatisation means the expression of psychological distress into bodily complaints for which medical help is sought. Other forms of persistent somatisation include hypochondriasis, dysmorphophobia and psychogenic pain. To meet the diagnostic criteria for somatisation disorder, the patient's physical complaints must not be intentionally induced and must result in medical attention or significant impairment in social, occupational, or other important areas of functioning. By definition, the first symptoms appear in adolescence and the full criteria are met by 30 years of age.

These points are especially worth noting:

+ Knowledge of early childhood experiences is not necessary.

+ Depression is often found, so antidepressives are useful.

+ Relatives should be involved.

+ Empathy, not persuasion, is the key to management.

2. Hypochondrial disorder

+ persistent belief in the presence of an underlying serious disease, e.g. cancer

+ patient refuses to accept reassurance or negative test results

3. Conversion disorder

+ typically involves loss of motor or sensory function

+ some patients may experience secondary gain from loss of function

+ patients may be indifferent to their apparent disorder

4. Dissociative disorder

+ dissociation is a process of 'separating off' certain memories from normal consciousness

+ in contrast to conversion disorder, involves psychiatric symptoms, e.g. amnesia, fugue, stupor

+ dissociative identity disorder (DID) is the new term for multiple personality disorder as it is the most severe form of dissociative disorder

5. Munchausen's syndrome

+ also known as factitious disorder

+ the intentional production of physical or psychological symptoms

6. Malingering

+ fraudulent simulation or exaggeration of symptoms often with the intention of financial or other gain

H. Depersonalisation

Depersonalisation is a change in an individual's experience of the environment where the world around them feels unreal and unfamiliar. The feeling that other people have changed is derealisation.

Depersonalisation is not exclusively seen in patients with schizophrenia. Depersonalisation may occur in:

- almost all major psychiatric disorders
- drug abuse
- migraine
- epilepsy
- systemic lupus erythematosus (SLE)

and, transiently, in:

- normal individuals

ECT has been tried in the past. Selective serotonin reuptake inhibitor (SSRI) antidepressants and coping strategies are useful.

I. Post-concussion syndrome

Post-concussion syndrome is seen after even minor head trauma.

Typical features include:

- headache
- fatigue
- anxiety/depression
- dizziness

J. Post-partum mental health problems

Post-partum mental health problems range from the '*baby blues*' to puerperal psychosis.

TABLE 10.1 Overview of types of post-partum mental health problems

'Baby blues'	Post-natal depression	Puerperal psychosis
Seen in around 60%–70% of women	Affects around 10% of women	Affects approximately 0.2% of women
Typically seen 3–7 days following birth and is more common in primips	Most cases start within a month and typically peak at 3 months	Onset usually within the first 2–3 weeks following birth
Mothers are characteristically anxious, tearful and irritable	Features are similar to depression seen in other circumstances	Puerperal psychosis is a mood disorder with features of loss of contact with reality, hallucinations, thought disorder and abnormal behaviour; it usually presents rapidly in the first month but most often starts in the first week
Reassurance and support; the health visitor has a key role	As with the baby blues, reassurance and support are important	Admission to hospital is usually required
	Cognitive behavioural therapy may be beneficial	There is around a 20% risk of recurrence following future pregnancies

Puerperal psychosis is a relatively rare complication of childbirth, affecting 1–2 per 1000 births. (Postnatal depression is much commoner, affecting 100–150 women per 1000 births.) Prognosis is good.

SIGN guideline 60 on post-natal depression and puerperal psychosis is an excellent guide to this topic.

K. Psychiatric features of medical disease

You should be aware of the psychiatric presentations of physical disease, including:

1. Effects of metabolic, biochemical and endocrine disorders

Endocrinopathies

* hyperthyroidism
* hypothyroidism
* Cushing's syndrome
* adrenocortical deficiency
* hyperparathyroidism
* hypoparathyroidism
* acromegaly
* hypopituitarism
* diabetes mellitus
* diabetes insipidus
* insulinoma
* phaeochromocytoma
* hepatic dysfunction
* deficiency of substrates of cerebral metabolism
* cerebral anoxia
* carbon monoxide poisoning
* hypoglycaemia

Disorders of electrolyte, acid-base and fluid balance

* uraemia
* hypernatraemia
* hyponatraemia
* hyperkalaemia
* hypokalaemia
* hypercalcaemia
* hypocalcaemia
* hypermagnesaemia

- hypomagnesaemia
- zinc deficiency
- alkalosis
- water intoxication
- water depletion
- disorders of vitamins
- vitamin B deficiency
- pellagra (nicotinic acid deficiency)
- alcoholic pellagra encephalopathy
- Wernicke's encephalopathy
- Korsakoff's psychosis
- folic acid deficiency
- vitamin excess

Miscellaneous disorders (*very rare*)

- Wilson's disease
- porphyria
- pantothenate kinase-associated neurodegeneration (PKAN)
- neuroacanthocytosis
- Niemann-Pick disease
- Tay-Sachs disease (GM2 gangliosidosis)
- the leucodystrophies

2. Epilepsy

- increasing tension, irritability and depression are sometimes apparent as prodromata for several days before a seizure
- transient confusional states and automatisms may occur during seizures (especially complex partial) and after seizures (usually those involving generalised convulsions, and complex partial seizures)
- occasionally, non-convulsive seizures may continue for days or even weeks (absence status and complex partial status)
- automatic behaviour is most commonly due to abnormal electrical discharge originating in the periamygdaloid region
- pain

3. Chronic fatigue syndrome

In general, in order to receive a diagnosis of **chronic fatigue syndrome**, a patient must satisfy two of the following criteria:

◆ a history of severe chronic fatigue of 6 months' or longer duration with other known medical conditions excluded by clinical diagnosis

◆ concurrently have four or more of the following symptoms:

  ● substantial impairment in short-term memory or concentration

  ● sore throat

  ● tender lymph nodes

  ● muscle pain

  ● multi-joint pain without swelling or redness

  ● headaches of a new type

  ● appropriate pattern or severity for this condition

  ● unrefreshing sleep

  ● post-exertional malaise lasting more than 24 hours (source: **CDC**)

There is an RCP report on CFS from 1996. Low-dose antidepressants are used in the treatment of CFS, but the suggested first-line therapy should include cognitive behavioural therapy, if access to this service is available.

4. Alcohol dependence

DCR-10

At least three of the following:

◆ a strong desire or sense of compulsion to drink

◆ difficulty in controlling the amount drunk

◆ physiological withdrawal state after drinking stops, with the possible use of alcohol to relieve this

◆ evidence of tolerance may appear

◆ progressive neglect of alternative pleasures and interests

◆ persistence of drinking in spite of evidence of harmful effects

Aetiology
Genetic
1. family studies:

   sevenfold increase in risk of alcoholism among first-degree relatives of alcoholics
2. twin studies:

   $MZ : DZ =$ 70% : 43% for males

   47% : 32% for females
3. adoption studies:
   a) sons of alcoholics are four times more likely to be alcoholic than sons of non-alcoholics, regardless of the drinking patterns of adoptive parents
   b) sons of alcoholics raised by non-alcoholic adoptive parents are no more susceptible to other non-alcoholic adult psychiatric disorder
4. chromosomal abnormalities
5. vulnerability markers
6. risk factors

Complications of alcohol abuse
Hepatic
1. may be due to toxic effects of acetaldehyde/damage to immune system by alcohol
2. women are more susceptible than men
3. fatty liver:
   a) may be present in 90% of drinkers
   b) reversible with abstinence
4. alcoholic hepatitis:
   a) abstinence aids resolution, but cirrhosis may follow
5. cirrhosis:
   a) 10% of chronic alcoholics
   b) more common in women
   c) vulnerability may be due to HLA-B8 antigen, found in 25% of population
   d) HLA-A28 may have a protective effect
   e) fibrosis of the liver and decompensation of liver function
   f) stigmata of liver disease may be present
6. carcinoma:
   a) 15% of patients with cirrhosis go on to develop hepato-cellular carcinoma
7. portal hypertension

Gastrointestinal

1. Barrett's oesophagitis
2. oesophageal varices
3. Mallory-Weiss tears
4. gastritis and gastric erosions
5. peptic ulceration – 20% of alcoholics' bleeding may be exacerbated by vitamin K deficiency secondary to cirrhosis
6. pancreatitis – both acute and chronic
7. gastric carcinoma
8. possible association with colorectal carcinoma
9. diabetes mellitus

Haematological

1. alcoholism is the commonest cause of macrocytosis
2. thrombocytopaenia and anaemia may also occur
3. Zieve's syndrome is a rare form of alcoholic haemolysis

Neurological

1. delirium tremens
2. alcoholic hallucinosis:
   a) rare conditions in which auditory hallucinations occur alone in clear consciousness
   b) usually clears in a few days, but may be followed by secondary delusional misinterpretation
   c) up to 50% go on to develop symptoms of schizophrenia (Benedetti, 1952)
3. epilepsy of late onset (>25 years) is the most common neurological complication
   a) trauma
   b) alcohol withdrawal
   c) brain damage
4. peripheral neuropathy is probably due to thiamine deficiency (dry beriberi)
5. optic atrophy:
   a) loss of visual acuity
   b) blindness associated with methanol poisoning, thiamine and B_{12} deficiency, and heavy tobacco smoking
6. Korsakoff's syndrome is caused by global cortical brain impairment
7. Wernicke's encephalopathy
8. central pontine myelinolysis

9. cerebellar atrophy/degeneration
10. widening of sulci on CT scan
11. EEG abnormalities – P_{300} is decreased, and other wave abnormalities have been reported in detoxified alcoholics

Cardiovascular

◆ moderate drinking is considered beneficial, due to changes in the lipoprotein profile

◆ heavy drinking has the following effects:

- increase in blood pressure
- weakened contraction of myocardium, leading to heart failure
- cardiac arrhythmia
- cardiomyopathy

Laboratory tests

◆ MCV may be raised

◆ γGT may be raised after a single heavy drinking bout

◆ CDT (*carbohydrate deficient transferrin*) can detect if someone has been drinking more than seven units a day for a week

◆ AST > ALT in alcoholism

Psychiatric disorders associated with alcoholism

◆ affective disorders

◆ anxiety

◆ schizophrenia

◆ personality disorder

◆ morbid jealousy

◆ delirium tremens

Treatment

◆ group therapy

◆ individual counselling

◆ inpatient detoxification

◆ Alcoholics Anonymous/recovery groups

Pharmacotherapy

◆ antabuse/disulfiram

◆ naltrexone

◆ acamprosate

References

Benedetti G. Die Alkohol halluzinosen (Stuttgart Thieme); 1952.

Scottish Intercollegiate Guidelines Network (SIGN). Postnatal depression and puerperal psychosis: guideline number 60. Edinburgh: SIGN; June 2002. Available at www.sign.ac.uk/pdf/sign60.pdf (accessed 23 September 2011).

Chapter 11

Renal medicine

The Foundation Programme and MRCP(UK) Part 1 syllabus (from the JRCPMTB) specify what is required in terms of competencies, skills and knowledge from junior physicians in core medical training in renal medicine. You are advised to consult carefully this syllabus, which emphasises the importance of basic medical sciences as well as a competent level of applied clinical practice.

INTRODUCTION

The purpose of the MRCP(UK) examination is not to examine in depth the basic anatomy and the physiology of the kidneys. However, you are supposed to be aware of some basic facts, at least.

A. Basic physiology

1. Renal blood flow

Renal blood flow (RBF) is approximately 25% of cardiac output. The 'Fick principle' can be used to estimate RBF through clearance. RBF is higher in the cortex than medulla, as one might expect with the increasing glomeruli in this region. Sympathetic stimuli produce vasoconstriction and RBF should be increased in response to hypoxia.

B. Clinical symptoms

1. Haematuria

The management of patients with haematuria is often difficult due to the absence of widely followed guidelines. It is sometimes unclear whether patients are best managed in primary care, by urologists or by nephrologists.

The terminology surrounding haematuria is changing. Microscopic or dipstick positive haematuria is increasingly termed non-visible haematuria whilst macroscopic haematuria is termed visible haematuria.

Causes of transient or spurious non-visible haematuria

◆ urinary tract infection

◆ menstruation

◆ vigorous exercise

◆ sexual intercourse

Causes of persistent non-visible haematuria

◆ cancer (bladder, renal, prostate)

◆ stones

◆ benign prostatic hyperplasia

◆ prostatitis

◆ urethritis, e.g. chlamydia

◆ renal causes: IgA nephropathy, thin basement membrane disease

Management

Current evidence, taken as a whole, does not support screening for haematuria. The incidence of non-visible haematuria is similar in patients taking aspirin/warfarin to the general population, hence these patients should also be investigated.

Testing

◆ Urine dipstick is the test of choice for detecting haematuria.

◆ Urine microscopy may be used but time to analysis significantly affects the number of red blood cells detected.

Guidelines

The guidelines for urgent referral are subject to change. You must consult the up-to-date guidelines in full, available from NICE.

The Joint Consensus Statement on the Initial Assessment of Haematuria (2008) predates the NICE guidelines (2008). These guidelines are very useful as they set out the conditions for the long-term monitoring of patients with haematuria (visible or non-visible) of undetermined aetiology.

Patients not meeting criteria for referral to urology or nephrology, or who have had negative urological or nephrological investigations, need long-term monitoring due to the uncertainty of the underlying diagnosis.

Patients should be monitored for the development of:

◆ voiding lower urinary tract symptoms

◆ visible haematuria

◆ significant or increasing proteinuria

◆ progressive renal impairment (falling eGFR)

◆ hypertension (noting that the development of hypertension in older people may have no relation to the haematuria and therefore not increase the likelihood of underlying glomerular disease)

It is definitely worth you consulting these guidelines for yourself.

C. Molecular biology and genetics

You are expected to possess a basic knowledge of genetic defects of common kidney disorders. Please note that this is a very popular topic in the MRCP(UK) Part 1.

1. Adult polycystic kidney disease

Autosomal dominant polycystic kidney disease (ADPKD) is the most common inherited cause of kidney disease, affecting one in 1000 Caucasians. Two disease loci have been identified, *PKD1* and *PKD2*, which code for polycystin-1 and polycystin-2, respectively.

TABLE 11.1 Types of ADPKD

ADPKD type 1	ADPKD type 2
85% of cases	15% of cases
Chromosome 16	Chromosome 4
Presents with renal failure earlier	

Increasingly, asymptomatic patients with a family history of AKPD have been diagnosed by screening. Patients without a family history are called *'sporadic'*. The screening investigation for relatives is abdominal ultrasound, although this is not normally done before the third decade because of the high potential rate of false positives.

Ultrasound diagnostic criteria (in patients with positive family history):

◈ two cysts, unilateral or bilateral, if aged <30 years

◈ two cysts in both kidneys if aged 30–59 years

◈ four cysts in both kidneys if aged >60 years

Polycystic liver disease is seen in 80% of patients but is usually asymptomatic. Abdominal ultrasound has a sensitivity approaching 100% for patients above 20 years of age. Renomegaly is not always a feature as such, but is actually present in many patients.

Genetic screening is also possible.

Hypertension should be aggressively managed, with ACE inhibitors the therapy of choice.

2. Alport's syndrome

Alport's syndrome is usually inherited in an X-linked dominant pattern. It is due to a defect in the gene which codes for type IV collagen resulting in an abnormal glomerular-basement membrane (GBM). The disease is more severe in males, with females rarely developing renal failure.

A favourite question in the MRCP(UK) concerns the patient with Alport's syndrome with a failing renal transplant. This may be caused by the presence of anti-GBM antibodies leading to a Goodpasture's syndrome-like picture.

Alport's syndrome usually presents in childhood. The following features may be seen:

◈ microscopic haematuria

◈ progressive renal failure

◈ bilateral sensorineural deafness

◈ lenticonus: protrusion of the lens surface into the anterior chamber

◈ retinitis pigmentosa

Note though: 10%–15% of cases are inherited in an autosomal recessive fashion, with rare autosomal dominant variants existing.

3. Hypophosphataemic rickets

Hypophosphataemic rickets due to decreased intestinal absorption either because of a low dietary intake or the prolonged ingestion of antacids will not be discussed further, as these do not involve a primary defect in renal phosphate handling.

The best known and most common of the inherited isolated proximal tubular defects associated with rickets is X-linked hypophosphataemic rickets (XLH).

This disease usually presents clinically in the first 2 years of life with short stature, bowing of the legs, osteomalacia and rickets, hypophosphataemia, phosphaturia, normocalcaemia and normal or nearly normal PTH with inappropriately low or normal $1,25\text{-}(OH)_2D$ concentrations.

Hypophosphataemia develops within the first few months of life and is, thus, a useful biochemical test in young infants who might be suspected of inheriting the abnormal gene from an affected parent.

D. Examples of glomerular and tubular diorders

1. When to suspect glomerular pathology

The presence of long-standing hypertension, haematuria and significant non-nephrotic proteinuria is highly suspicious of glomerular pathology such as IgA nephropathy, which is best characterised by a renal biopsy.

In the absence of obstruction on ultrasound, intravenous urography, retrograde pyelography and isotope renography are not appropriate.

Renal size asymmetry in the presence of hypertension and renal impairment might prompt the search for renovascular disease. However, in this condition, the kidneys tend to be of similar and normal size.

Casts containing erythrocytes (red cell casts) are an indication of renal bleeding and are typically found when there is acute glomerular inflammation caused by glomerulonephritis or vasculitis.

2. Diabetes mellitus

Kimmelstiel-Wilson nodules (focal glomerular sclerosis) are characteristic, but mesangial matrix deposition and diffuse glomerular sclerosis with vascular changes are more common. Diabetic nephropathy is one of the most common causes of end-stage renal failure.

The earliest sign is microalbuminuria (albumin excretion of 20–100 mcg/ min). A majority of patients with microalbuminuria will develop overt diabetic nephropathy with protein, and go on to develop hypertension and chronic renal failure.

Diabetic nephropathy usually takes five or more years to evolve; a typical patient is likely to have had the condition for many years prior to it even being diagnosed. Proteinuria heralds onset of loss of GFR and eventually to ESRD. A minor point is that up to 5% of patients with overt severe proteinuria will also have associated microscopic haematuria.

Microalbuminuria is defined as a urine albumin excretion of between 30 and 300 mg per 24 hours. A concentration above 300 mg/24 hours signifies albuminuria and a concentration above 3.5 g/24 hours signifies overt proteinuria. Microalbuminuria is not just an indicator of early renal involvement but it also identifies increased cardiovascular risk with an approximate twofold cardiovascular risk above the already increased risk in the diabetic population.

A useful surrogate of the total albumin excretion is the albumin : creatinine ratio. The urinary albumin : creatinine ratio is measured using the first morning urine sample where practicable. Microalbuminuria is indicated where there is an albumin : creatinine ratio ≥ 2.5 mg/mmol (men) or 3.5 mg/mmol (women). Proteinuria is indicated by a ratio of ≥ 30 mg/mmol.

3. Systemic lupus erythematosus (SLE)

WHO classification

+ class I: normal kidney
+ class II: mesangial glomerulonephritis
+ class III: focal (and segmental) proliferative glomerulonephritis
+ class IV: diffuse proliferative glomerulonephritis
+ class V: diffuse membranous glomerulonephritis
+ class VI: sclerosing glomerulonephritis

Class IV (diffuse proliferative glomerulonephritis) is the most common and severe form.

Management

◆ treat hypertension

◆ corticosteroids if clinical evidence of disease

◆ immunosuppressants, e.g. azathiopine/cyclophosphamide

◆ (**Note:** there is good evidence that immunosuppression could alter outcome in the presence of proliferative glomerulonephritis but not in mesangial or membranous glomerulonephritis. Therefore the best line of treatment in a patient with a mesangial lupus nephritis would be a conservative approach to address risk factors for progression of renal impairment such as uncontrolled hypertension.)

Diffuse proliferative glomerulonephritis is the most common and severe form of renal disease in SLE patients. Note also that SLE is associated with low complements. The established and widely used regimen of long-term high-dose monthly or quarterly intravenous 'pulse' cyclophosphamide pioneered by the National Institutes of Health (NIH) has been challenged on several fronts. Recent studies have shown that short courses of low-dose pulse cyclophosphamide followed by azathioprine achieve similar results to the NIH regimen with less toxicity.

Also note that systemic lupus erythematosus (SLE) can also present with antiphospholipid syndrome, possibly due to renal vein thrombosis (flank pain with blood and protein in urine). The diagnosis would be supported by the thrombocytopaenia, history of hypertension and the *livedo reticularis*.

BOX 11.1   A note on complement and renal failure

Causes of renal failure and low C3

- systemic lupus erythematosus
- mesangiocapillary glomerulonephritis
- post-streptococcal glomerulonephritis
- infective endocarditis

Causes of renal failure and low C3

- Cryoglobulinaemia

4. Hypertensive nephrosclerosis

In essential hypertension, renal damage is manifested by vascular wall thickening and luminal obliteration with interstitial fibrosis and glomerulosclerosis (*hypertensive nephrosclerosis*).

5. Focal segmental glomerulosclerosis

Approximately 50% of subjects with focal segmental glomerulosclerosis do not respond to steroid therapy but ACE inhibitors are a recognised strategy to slow the progression of renal disease. Such a patient is in fact at high risk of cardiovascular disease with a very high cholesterol but the question specifically asks about renal disease.

6. Membranous glomerulonephritis

Most cases of membranous glomerulonephritis are idiopathic, but in some patients there is a history of an infection or a malignancy (usually lung) with antigenemia.

7. Vasculitis: Wegener's granulomatosis

Wegener's granulomatosis is an autoimmune condition associated with a necrotising granulomatous vasculitis, affecting both the upper and lower respiratory tract as well as the kidneys.

Features

- upper respiratory tract: epistaxis, sinusitis, nasal crusting
- lower respiratory tract: dyspnoea, haemoptysis
- glomerulonephritis ('pauci-immune', 80% of patients)
- saddle-shape nose deformity
- also: vasculitic rash, eye involvement (e.g. proptosis), cranial nerve lesions

Investigations

- cANCA positive in >90%, pANCA positive in 25%
- chest X-ray: wide variety of presentations, including cavitating lesions
- renal biopsy: crescenteric glomerulonephritis

Management

- steroids

◆ cyclophosphamide (80% go into remission with cyclophosphamide IV better than oral in terms of side effects and total dose exposure)

◆ plasma exchange (plasma exchange indications include pulmonary haemorrhage creatinine greater than 500 at presentation)

◆ median survival = 8–9 years

◆ **rituximab** is now used for recalcitrant or frequently relapsing disease

8. Pulmonary renal syndrome

A patient with **pulmonary renal syndrome** is typically a young patient who may present with a history of pulmonary haemorrhage and acute renal failure requiring dialysis, and crescenteric glomerulonephritis on renal biopsy. This syndrome is most commonly due to an anti-neutrophil cytoplasmic antibody (ANCA) test positive vasculitis and less commonly due to Goodpasture's syndrome (anti-glomerular basement membrane (GBM) antibodies).

ANCA antibodies are of two types:

◆ c-ANCA which correlates with anti-proteinase 3 antibodies (PR3)

◆ p-ANCA which correlates with anti-myeloperoxidase antibodies; p-ANCA/ MPO antibodies are highly sensitive and specific for rapidly progressive glomerulonephritis and haemorrhagic alveolar capillaritis

9. Amyloidosis

Types
AL amyloid

◆ L for immunoglobulin **Light chain fragment**

◆ due to myeloma, Waldenström's, MGUS

◆ features include: cardiac and neurological involvement, macroglossia, periorbital eccymoses

AA amyloid

◆ A for precursor serum amyloid A protein, an acute phase reactant

◆ seen in chronic infection/inflammation

◆ possible causes: TB, bronchiectasis, rheumatoid arthritis

◆ features: renal involvement most common feature

β-2 microglobulin amyloidosis

◆ precursor protein is β-2 microglobulin, part of the major histocompatibility complex

◆ associated with patients on renal dialysis

10. Goodpasture's syndrome

Goodpasture's syndrome is a rare condition associated with both pulmonary haemorrhage and rapidly progressive glomerulonephritis. It is caused by anti-glomerular basement membrane (anti-GBM) antibodies against type IV collagen. Goodpasture's syndrome is more common in men (sex ratio 2 : 1) and has a bimodal age distribution (peaks in 20–30 and 60–70 age brackets). It is associated with HLA DR2.

Features

◆ pulmonary haemorrhage

◆ followed by rapidly progressive glomerulonephritis

Factors which increase likelihood of pulmonary haemorrhage

◆ young males

◆ smoking

◆ lower respiratory tract infection

◆ pulmonary oedema

◆ inhalation of hydrocarbons

Investigations

◆ renal biopsy: linear IgG deposits along basement membrane

◆ raised transfer factor secondary to pulmonary haemorrhages

Management

◆ plasma exchange

◆ steroids

◆ cyclophosphamide

Studies reveal that without treatment, mortality is as high as 90% in association with Goodpasture's syndrome. However, the prognosis is drastically improved with the removal of antigen through plasmapheresis, immunosuppression with corticosteroids and cyclophosphamide.

There are some studies revealing the potential of mycophenolate mofetil but the evidence is rather anecdotal.

11. Drug-induced interstitial nephritis

Drug-induced interstitial nephritis (DIN) is characterised by a sudden impairment of renal function and is mainly a result of an immune-mediated reaction after intake of a drug.

Causes

Many different drugs, such as antibiotics (such as flucloxacillin), anticonvulsants, diuretics, proton pump inhibitors (such as omeprazole), NSAIDs and many others, are known to cause DIN.

Features

The clinical manifestations are characterised by arthralgias, macular or maculo-papular exanthema and fever, together with mild proteinuria, sterile pyuria and eosinophilia. In many cases the only sign is an asymptomatic increase in serum creatinine.

Diagnosis

Histopathological analysis shows inflammatory infiltrates in the interstitium. Often, plasma cells are present, while glomeruli and vessels are spared.

The lymphocyte transformation test can demonstrate sensitisation to a certain drug, but it is often negative.

Treatment

The mainstay of treatment is drug discontinuation; the role of steroids is controversial.

12. Nephrotic syndrome

The hallmarks of the triad of the **nephrotic syndrome** are:

- proteinuria (>3 g/24 hours), causing:
- hypoalbuminaemia (<30 g/L) and
- oedema

Loss of antithrombin-III, proteins C and S and an associated rise in fibrinogen levels predispose to thrombosis. Loss of thyroxine-binding globulin lowers the total, but not free thyroxine levels.

A young patient (say, aged about 16 years) and a previous good response to corticosteroids would be very suggestive of an underlying diagnosis of minimal change nephropathy. As such, a further course of corticosteroids would be the treatment of choice. You should note that, given the inherent but low risks associated with renal biopsy, it is usually only attempted when three or more episodes of oedema have occurred. Eighty per cent of adults with minimal change glomerulonephritis will respond to steroids, although remissions can take up to 16 weeks.

Very few patients with minimal change disease actually progress to end-stage renal disease, and only around 10% of children with the disease suffer from hypertension.

Complications

- increased risk of infection due to urinary immunoglobulin loss
- increased risk of thromboembolism related to loss of antithrombin III and plasminogen in the urine
- hyperlipidaemia
- hypocalcaemia (vitamin D and binding protein lost in urine)
- acute renal failure

Amyloidosis is a cause of the nephrotic syndrome, for example in patients with rheumatoid disease. It is therefore worth reviewing the topic of amyloidosis at this point.

You especially should have an understanding of disturbed renal and metabolic functions in nephrotic syndrome from a variety of causes.

Causes

The most common primary causes are the following:

◆ minimal change disease

◆ focal segmental glomerulosclerosis

◆ membranous nephropathy

Secondary causes account for <10% of childhood cases but >50% of adult cases, most commonly the following:

◆ diabetic nephropathy

◆ pre-eclampsia

Amyloidosis, an under-recognised cause, is responsible for 4% of cases.

Physiology

Proteinuria occurs because of changes to capillary endothelial cells, the glomerular basement membrane (GBM) or podocytes, which normally filter serum protein selectively by size and charge. The mechanism of damage to these structures is unknown in primary and secondary glomerular diseases.

Nephrotic syndrome predisposes to thrombotic episodes, possibly due to loss of antithrombin III. These commonly occur in the renal veins and may be bilateral. Common symptoms include loin pain and haematuria.

A greater rise in the ESR would be expected if the renal failure was due to an exacerbation of SLE.

13. Papillary necrosis

Causes

◆ chronic analgesia use

◆ sickle cell disease

◆ TB

◆ acute pyelonephritis

◆ diabetes mellitus

Features

◆ fever, loin pain, haematuria

◆ IVU: papillary necrosis with renal scarring – *'cup and spill'*

14. Renal tubular acidosis

All three types of renal tubular acidosis (RTA) are associated with hyperchloraemic metabolic acidosis (normal anion gap).

Type 1 RTA (distal)

- inability to generate acid urine (secrete H+) in distal tubule
- causes hypokalaemia
- complications include nephrocalcinosis and renal stones
- causes include idiopathic, RA, SLE, Sjögren's syndrome

Type 2 RTA (proximal)

- decreased HCO_3^- reabsorption in proximal tubule
- causes hypokalaemia
- complications include osteomalacia
- causes include idiopathic, as part of Fanconi syndrome, Wilson's disease, cystinosis, outdated tetracyclines

Type 4 RTA (hyperkalaemic)

- causes hyperkalaemia
- causes include hypoaldosteronism, diabetes
- H+ secretion, sodium reabsorption and ammonia production diminishes

RTA Type 4 is, in effect, **hyporeninaemic hypoaldosteronism** or failure of aldosterone action, and thus helped treated with mineralocorticoids. It is usually seen in chronic renal disease and hence low GFR and particularly.

15. IgA nephropathy

IgA nephropathy (**Berger's disease**) is the most common glomerulonephritis worldwide and characteristically affects young males, presenting with frank haematuria after an episode of pharyngitis. This usually develops 1–2 days after a sore throat. It is most common in the second and third decades of life.

However, it may also present with proteinuria, microscopic haematuria, renal failure or hypertension.

It is probably part of a spectrum of disease with Henoch-Schönlein purpura, which presents with arthritis, rash, abdominal pain and nephritis. In both there are mesangial IgA deposits in the kidney.

The urine may be frankly bloody or may be the colour of cola. There are no clots in the urine and the haematuria is generally painless, although some patients complain of mild loin pain.

It tends to settle spontaneously within 5 days, although the episodes may be recurrent, lasting for 1–2 years. Thirty per cent of children will have a spontaneous remission within 10 years, but 25% will go on to develop ESRF within 20 years.

Renal biopsy will show mesangial IgA deposition on immunofluorescence and light microscopy will show mesangial hypercellularity and matrix expansion.

The treatment of IgA nephritis is variable. In a patient with haematuria only, the treatment is conservative. When there is nephrotic range proteinuria (>3 g/day, as in this case) an 8- to 12-week course of prednisolone should be prescribed. If the proteinuria is <3 g/day, an ACE inhibitor can be used. In all patients, careful control of blood pressure should be achieved, by using ACE inhibitors in the first instance, and regular follow-up of renal function and urinalysis.

E. Infections of the kidney

1. Urinary tract infection

Infection usually enters the urinary tract through the urethra, but blood-borne infection can deposit in the kidney. The higher incidence in women is attributed to the easier access for pathogens through the shorter female tract.

The usual organisms are Gram-negative *Escherichia coli*, *Klebsiella* and *Proteus* infections.

Lower urinary tract infection is restricted to the bladder and urethra; it usually involves only the superficial mucosa and has no-long term effects. Upper urinary tract infection, affecting the kidney or ureters, involves the deep medullary tissue and can permanently damage the kidneys.

Infection of the urinary tract by *Mycobacterium tuberculosis* is uncommon in the UK, but is a cause of sterile pyuria (white cells in the urine, but no organism grown under standard culture conditions). Early morning urine samples should be cultured specifically for mycobacteria when this diagnosis is considered.

The clinical presentation is variable. Lower UTI can produce discomfort or burning on micturition, increased urinary frequency and offensive-smelling urine. Upper UTI can produce loin pain, fever, frank tenderness and rigors. Physical signs include fever and tenderness over the kidneys or bladder.

Management

Lower urinary tract infections in women (cystitis). Local antibiotic guidelines should be followed if available. **The NHS Clinical Knowledge Summaries** (CKS) recommend trimethoprim or nitrofurantoin for 3 days.

Lower urinary tract infections in pregnancy

◆ Asymptomatic bacteriuria is screened for on the booking visit and should be treated with an antibiotic for 7 days (sensitivities should already be available).

◆ For acute lower urinary tract infections, consider amoxicillin or an oral cephalosporin for 7 days.

◆ For patients with sign of acute pyelonephritis, hospital admission should be considered.

◆ Local antibiotic guidelines should be followed if available. The BNF currently recommends a broad-spectrum cephalosporin or a quinolone for 10–14 days. Clinical Knowledge Summaries currently recommend ciprofloxacin for 7 days or co-amoxiclav for 14 days.

BOX 11.2   A note on trimethoprim and nitrofurantoin

The NHS Clinical Knowledge Summaries also mention the use of trimethoprim and nitrofurantoin. Trimethoprim is a folate antagonist and concerns have been raised regarding the potential risk of neural tube defects. Whilst short-term trimethoprim use is unlikely to cause folate deficiency it would seem reasonable to use an antibiotic such as amoxicillin first-line. Nitrofurantoin should be avoided at term because of the risk of neonatal haemolysis.

---

2. Predisposing factors of UTIs

After the flu and common cold, urinary tract infections (UTIs) are the most common medical complaint among women in their reproductive years. UTIs are far more common among women than among men.

Most women will develop a UTI at some time in their lives, and many will have recurrences. Men become more susceptible to UTIs after 50 years of age, when they begin to develop prostate problems.

Benign prostatic hyperplasia can produce obstruction in the urinary tract and increase the risk for infection. In men, recurrent urinary tract infections are also associated with prostatitis, an infection of the prostate gland.

Although only about 20% of UTIs occur in men, these infections can cause more serious problems than they do in women. Men with UTIs are far more likely to be hospitalised than women.

F. Reflux nephropathy

1. Reflux nephropathy (RN)

Reflux nephropathy (RN) is a term applied when small and scarred kidneys are associated with vesico-ureteric reflux. CPN being the commonest cause, there are other causes including analgesic nephropathy and obstructive injury.

Scarring is essential in developing RN and is said often to occur almost always during the first 5 years of life. The end results of RN are hypertension, proteinuria, CRF and eventually end-stage renal disease.

The patient usually has a long history of urinary tract infections, and this could predispose a female patient to developing pyelonephritis in pregnancy.

Diagnosis

It is diagnosed by micturating cystography; scarring can of course be demonstrated by ultrasound or DMSA.

Treatment

The aim of treatment is to reduce renal scarring.

Those children with grade II or worse should receive low-dose prophylactic antibiotics (nitrofurantoin, trimethoprim, cotrimoxazole, cephalexin in those with CRF).

Other treatment modalities also include surgery (e.g. endoscopic injection of collagen behind the intravesical ureter, ureteric reimplantation or lengthening of the submucosal ureteric tunnel).

G. Calculus formation within the urinary tract

You should possess a knowledge of metabolic disorders predisposing to **stone or calculus formation**, their investigation, prevention and medical management (prevention).

1. Risk factors

◆ dehydration

◆ hypercalciuria, hyperparathyroidism, hypercalcaemia

◆ cystinuria

◆ high dietary oxalate

◆ renal tubular acidosis

◆ medullary sponge kidney, polycystic kidney disease

◆ beryllium or cadmium exposure

Risk factors for urate calculi

◆ gout

◆ ileostomy: loss of bicarbonate and fluid results in acidic urine, causing the precipitation of uric acid

2. Drug causes

◆ drugs that promote calcium stones: loop diuretics, steroids, acetazolamide, theophylline

◆ thiazides can prevent calcium stones (increase distal tubular calcium resorption)

3. Genetic causes

Some causes are known now to be genetic. **Cystinuria/nephropathic cystinosis** is an autosomal recessive genetic defect in membrane transport for cystine, lysine, ornithine and arginine in epithelial cells. The disease is characterised by recurrent nephrolithiasis.

Idiopathic hypercalciuria has a familial or sporadic pattern. In the familial pattern an autosomal dominant inheritance is present. The type of the disease is identical in affected members of the same family and the typical presentation is of recurrent urinary calculi.

4. Imaging

TABLE 11.2 Appearance of renal or urinary stones on X-ray

Type	Frequency	Radiograph appearance
Calcium oxalate	40%	Opaque
Mixed calcium oxalate/phosphate stones	25%	Opaque
Triple phosphate stones	10%	Opaque
Calcium phosphate	10%	Opaque
Urate stones	5%–10%	Radiolucent
Cystine stones	1%	Semi-opaque, 'ground-glass' appearance
Xanthine stones	<1%	Radiolucent

5. Management

Acute management of renal colic

Diclofenac, 75 mg by intramuscular injection, is the analgesia of choice for **renal colic** (though not if the patient has renal failure). A second dose can be given after 30 minutes if necessary.

Medical management (prevention) of renal stones
Calcium stones

◆ high fluid intake

◆ low animal protein, low-salt diet (a low-calcium diet has not been shown to be superior to a normocalcaemic diet)

◆ thiazide diuretics (increase distal tubular calcium resorption)

◆ stones <5 mm will usually pass spontaneously

◆ lithotripsy, nephrolithotomy may be required

Oxalate stones

◆ cholestyramine reduces urinary oxalate secretion

◆ pyridoxine reduces urinary oxalate secretion

Uric acid stones

◆ allopurinol

◆ urinary alkalinisation, e.g. oral bicarbonate

H. Renal failure

1. Acute renal failure

Renal failure is abnormal renal function, identified by a high creatinine or oliguria (<10 mL/h), is frequent and caused by a wide range of processes. When it develops over hours or days, the term **acute renal failure (ARF)** is used. The majority (55%) of cases of ARF result from renal hypoperfusion and ischaemic damage. The resulting renal histopathological lesion is **acute tubular necrosis**.

Causes of acute renal failure

The causes of ARF, with approximate relative frequency, are as follows:

◆ prerenal factors leading to renal hypoperfusion and ATN (55%)

◆ toxic ATN (5%)

◆ structural abnormalities of renal vasculature (5%)

◆ acute glomerulonephritides and vasculitides (15%)

◆ interstitial nephritis (5%)

◆ myeloma/tubular cast nephropathy (5%)

◆ urinary tract obstruction (10%)

Acute tubular necrosis compared to prerenal uraemia

Regarding acute renal failure, you will be expected to differentiate acute tubular necrosis compared to prerenal uraemia.

In **prerenal uraemia**, the kidneys hold on to sodium to preserve volume. A comparison between prerenal uraemia and acute tubular necrosis is shown in Table 11.3.

TABLE 11.3 Types of acute renal failure (ARF)

	Pre-renal uraemia	Acute tubular necrosis
Urine sodium	<20 mmol/L	>30 mmol/L
Urine: plasma osmolality	>1.5	<1.1
Urine: plasma urea	>10 : 1	<8 : 1
Specific gravity	>1020	<1010
Urine	'bland' sediment	brown granular casts
Response to fluid challenge	Yes	No

Causes of acute tubular necrosis

Renal failure from ATN occurs in 25% of patients with severe hepatic damage.

Accelerated hypertension can cause small vessel obstruction with proliferative endarteritis of intralobular arteries and fibrinoid necrosis of afferent arterioles and glomerular capillary tuft.

Other causes of ATN include:

◆ hypotension

◆ hepatic failure

◆ eclampsia

◆ drugs such as aminoglycosides, cephalosporins, cisplatin, amphotericin

2. Chronic renal failure

Chronic renal failure is the irreversible loss of glomerular filtration rate (GFR). This is important as there may be direct consequences of impaired renal function; secondly, loss of GFR tends to be progressive, ultimately leading to end-stage renal failure.

Aetiology of chronic renal failure

Diverse primary processes result in loss of GFR. The commonest causes in the UK are as follows:

A. glomerulonephritides (the most common is the IgA nephropathy)
B. diabetes mellitus
C. chronic pyelonephritis/reflux nephropathy
D. obstructive neuropathy
E. autosomal dominant polycystic kidney disease
F. vascular disease/renal hypertension

 Features of chronic kidney disease

Major pathophysiological abnormalities of chronic renal failure include the following:

◆ accumulation of nitrogenous waste products

◆ acidosis: bicarbonate wasting, decreased ammonia secretion, decreased acid excretion

◆ sodium wasting: solute diuresis, tubular damage

◆ sodium retention: nephrotic syndrome, CCF, anuria, excess sodium intake

◆ urinary concentrating defect: nephron loss, solute diuresis

+ hyperkalaemia: decreased glomerular filtration rate (GFR), acidosis, hyperaldosteronism

+ renal osteodystrophy: decreased intestinal calcium absorption, impaired 12-dihydroxy vitamin D production, secondary hyperparathyroidism

+ growth retardation: protein calorie deficiency, renal osteodystrophy, acidosis, anaemia

+ anaemia: decreased erythropoietin production, low-grade haemolysis, inadequate intake (it is now hypothesised that improvement in haemoglobin level results with erythropoietin in increased well-being and better appetite)

+ bleeding tendency: thrombocytopaenia, decreased platelet function

+ infection: defective granulocyte function

+ neurology: uraemia, aluminium toxicity results in fatigue, poor concentration, headache, memory loss, slurred speech, muscle weakness and cramps, seizures and coma

+ GI ulceration: gastric acid hypersecretion

+ hypertension: sodium and water overload, hyperammonaemia

+ hypertriglyceridaemia: decreased plasma lipoprotein lipase activity

+ pericarditis and cardiomyopathy: cause unknown

+ glucose intolerance: tissue insulin resistance

3. Drugs in chronic kidney disease

If a patient has renal artery stenosis, any ACE inhibitor should be stopped.

Metformin is excreted unchanged in the urine with the half-life prolonged and renal clearance decreased in proportion to any decrease in creatinine clearance. This may occur chronically in chronic renal impairment, or acutely with dehydration, shock and intravascular administration of iodinated contrast agents, all of which have the potential to alter renal function.

Tissue hypoxia also has a significant role, and acute or chronic conditions that may predispose to this condition, such as sepsis, acute myocardial infarction, pulmonary embolism, cardiac failure and chronic liver disease, may act as triggers.

Also, in chronic kidney disease, guidelines currently suggest that metformin should be stopped if creatinine is above 150 µmol/L. The estimated prevalence of life-threatening lactic acidosis is one to five cases per 100 000, with mortality in reported cases up to 50%. Traditionally this complication has been thought of as secondary to an accumulation of the drug.

BOX 11.3 A note on renal artery stenosis

The gold standard for establishing a diagnosis of renal artery stenosis is **renal arteriography**, and this is commonly performed with magnetic resonance angiography. In one-third of cases the disease is bilateral, 40% may have peripheral vascular disease and there may be proteinuria. Investigations also include captopril renography and magnetic resonance (MR) angiography, which is virtually as good as renal arteriography. An ultrasound diagnosis is likely to be atherosclerotic renal artery stenosis (RAS), as suggested by the asymmetric reduction in renal size, with mild proteinuria quite common in the condition.

---

4. Rhabdomyolysis

Rhabdomyolysis will typically feature in the exam as a patient who has had a fall or prolonged epileptic seizure and is found to have acute renal failure on admission.

Features

◆ acute renal failure with disproportionately raised creatinine
◆ elevated creatine kinase
◆ myoglobinuria
◆ hypocalcaemia (myoglobin binds calcium)
◆ elevated phosphate (released from myocytes)

Causes

◆ seizure
◆ collapse/coma (e.g. elderly patient collapses at home, found eight or so hours later)
◆ ecstasy (MDMA)
◆ crush injury
◆ McArdle's syndrome
◆ drugs: statins

Management

◆ IV fluids to maintain good urine output

◆ urinary alkalinisation is sometimes used, but very hard to achieve in reality

◆ **dialysis is used in oliguric patients**

I. Other important clinical syndromes

1. The overlap between haemolytic uraemic syndrome and thrombotic thrombocytopaenic purpura

According to Miha Furlan and Bernhard Lämmle in a relatively recent review (2000), **haemolytic uraemic syndrome (HUS) and thrombotic thrombocytopaenic purpura (TTP)** are two clinically similar disorders, characterised by severe microangiopathic haemolytic anaemia and thrombocytopaenia. HUS is characterised by thrombocytopaenia, anaemia and renal insufficiency, whereas the pentad of signs and symptoms including thrombocytopaenia, anaemia, neurological deficit, renal dysfunction and fever is observed in TTP. However, about 60% of patients diagnosed with acute TTP lack one or more of these criteria, while about 30% of those receiving a diagnosis of HUS exhibit neurological symptoms and fever. Thus, the two disorders are often difficult to distinguish.

2. Haemolytic uraemic syndrome

Haemolytic uraemic syndrome is generally seen in young children and produces a triad of:

◆ acute renal failure

◆ microangiopathic haemolytic anaemia

◆ thrombocytopaenia

Causes

◆ post-dysentery – classically *E coli* 0157:H7 ('verotoxigenic', 'enterohaemorrhagic')

◆ tumours

◆ pregnancy

◆ drugs, e.g. cyclosporin, oral contraceptive pill

◆ systemic lupus erythematosus

◆ HIV

Management

+ Treatment is supportive, e.g. fluids, blood transfusion and dialysis if required.

+ There is no role for antibiotics, despite the preceding diarrhoeal illness in many patients.

+ The indications for plasma exchange in HUS are complicated. As a general rule, plasma exchange is reserved for severe cases of HUS not associated with diarrhoea.

3. Thrombotic thrombocytopaenic purpura

Pathogenesis of thrombotic thrombocytopaenic purpura (TTP)

+ abnormally large and sticky multimers of von Willebrand's factor cause platelets to clump within vessels

+ in TTP there is a deficiency of caspase which breaks down large multimers of von Willebrand's factor

+ overlaps with haemolytic uraemic syndrome (HUS)

Features

+ *rare*, typically adult females

+ fever

+ fluctuating neurological signs (microemboli)

+ microangiopathic haemolytic anaemia

+ thrombocytopaenia

+ renal failure

Causes

+ post-infection, e.g. urinary, gastrointestinal

+ pregnancy

+ drugs: cyclosporin, oral contraceptive pill, penicillin, clopidogrel, acyclovir

+ tumours

+ SLE

+ HIV

4. Hypertension and renal problems in pregnancy

In normal pregnancy, urinary protein excretion increases substantially, due to a combination of increased glomerular filtration rate and increased permeability of the glomerular basement membrane. Hence, total protein excretion is considered abnormal in pregnant women when it exceeds 300 mg/24 hours.

Pre-eclampsia

Pre-eclampsia is a condition seen after 20 weeks' gestation character-ised by pregnancy-induced hypertension in association with proteinuria (>0.3 g/24 hours).

Oedema used to be the third element of the classic triad but is now often not included in the definition as it is not specific.

Pre-eclampsia is very important as it predisposes to the following problems:

- foetal: prematurity, intrauterine growth retardation
- eclampsia
- haemorrhage: placental abruption, intra-abdominal, intra-cerebral
- cardiac failure
- multi-organ failure

Risk factors

- >40 years old
- nulliparity (or new partner)
- multiple pregnancy
- body mass index >30 kg/m^2
- diabetes mellitus
- pregnancy interval of more than 10 years
- family history of pre-eclampsia
- previous history of pre-eclampsia
- pre-existing vascular disease such as hypertension or renal disease

Features of severe pre-eclampsia

- hypertension: typically >170/110 mmHg and proteinuria as above
- proteinuria: dipstick ++/+++
- headache
- visual disturbance

◆ papilloedema

◆ RUQ/epigastric pain

◆ hyperreflexia

◆ platelet count <100 × 10^6/L, abnormal liver enzymes or HELLP syndrome

Management

◆ Consensus guidelines recommend treating blood pressure >160/110 mmHg although many clinicians have a lower threshold.

◆ Oral methyldopa is often used first-line with oral labetalol, nifedipine and hydralazine also being used.

◆ For severe hypertension IV labetalol and IV hydralazine are used in addition to the above.

◆ Delivery of the baby is the most important and definitive management step. The timing depends on the individual clinical scenario.

J. Renal replacement therapy

1. Different types of dialysis and their complications

Dialysis is a treatment for kidney failure that removes waste and extra fluid from the blood, using a filter. In peritoneal dialysis (PD), the filter is the lining of the abdomen, called the peritoneum. In haemodialysis (HD), the filter is a plastic tube filled with millions of hollow fibres, called a dialyser.

Different forms: Each of the five modalities of dialysis offers different things, and it is essential to match the modality correctly to the patient.

◆ chronic ambulatory peritoneal dialysis (CAPD) – a manual form of peritoneal dialysis, with no machine

◆ chronic cycling peritoneal dialysis (CCPD) – a form of peritoneal dialysis using a cycler at night

◆ conventional home haemodialysis – dialysis at home three times a week

◆ daily home haemodialysis – short (2–3 hour) treatments, 5–6 days a week

◆ nocturnal home dialysis – nightly 6- to 8-hour treatments, 3+ days a week

Haemodialysis is favoured in the following situations:

◆ recurrent abdominal surgery or irreducible hernia

◆ recurrent or persistent peritonitis

◆ peritoneal membrane failure

◆ severe malnutrition

◆ intercurrent severe illness with hypercatabolism

◆ chronic severe respiratory disease

◆ loss of residual renal failure

Mechanism: Haemodialysis often involves fluid removal through ultrafiltration, because most patients with renal failure pass little or no urine.

Side effects caused by removing too much fluid and/or removing fluid too rapidly include low blood pressure, fatigue, chest pains, leg cramps, nausea and headaches. Symptoms can occur during the treatment and can persist post-treatment.

Complications: Since haemodialysis requires access to the circulatory system, patients undergoing haemodialysis may expose their circulatory system to infection and sepsis, including endocarditis or osteomyelitis. Bleeding may also occur; again, the risk varies depending on the type of access used. Long-term complications of haemodialysis include amyloidosis, neuropathy and ventricular enlargement.

2. Criteria for urgent renal replacement therapy

◆ severe hyperkalaemia

◆ fluid overload leading to acute pulmonary oedema

◆ acidosis resulting in circulatory collapse

◆ uraemia causing encephalopathy, pericarditis or bleeding

3. Chronic graft rejection of a renal transplant

Chronic rejection of a renal transplant is characterised by fibrosis of normal organ structures.

The pathogenesis of chronic rejection is not clear – some prefer the term *'chronic allograft dysfunction'* since both immunological (antigen-dependent and antigen-independent) and non-immunological factors have been identified.

Cell-mediated and humoral immune mechanisms have been implicated in this form of graft rejection.

It has also been suggested that rejection is a response to chronic ischaemia caused by injury to endothelial cells.

Proliferation of intimal smooth muscle is observed leading to vascular occlusion.

The fact that chronic rejection is rare in transplants between human leucocyte antigen (HLA)-identical siblings suggests that HLA-antigen dependent immunological factors are important.

Risk factors include:

◆ number of previous acute rejection episodes

◆ presence of anti-HLA antibodies

◆ anti-endothelial antibodies

◆ cytomegalovirus (CMV) infection

◆ dyslipidaemia

◆ hypertension

◆ functional mass of the donor kidney

◆ delayed graft function (a clinical manifestation of ischaemia/reperfusion injury)

You should also understand the complications related to immunosuppressive therapy following renal transplantation.

4. Cyclosporin

Cyclosporin is an immunosuppressant which decreases clonal proliferation of T cells by reducing IL-2 release. It acts by binding to cyclophilin, forming a complex which inhibits calcineurin, a phosphotase that activates various transcription factors in T cells.

It is used following a renal transplant. It is also used in glomerulonephritis: resistant minimal change and membranous glomerulonephritis.

Formulations include neoral and sandimmune.

Adverse effects of cyclosporin

◆ nephrotoxicity

◆ hepatotoxicity

◆ fluid retention

◆ hypertension

◆ hyperkalaemia

◆ hypertrichosis

◆ gum hyperplasia

◆ tremor

◆ impaired glucose tolerance

Indications

◆ Crohn's disease

◆ rheumatoid arthritis

◆ psoriasis (has a direct effect on keratinocytes as well as modulating T cell function)

◆ following organ transplantation

◆ pure red cell aplasia

5. Cyclophosphamide

Cyclophosphamide is an alkylating agent used in the management of cancer and autoimmune conditions. It works by causing cross-linking of DNA.

Adverse effects

◆ haemorrhagic cystitis: incidence reduced by the use of hydration and mesna

◆ myelosuppression

◆ transitional cell carcinoma

K. Renal cell carcinoma

Renal cell carcinomas may present in a variety of ways, with only a minority being diagnosed with the classical triad of:

◆ haematuria

◆ loin pain

◆ a palpable mass

Relatively *common* presentations include:

◆ anaemia

◆ hypertension

◆ pyrexia of unknown origin

◆ fatigue

◆ increased plasma viscosity

Less common presentations include:

+ hypercalcaemia
+ polycythaemia
+ liver dysfunction
+ enteropathy
+ myopathy

Urinalysis may show sterile pyuria.
   Other causes of sterile pyuria are:

+ partially treated urinary tract infections (UTI)
+ tuberculosis (TB) of the renal tract
+ urethritis and sexually transmitted diseases
+ acute glomerulonephritis
+ tubulo-interstitial diseases
+ adult polycystic kidney disease
+ renal stones

Ultrasound scan of the renal tract would be the first investigation of choice, as it is able to pick up 95% of renal cell carcinomas greater than 1 cm in diameter. It would also exclude infective or inflammatory collections within the renal tract.

   If required **a computerised tomography** (CT) +/− guided biopsy could be obtained to prove the diagnosis.

   An intravenous urogram (IVU) was considered the investigation of choice before the advent of ultrasound.

   A **chest X-ray** and **bone scan** would be required to complete the basic investigations.

References

Furlan M, Lämmle B. Haemolytic-uraemic syndrome and thrombotic thrombocyto-paenic purpura – new insights into underlying biochemical mechanisms. *Nephrol Dial Transplant.* 2000; **15**(8): 1112–14.

Mason PD, Pusey CD. Glomerulonephritis: diagnosis and treatment [review]. *BMJ.* 1994; **309**(6968): 1557–63.

Chapter 12

Respiratory medicine

The Foundation Programme and MRCP(UK) Part 1 syllabus (from the JRCPMTB) specify what is required in terms of competencies, skills and knowledge from junior physicians in core medical training in respiratory medicine. You are advised to consult carefully this syllabus, which emphasises the importance of basic medical sciences as well as a competent level of applied clinical practice.

INTRODUCTION

The clinical features, investigation and management of respiratory disease likely to be encountered by a general physician must be known.

A. Important cases

1. Pleural effusion

You should have an understanding of the key points of the BTS guidelines on the management of a unilateral pleural effusion in adults.

Figure 12.1 gives a list of the causes of a transudative and exudative pleural effusion. The classical way of separating a transudate from an exudate is by pleural fluid protein, with exudates having a protein level of >30 g/L and transudates a protein level of <30 g/L. Care should be taken in interpreting this result if the serum total protein is abnormal. Unfortunately, the protein level often lies very close to the 30 g/L cut-off point, making clear differentiation difficult.

In these cases, measurement of serum and pleural fluid lactate dehydrogenase (LDH) and total protein levels will allow the use of **Light's criteria** to distinguish between these two more accurately. The pleural fluid is an exudate if one or more of the following criteria are met: the pleural fluid protein divided by serum protein >0.5, the pleural fluid LDH divided by serum LDH >0.6, and pleural fluid LDH more than two-thirds the upper limits of normal serum LDH.

CAUSES OF TRANSUDATE PLEURAL EFFUSIONS	CAUSES OF EXUDATE PLEURAL EFFUSIONS
Very common causes • left ventricular failure • liver cirrhosis • hypoalbuminaemia • peritoneal dialysis **Less common causes** • hypothyroidism • nephrotic syndrome • mitral stenosis • pulmonary embolism **Rare causes** • constrictive pericarditis • urinothroax • superior vena cava obstruction • ovarian hyperstimulation • Meigs' syndrome	**Common causes** • malignancy • parapneumonic effusions **Less common causes** • pulmonary infarction • rheumatoid arthritis • autoimmune diseases • benign asbestos effusion • pancreatitis • post-myocardial infarction syndrome **Rare causes** • yellow nail syndrome • drugs • fungal infections

FIGURE 12.1 Causes of pleural effusion

2. 'Respiratory' chest pain

[Note that, whilst this appears in the Respiratory syllabus for MRCP(UK), chest pain is clearly obvious relevant to other systems of the body.]

Points in the history

An accurate history of the chest pain is vital. This includes:

◆ Where – ischaemic pain is poorly localised, retrosternal discomfort often described as tightness, pressure or burning

◆ Nature – ischaemic pain is heavy or tight; often patients deny the symptom of pain and refer to it as discomfort

◆ Radiation – may radiate to the arms, neck, jaw, gums or abdomen, and sometimes these may be the only sites

◆ Exacerbating factors – including exertion effects, posture, meals

Cardiac risk factors

Cardiac pain tends to be heaviness, band-like, gripping and a dull ache. Precipitants are exertion, cold weather or stress.

Non-cardiac pain tends to be a dull ache, sharp, shooting and precipitated by specific body motion. Enquire about rest and nocturnal pain. A history of hot and shivery symptoms, central chest pain comfortable when sitting upright, inability to sleep lying down, no effect of exertion and eating is suggestive of pericarditis, maybe on the background of autoimmune disease. Pericarditis is pleuritic chest pain, varying with posture, classically relieved by sitting forward. Consider pre-disposing factors to angina, including obesity, hyperlipidaemia, hypertension, hyperthyroidism, anaemia.

Enquire about previous medical history: cardiovascular or cerebrovascular disease, cholesterol, diabetes, hypertension, risk factors for PE/DVT, pericarditis risk factors (pyogenic, TB, malignant, uraemia, hypothyroid, autoimmune disorders). Include a drug history, family history of peripheral vascular disease, thrombophilia, familial hypercholesterolaemia and social history (smoking, occupational lifestyle, recent travel).

Differential diagnosis: (1) chronic stable angina, predictable on exercise and may be relieved by rest, worse in cold or windy weather, induced by stress, rapidly improved by GTN; (2) unstable angina, at rest; (3) pericarditis – localised anterior central pain, worse on breathing and lying flat; (4) aortic dissection, sudden onset radiating to the back; (5) pleural pain, lateralised and worse on breathing and associated with cough; (6) oesophageal pain, may be worse on eating and associated with vomiting, oesophagitis, may be pain after meals, particularly citrus juices or spirits, with relief on sitting or standing up; (7) spinal pain, mainly in the back but may radiate round to front in a nerve root distribution; (8) skin pain, usually due to shingles; (9) musculoskeletal pain, usually tender to palpation (10) pulmonary embolism which may cause sudden chest pain, hypotension, dyspnoea, collapse and right heart strain.

Investigations: FBC (neutrophil leucocytosis and thrombocytosis in MI), ECG (resting rhythm, evidence of previous MI, LVH, right heart strain), glucose, lipids, CK/troponin I, exercise testing, CXR (focal lung disease, masses, pruning of pulmonary vessels as in pulmonary hypertension), Hb/TFTs (thyroid function can exacerbate pain as can anaemia), V/Q scan (if PE suspected), echocardiogram (structural heart disease), *H. pylori* if suspicion of oesophageal pain (also consider upper GI endoscopy and oesophageal manometry).

3. Haemoptysis

Points in the history

Confirm **haemoptysis** is not a fleck of blood, and is *not* haematemesis! Check it isn't coming from the mouth (poor dentition, gum disease, nasal problems).

Ask therefore about the nature of the haemoptysis: fresh red blood or mixed in with sputum? If from the mouth, a nasopharyngeal source is likely. Blood from the chest is usually red, not brown. Any history of recent trauma, such as a sports injury?

When did the haemoptysis develop? How often? What is the approximate volume? Egg cup, tablespoon or teaspoonful (any cause)?

Ask about related symptoms suggestive of an underlying disorder:

◆ Pleuritic chest pain, dyspnoea, fever and recent leg swelling (i.e. DVT) may suggest a PE. If so, elicit relevant risk factors for PE.

◆ A long history of dyspnoea may be associated with chronic lung disease or mitral stenosis.

◆ Progressive weight loss is suggestive of TB or bronchial carcinoma.

◆ Cough and purulent sputum imply infection – tuberculosis can present with fever, night sweats and haemoptysis.

◆ Lung cancer is suggested by lethargy, weight loss, lymphadenopathy, bone pain and paraneoplastic syndromes.

◆ Vasculitis is suggested by fevers, joint pains, haematuria, rash. Epistaxis and haemoptysis occur together with Wegener's granulomatosis and hereditary haemorrhagic telangiectasia.

Past history of cardiac or pulmonary (e.g. COPD, pneumonia, tuberculosis, recurrent infections suggesting bronchiectasis), history of vasculitis and specifically any history of rheumatic fever as a child which may have caused mitral stenosis. Recurrent haemoptysis over several years is common in bronchiectasis, but consider also TB, aspergilloma and lung malignancy.

Drug history (anticoagulants), contact history (areas endemic with TB, air travel), family history (e.g. haemorrhagic telangiectasia or a disorder of coagulation/thrombophilia), smoking history, occupational history (exposure to asbestosis).

Differential diagnosis

Pneumonia, lung cancer, bronchiectasis, pulmonary emboli, TB, overanticoagulation, rare causes (arteriovenous malformation, amyloidosis, sarcoidosis, foreign body, benign tumour, vasculitides, aspergilloma, mitral stenosis).

Investigations

These should be targeted at what is most likely. Possibilities include:

+ CXR (lung cancer, COPD, bronchiectasis, TB, pneumonia)
+ sputum (cytology if there is a suggestion of bronchial carcinoma, AFBs in the sputum for TB, respiratory culture for pneumonia)
+ blood tests (FBC, U/Es, anti-GBM antibodies, LFTs, clotting screen, cANCA, D-dimers, calcium)
+ ECG (right heart strain (PE), atrial fibrillation, urinary microscopy for red cell casts)
+ spirometry
+ oxygen saturation
+ CT scan of thorax (useful especially for bronchiectasis, PE and lung cancer)
+ bronchoscopy (lung cancer useful also for other sources of bleeding such as arteriovenous malformations)
+ aspirate of pleural effusion, biopsy of any tumour or relevant organ (e.g. kidney)
+ radioisotope scan (e.g. Q scan for pulmonary embolus)
+ previous investigations and treatment (e.g. surgical, radiotherapy, chemotherapy, palliative care)
+ echocardiogram (useful for both left and right ventricular failure, as well as mitral stenosis)

4. Breathlessness

Points in the history

Assessment of the premorbid state.

Account of symptoms (acute or chronic/progressive, sudden or insidious episodic, stepwise or continuous?).

+ Could the breathlessness be due to a cardiac complaint as well as a respiratory one? (Is the patient on a medication for chronic heart failure?)
+ Is the breathlessness progressive as in lung fibrosis, COPD or does it follow a diurnal rhythm such as in asthma?

◆ Is the breathlessness of rapid onset (e.g. foreign body, anaphylaxis, anxiety, pneumothorax or pulmonary embolism)?

◆ Is the onset of breathlessness associated with chest pain? Is the pain pleuritic?

◆ Does the breathlessness come on over a few minutes or hours? (If the onset lasts a few hours, consider asthma, COPD, chest infection, metabolic acidosis or left heart failure; asthma is distinguished by the absence of a history of chest pain, the absence of murmurs, and a previous history of asthma.)

◆ Is there a history of antecedent illness (e.g. pericardial tamponade)?

◆ Is there breathlessness sufficient to wake the patient at night, for example paroxysmal nocturnal dyspnoea, or noctural asthma?

◆ Does the breathlessness come on over several weeks (diffuse pulmonary fibrosis, chronic heart failure, recurrent pulmonary embolism, anaemia)?

◆ Is there dyspnoea at rest or exertion?

◆ Any difficulty sleeping because of symptoms? Usual symptoms during the day? Effects on daily activities? Effects of daily activities on symptoms? Concerns about illness?

◆ What is the impact of the disease, both physical and psychosocial?

Enquire about risk factors – past respiratory disease (recurrent pneumonias, previous pneumothorax TB), family history, smoking, hypertension, lipid profile, diabetes, atopy number of exacerbations per year.

Enquire about relevant triggers, including exercise, cold, smoking, occupational exposure (e.g. asbestos, compost), allergens (house dust mite, dog allergen, cat allergen, birds including parrots, pollen and moulds). Ask about any evidence of winter exacerbations (e.g. COPD).

Take a decent drug history (especially NSAIDs for wheeze, ACE for cough, drug-induced fibrosis, e.g. nitrofurantoin, busulphan), and occupational history (including asbestos and compost), social history (passive, pipe and cigarette smoking), travel history (atypical pneumonias and TB).

Differential diagnosis
Cardiovascular (LV systolic/diastolic failure), LVH, myocardial ischaemia, pericardial disease respiratory (COPD, asthma, upper respiratory tract obstruction, interstitial lung disease, respiratory infection, pleural effusion), other (anaemia, diabetic ketoacidosis, salicylate poisoning, hyperventilation syndrome). Features

of a hyperventilation syndrome include headaches, dizziness, palpitations and perioral paraesthesiae.

Investigations

These might include:

+ CXR (emphysema, asthma, consolidation, cardiac failure, pulmonary oedema, pneumothorax, bronchial carcinoma, foreign body)
+ FBC (to exclude anaemia, or polycythaemia)
+ ECG (especially arrhythmias)
+ PEFR
+ ABG (hypoxia, acidosis, hypocapnia, hypercapnia)
+ full lung function tests including spirometry, reversibility of forced expiratory volume in 1s, arteral blood gases (severity of disease and type of respiratory failure)
+ sputum and blood cultures should be taken if an infective aetiology is suspected; blood immunological investigations (if relevant)
+ bronchoscopy can be performed if a foreign body is aspirated; CT of thorax can evaluate masses of unknown aetiology
+ an echocardiogram is useful if cardiac failure or a valvular lesion is suspected; a Q scan or CTPA is useful if pulmonary emboli are suspected
+ demonstration of variable obstruction of the airways provides good evidence for asthma, with its characteristic morning dips. Failure to respond to bronchodilator therapy does not exclude asthma as response may be small in children, and in adults with persistent or more severe asthma. Those who fail to respond to inhaled bronchodilator require a steroid trial (either 4 weeks of high-dose inhaled steroids or 2 weeks of oral prednisolone).

Treatment

Consider the following approaches, but aim for diagnosis-driven treatment.

+ withdrawal of offending agent (e.g. fungus in hypersensitivity pneumonitis, drug in drug-induced lung fibrosis)
+ symptomatic treatment with bronchodilators and anticholinergics ?antibiotics
+ ?home oxygen therapy and inhaler technique (depends on degree of hypoxia and blood gases)

◆ consider also non-pharmacological treatments (e.g. postural adjustments and breathing exercises to relieve anxiety, fan cooling)

5. Pneumothorax

Management of a pneumothorax

A **pneumothorax** is termed primary if there is no underlying disease, and secondary if there is.

Primary pneumothorax

Recommendations include:

◆ If the rim of air is <2 cm and the patient is not short of breath then discharge should be considered.

◆ Otherwise, aspiration should be attempted.

◆ If this fails, then repeat aspiration should be considered.

◆ If this fails, then a chest drain should be inserted.

Secondary pneumothorax

Recommendations include:

◆ If the patient is >50 years old and the rim of air is >2 cm and the patient is short of breath, then a chest drain should be inserted.

◆ Otherwise, aspiration should be attempted. If aspiration fails, a chest drain should be inserted. All patients should be admitted for at least 24 hours.

6. Pulmonary embolism

You should have an understanding of the BTS guidelines for the treatment of a suspected thromboembolism.

Key points from these guidelines provide that:

◆ CTPA is now recommended as the initial lung-imaging modality for a non-massive PE. Advantages compared to a V/Q scan include: speed, easier to perform out of hours, a reduced need for further imaging and the possibility of providing a further diagnosis if PE is excluded.

◆ If the CTPA is negative, patients do not need further investigations or treatment for PE.

◆ Perfusion scanning may be used initially if appropriate facilities exist, the chest X-ray is normal and there is no significant concomitant cardiopulmonary disease.

✦ Anticoagulation: low molecular weight heparin (LMWH), rather than unfractionated heparin (UFH) should be used routinely in patients with suspected pulmonary embolism. This reflects the equal efficacy and safety of LMWHs as well as their ease of use. Exceptions include patients with a massive PE or in situations where rapid reversal of anticoagulation may be necessary. Warfarinisation: the standard duration of anticoagulation is 4–6 weeks if temporary risk factors are present, 3 months for the first idiopathic PE and at least 6 months for other situations.

Thrombolysis is now recommended as the first-line treatment for massive PE where there is circulatory failure (e.g. hypotension).

If a **massive PE** is suspected or confirmed PE with hypotension, collapse, hypoxia, evidence of right heart strain (ECHO/CT), raised troponin +/– raised BNP, then consider thrombolysis. Further management points are:

✦ stable patient: alteplase 100 mg in 90 minutes

✦ unstable/deteriorating patient: alteplase 50 mg stat as per BTS guidelines

✦ thrombolysis is followed by unfractionated heparin after 3 hours

Other invasive approaches should be considered where appropriate facilities exist.

7. Asthma

Points in the history

Questions relating to current symptoms: onset and duration of symptoms, nature of symptoms (cough, sputum, haemoptysis, worsening wheeze, fever, chest pain, disturbance of sleep, presence of nocturnal cough) any diurnal variation, precipitating factors – infection, contact with known allergens, stress, exercise, poor compliance with medication how the PEFR has changed.

Questions relating to where the diagnosis was made: underlying stability/severity of disease, reversibility associated with therapy, usual treatment – home nebulisers, steroids, previous exacerbations and their management (whether in hospital?), days taken off work, previous admissions to ITU and whether patient was ventilated in the past, primary or secondary care of management.

Previous medical history: eczema, atopy, nasal polyps, recent surgery.

Drug history: NSAIDs, beta-blockers, common allergies (including drug allergies).

Travel history: recent air travel (are the symptoms actually suggestive of a pulmonary embolus?).

Social history: anxiety and stress, smoking. Family history: asthma, clotting disorders.

Investigations
PEFR, pulse oximeter, arterial blood gases, CXR, FBC, U&E, CRP and ESR, sputum MC+S, spiral CT scan, lung funtion tests, serum precipitins.

Management
The British Thoracic Society guidelines take a practical approach to the diagnosis of asthma. If a patient has typical symptoms of asthma, a trial of treatment is recommended. Normal spirometry when the patient is well does not exclude a diagnosis of asthma. The 2009 British Thoracic Society guidelines marked a subtle change in the approach to diagnosing asthma.

It suggested dividing patients into a high, intermediate and low probability of having asthma based on the presence or absence of typical symptoms. A list can be found in the external link, but include typical symptoms such as wheeze, nocturnal cough, etc.

Example of features used to assess asthma are shown in Table 12.1.

TABLE 12.1 The diagnosis of asthma

Increase possibility of diagnosis of asthma	Decrease possibility of diagnosis of asthma
• Wheeze, breathlessness, chest tightness and cough, worse at night/early morning	• Prominent dizziness, light-headedness, peripheral tingling
• History of atopic disorder	• Chronic productive cough in the absence of wheeze or breathlessness
• Wheeze heard on auscultation	• Repeatedly normal physical examination
• Unexplained peripheral blood eosinophilia	• Significant smoking history (i.e. >20 pack-years)
	• Normal PEF or spirometry when symptomatic

Management is based on this assessment:

◈ high probability: trial of treatment

◈ intermediate probability: see below

◈ low probability: investigate/treat other condition

For patients with an intermediate probability of asthma, further investigations are suggested. The guidelines state that spirometry is the preferred initial test:

◆ FEV_1/FVC <0.7: trial of treatment

◆ FEV_1/FVC >0.7: further investigation/consider referral

Recent studies have shown the limited value of other 'objective' tests. It is now recognised that in patients with normal or near-normal pretreatment lung function there is little room for measurable improvement in FEV_1 or peak flow.

A >400 ml improvement in FEV_1 is considered significant:

◆ before and after 400 mcg inhaled salbutamol in patients with diagnostic uncertainty and airflow obstruction present at the time of assessment

◆ if there is an incomplete response to inhaled salbutamol, after either inhaled corticosteroids (200 mcg twice daily beclometasone equivalent for 6–8 weeks) or oral prednisolone (30 mg once daily for 14 days)

It is now advised to interpret peak flow variability with caution due to the poor sensitivity of the test:

◆ diurnal variation % = ((highest–lowest PEFR)/highest PEFR) × 100

◆ assessment should be made over 2 weeks

◆ greater than 20% diurnal variation is considered significant

Step-wise management in adults

The management of stable asthma is now well established with a step-wise approach, given in Table 12.2.

TABLE 12.2 Management of asthma

Step 1	Inhaled short-acting β2 agonist as required
Step 2	Add inhaled steroid at 200–800 mcg/day
	400 mcg is an appropriate starting dose for many patients; start at dose of inhaled steroid appropriate to severity of disease
Step 3	1. Add inhaled long-acting β2 agonist (LABA)
	2. Assess control of asthma:
	• good response to LABA: continue LABA
	• benefit from LABA but control still inadequate: continue LABA and increase inhaled steroid dose to 800 mcg/day (if not already on this dose)
	• no response to LABA: stop LABA and increase inhaled steroid to 800 mcg/day; if control still inadequate, institute trial of other therapies, leukotriene receptor antagonist or SR theophylline

(continued)

Step 4   Consider trials of:

  • increasing inhaled steroid up to 2000 mcg/day

  • addition of a fourth drug, *e.g.* leukotriene receptor antagonist, SR theophylline, β2 agonist tablet

Step 5   Use daily steroid tablet in lowest dose providing adequate control

Consider other treatments to minimise the use of steroid tablets

Maintain high-dose inhaled steroid at 2000 mcg/day

Refer patient for specialist care

ADDITIONAL NOTES

Leukotriene receptor antagonists, e.g. montelukast, zafirlukastchave both anti-inflammatory and bronchodilatory properties should be used when patients are poorly controlled on high-dose inhaled corticosteroids and a long-acting b2-agonist particularly useful in aspirin-induced asthma associated with the development of Churg-Strauss syndrome.

Fluticasone is more lipophilic and has a longer duration of action than beclometasone. Hydrofluoroalkane is now replacing chlorofluorocarbon as the propellant of choice. Only half the usual dose is needed with hydrofluoroalkane due to the smaller size of the particles.

Long acting β2-agonists act as bronchodilators but also inhibit mediator release from mast cells. Eformoterol has an onset of action similar to that of salbutamol. A recent meta-analysis showed adding salmeterol improved symptoms compared to doubling the inhaled steroid dose.

8. Acute severe asthma

Patients with acute severe asthma are stratified into moderate, severe or life-threatening. This is shown in Table 12.3.

TABLE 12.3 Features of acute severe asthma

Moderate	Severe	Life-threatening
• PEF >50% best or predicted	• PEF 33%–50% best or predicted	• PEF <33% best or predicted
• Speech normal	• Can't complete sentences	• Oxygen sats <92%
• RR <25/minute	• RR >25/minute	• Silent chest, cyanosis or feeble respiratory effort
• Pulse <110 bpm	• Pulse >110 bpm	• Bradycardia, dysrhythmia or hypotension
		• Exhaustion, confusion or coma

British Thoracic Society guidelines 2003 (updated 2004) suggested originally:

◆ magnesium sulphate recommended as next step for patients who are not responding (e.g. 1.2–2 g IV over 20 minutes)

◆ little evidence to support use of IV aminophylline (although still mentioned in management plans)

◆ if no response consider IV salbutamol

9. Chronic obstructive pulmonary disease

The NICE guideline CG12 sets out the principles of management of chronic obstructive airways disease (COPD). In this document, there is a very helpful algorithm for the initial diagnosis of COPD.

General principles of subsequent management

◆ smoking cessation advice

◆ pneumococcal vaccine

◆ annual influenza vaccine

Stages of therapy

◆ short-acting β2-agonist is first-line treatment

◆ if still symptomatic add a long-acting anti-cholinergic (e.g. tiotropium)

+ if severe COPD (FEV_1 <50% predicted or who are having two or more exacerbations requiring treatment with antibiotics or oral corticosteroids in a 12-month period) add a long-acting β2-agonist/inhaler corticosteroid combination inhaler (e.g. Seretide)

If the patient is symptomatic despite the above measures:

+ oral theophylline

Mucolytics

The role of mucolytics is still being evaluated but they appear to reduce exacerbation, frequency and duration.

Factors which may improve survival in patients with stable COPD

+ smoking cessation – the single most important intervention in patients who are still smoking
+ long-term oxygen therapy (>15 hours of use/day) in patients who fit criteria
+ lung volume reduction in selected patients by either surgery or bronchoscopically

The functions of oxygen therapy

The British Thoracic Society published guidelines on emergency oxygen therapy in 2008. The following selected points are taken from the guidelines. Please see the link provided for the full guidelines.

Oxygen saturation targets

+ acutely ill patients: 94%–98%
+ patients at risk of hypercapnia (e.g. COPD patients): 88%–92% (see below)
+ oxygen should be reduced in stable patients with satisfactory oxygen saturation

Management of COPD patients

+ prior to the availability of blood gases, use a 28% venturi mask at 4 L/min and aim for an oxygen saturation of 88%–92% for patients with risk factors for hypercapnia but no prior history of respiratory acidosis
+ adjust target range to 94%–98% if the pCO_2 is normal

Situations where oxygen therapy should **not** be used routinely if there is no evidence of hypoxia:

+ myocardial infarction and acute coronary syndromes
+ stroke
+ obstetric emergencies
+ anxiety-related hyperventilation

After smoking cessation, long-term oxygen therapy is one of the few interventions that has been shown to improve survival in COPD.

10. Bronchiectasis
Bronchiectasis describes a permanent dilatation of the airways secondary to chronic infection or inflammation.

Causes
There is a wide variety of causes:

+ post-infective: tuberculosis, measles, pertussis, pneumonia
+ cystic fibrosis
+ bronchial obstruction, e.g. lung cancer/foreign body
+ immune deficiency: selective IgA, hypogammaglobulinaemia
+ allergic bronchopulmonary aspergillosis (ABPA)
+ ciliary dyskinetic syndromes: e.g. Kartagener's syndrome
+ yellow nail syndrome

Management
After assessing for treatable causes (e.g. immune deficiency) management is as follows:

+ physical training (e.g. inspiratory muscle training) – has a reasonably good evidence base for patients with non-cystic fibrosis bronchiectasis
+ postural drainage/clearance techniques
+ antibiotics for exacerbations + long-term rotating antibiotics in severe cases
+ bronchodilators in selected cases
+ immunisations
+ surgery in selected cases (e.g. very localised disease)

Kartagener's syndrome

Kartagener's syndrome (also known as primary ciliary dyskinesia) was first described in 1933 and most frequently occurs in examinations due to its association with dextrocardia (e.g. 'quiet heart sounds', 'small volume complexes in lateral leads').

Features

- dextrocardia or complete situs inversus
- bronchiectasis
- recurrent sinusitis
- subfertility (secondary to diminished sperm motility and defective ciliary action in the Fallopian tubes)

11. Recognition of adverse prognostic features of pneumonia
The CURB-65 criteria of severe pneumonia are:

- confusion (abbreviated mental score $< \text{⁸⁄₁₀}$)
- urea >7 mmol/L
- respiratory rate = 30/minute
- bp: systolic <90 mmHg or diastolic <60 mmHg
- age >65 years

Patients with three or more of these factors are regarded as having a severe pneumonia. Other poor prognostic factors include:

- presence of co-existing disease
- hypoxaemia independent of FiO_2

12. Occupational lung disease
Occupational asthma
Causes

- isocyanates
- platinum salts
- soldering flux resin
- glutaraldehyde
- flour

- epoxy resins
- proteolytic enzymes

Diagnosis

Specific recommendations are made in the 2007 joint British Thoracic Society and SIGN guidelines. You are recommended to read these.

Please note, however, that serial measurements of peak expiratory flow are recommended at work and away from work.

13. Extrinsic allergic alveolitis

Extrinsic allergic alveolitis (EAA) is a condition caused by hypersensitivity-induced lung damage due to a variety of inhaled organic particles. It is thought to be largely caused by immune-complex mediated tissue damage (type III hypersensitivity) although delayed hypersensitivity (type IV) is also thought to play a role in EAA, especially in the chronic phase.

Examples

- bird fancier's lung (avian proteins)
- farmer's lung (spores of *Micropolyspora faeni*)
- malt worker's lung (*Aspergillus clavatus*)
- mushroom worker's lung (thermophilic actinomycetes)

Presentation

- acute: occurs 4–8 hours after exposure with SOB, dry cough and fever
- chronic symptoms of SOB and dry cough but usually without fever

Investigation

- CXR: upper lobe fibrosis
- BAL: lymphocytosis
- blood: NO eosinophilia

14. Farmer's lung

Farmer's lung is an example of extrinsic allergic alveolitis (EAA) caused by hypersensitivity-induced lung damage due to a variety of inhaled organic particles. It is thought to be largely caused by immune-complex mediated tissue damage (type III hypersensitivity) although delayed hypersensitivity (type IV) is also thought to play a role in EAA, especially in the chronic phase. Farmer's lung is caused by spores of *Micropolyspora faeni*. Presentation can be acute (this occurs 4–8 hrs after exposure and causes SOB, dry cough, fever) or can be chronic. Investigation shows upper lobe fibrosis on the CXR, lymphocytosis on the BAL and NO eosinophilia in the blood.

15. Pneumoconiosis

Examples

✦ coal – upper-zone fibrosis as well as the formation of nodular lesions within the lungs

✦ silicosis – upper-zone fibrosis with eggshell hilar calcification that predisposes to TB infection

✦ berylliosis – granulomatous lesions resulting in fibrosis, similar to sarcoid

16. Asbestos-related lung disease

The severity of asbestosis is related to the length of exposure. This is in contrast to mesothelioma where even very limited exposure can cause disease. Asbestosis typically causes lower lobe fibrosis. Crocidolite (blue) asbestos is the most dangerous form.

Usually the disease occurs >20 years after exposure, proportional to the intensity of exposure. It is characterised by exertional dyspnoea, dry cough, and inspiratory crackles in lower zones.

Chest X-ray may show irregular opacities, and with more advanced disease, honeycombing. Pulmonary function tests reveal restrictive lung disease with a reduced transfer factor.

Lung cancer is increased synergistically with smoking, and the risk of mesothelioma is markedly increased.

Patients are eligible for industrial injury benefit. Benign pleural disease involves plaques, diffuse pleural thickening, effusion and calcification. Benign pleural disease is usually asymptomatic and detected on CXR. Patients are usually not eligible for industrial injury benefit. Mesothelioma normally occurs >30 years and is almost always caused by asbestosis. High-risk asbestosis is crocidolite (blue asbestos). Diagnosis is confirmed by pleural biopsy.

17. Sleep disorders

The most important sleep disorder for the MRCP(UK) is obstructive sleep apnoea. You should have a thorough knowledge of the **current NICE guidance on this, TA139.**

Predisposing factors

- obesity
- macroglossia: acromegaly, hypothyroidism, amyloidosis
- large tonsils
- Marfan's syndrome
- acromegaly
- hypothyroidism
- Cushing's syndrome

Consequences

- daytime somnolence
- multiple nocturnal wakenings
- hypertension
- right heart strain
- polycythaemia

Please see the SIGN guidelines for the diagnosis and management of patients with OSAHS, published in 2003.

Assessment of sleepiness

- Epworth Sleepiness Scale – questionnaire completed by patient +/– partner
- STOP-BANG questionnaire

Diagnostic tests

- sleep studies – ranging from monitoring of pulse oximetry at night to full polysomnography where a wide variety of physiological factors are measured including EEG, respiratory airflow, thoraco-abdominal movement, snoring and pulse oximetry
- Multiple Sleep Latency Test (MSLT) – measures the time to fall asleep in a dark room (using EEG criteria)

Management

◈ weight loss

◈ CPAP is first-line for moderate or severe OSAHS

◈ intra-oral devices (e.g. mandibular advancement) may be used if CPAP is not tolerated or for patients with mild OSAHS where there is no daytime sleepiness

◈ limited evidence to support use of pharmacological agents

BOX 12.1   A note on cor pulmonale secondary to OSA

Cor pulmonale secondary to diurnal respiratory failure can occur in patients with severe obstructive sleep apnoea (OSA). Typically, this might be an elderly patient with a high BMI, but presents with impotence, nocturia and depression. He might be hypoxic at rest on air and have ankle oedema. Most patients who develop this complication have lower airway obstruction (from smoking), gross obesity or respiratory muscle weakness.

---

18. Bronchial carcinoid

Bronchial carcinoid is a highly vascular 'cherry-like' tumour causing recurrent haemoptysis and bronchial obstruction. It may rarely produce the classical symptoms of carcinoid syndrome, such as cyanotic flushings, intestinal cramps and diarrhoea following liver metastases in 5% of cases.

Bronchoscopy identifies up to 80% of carcinoid tumours in the main bronchi. Biopsy is usually followed with brisk bleeding and should be done via rigid bronchoscopy.

19. Tuberculosis

Points in the history

Ask about the duration of symptom relevant to a putative diagnosis of tuberculosis.

?is the cough productive, ?sputum – quantity and colour, ?is there haemoptysis (see above), ?is there chest pain often related to pleurisy, ?is there shortness of breath, ?is there a temperature, ?is there loss of weight

Pulmonary TB: typically causes a slow onset of symptoms including productive cough, haemoptysis, weight loss and night sweats.

Neurological TB: cranial nerve palsies, meningitis, spinal cord involvement.

Rashes: e.g. lupus vulgaris, erythema nodosum. Adrenals: lethargy, anorexia and dizziness. Atypical pneumonias. Sarcoidosis.

Previous medical history: BCG vaccination or recent Mantoux/Heaf test immunosuppression – HIV, immunosuppressive drugs, other recent infections, e.g. shingles.

Drug history: previous treatment for TB. Family history: TB and contacts with them. Travel history: especially to areas endemic of TB. Social history: occupational, crowded accommodation, contacts, alcohol dependence syndrome, living rough. Sexual history: HIV/AIDS.

Investigations

Repeat CXR, sputum smear and microscopy, Gram's stain, Ziehl-Neelsen stain, blood cultures, FBC, film – haemolysis. LFTs prior to anti-TB therapy, hepatitis, U&E – hyponatraemia, complement fixation test, HIV test, interferon-γ (interferon-gamma) release assays (IGRAs, e.g. ELISpot), Mantoux test serum, ACE sputum culture for TB, pulmonary function tests, consider pleural biopsy CT and biopsy.

The presence of acid-fast bacilli yet absence of TB suggests an atypical acid-fast bacilli such as *Mycobacterium avium-intracellulare*.

Management

Hepatotoxicity is a feature of antituberculous treatment. Liver function should be checked before treatment for clinical cases.

Quadruple therapy, side effects (rifampicin – red urine, tears; isoniazid – impaired LFTs, peripheral neuropathy; pyrazinamide – arthralgia and sideroblastic anaemia; ethambutol – optic neuritis and peripheral neuropathy) for 2 months then dual therapy (rifampicin and isoniazid) for 4 months. TB is a notifiable disease. Regular f/u. Rifampicin results in less effective oral contraception.

20. Sarcoidosis

Sarcoidosis is a multi-system disorder of unknown aetiology characterised by non-caseating granulomas. It is more common in young adults and in people of African descent.

Affects:

- lungs
- joints
- eyes (uveitis, uveoparotitis and retinal inflammation)
- skin (granuloma lesions, erythema nodosum, lupus pernio)

✦ heart (arrhythmias, sudden death)

✦ nervous system

✦ systemic symptoms (night sweats, lethargy, weight loss)

Indications for steroids include:

✦ hypercalcaemia

✦ worsening lung function

✦ eye, heart or neurological involvement

21. Pulmonary eosinophilia

Causes of pulmonary eosinophilia

✦ Churg-Strauss syndrome

✦ allergic bronchopulmonary aspergillosis (ABPA)

✦ Loeffler's syndrome

✦ eosinophilic pneumonia

✦ hypereosinophilic syndrome

✦ tropical pulmonary eosinophilia

✦ drugs: nitrofurantoin, sulphonamides

✦ less common: Wegener's granulomatosis

Loeffler's syndrome

✦ transient CXR shadowing and blood eosinophilia

✦ thought to be due to parasites such as *Ascaris lumbricoides* causing an alveolar reaction

✦ presents with a fever, cough and night sweats which often last for less than 2 weeks

✦ generally a self-limiting disease

Tropical pulmonary eosinophilia

✦ associated with *Wuchereria bancrofti* infection

Allergic bronchopulmonary aspergillosis (ABPA)

✦ Immediate (type I) reactions occur in virtually all patients with ABPA following intradermal injections of *A. fumigatus* extracts, with only 16% developing delayed (type IV) reactions.

◆ Precipitating IgG antibodies are present in 70% of patients.

◆ Transfer factor may be affected in the later fibrotic stage of the disease.

◆ Haemoptysis is a symptom of aspergilloma and bronchiectasis, but is not characteristic of ABPA.

22. Fat embolism

Fat embolism is thought to occur as a result of release of lipid globules from damaged bone marrow fat cells. Another mechanism that has been suggested is the increased mobilisation of fatty acids peripherally.

The effects that are seen clinically depend on what part of the microvasculature is affected by the lipid globules.

Pulmonary symptoms are caused by ventilation perfusion mismatch. Confusion (cerebral effects) may be seen, as well as a petechial rash caused by capillary damage in the skin.

23. Methaemoglobinaemia

A patient with methaemoglobinaemia may typically appear desaturated with saturations of 85%, yet good pO_2. This is a typical description of methaemoglobinaemia, which is the accumulation of reversibly oxidised methaemoglobin causing reduced oxygen affinity of the Hb molecule with consequent cyanosis. It can occur due to an inherited condition or as a consequence of drugs such as nitrites.

24. Cystic fibrosis (CF)

Importance

Over 7000 people have cystic fibrosis in the United Kingdom. It is the commonest genetically inherited disease in white populations (one in 2500 newborns), although it is increasingly recognised as being important in non-white populations.

Genetics

Cystic fibrosis is an autosomal recessive disease.

It is caused by mutations in the *CFTR* (cystic fibrosis transmembrane conductance regulator) gene. The commonest mutation is the deletion of phenylalanine at codon 508 (phe508del, until recently known as ΔF508). This occurs in about 70% of patients with cystic fibrosis. Over 1600 mutations of the *CFTR* gene have been described.

Different mutations in this gene have varying effects on CFTR function and can result in different phenotypes of the disease. Some mutations will result in milder forms of the disease. The CFTR protein is expressed in many cells and has several functions, not all of which have been linked with disease. The primary function of the CFTR protein is as an ion channel that regulates liquid volume on epithelial surfaces through chloride secretion and inhibition of sodium absorption.

Clinical features

Disease manifests in many organs, but most notably the upper and lower airways, pancreas, bowel and reproductive tracts. For most patients, lung disease is the most important problem in terms of symptoms, treatment required and the fact that it is the most likely cause of death.

Diagnosis

The optimal diagnostic test for cystic fibrosis is the measurement of sweat electrolyte levels. Patients with the disease have raised concentrations of sodium and chloride (>60 mmol/L, diagnostic; 40–60 mmol/L, intermediate (but more likely to be diagnostic in infants); <40 mmol/L, normal).

Newer techniques have reduced the amount of sweat needed. The test needs to be done by someone trained and experienced. For this reason the diagnosis will usually be made in secondary and tertiary centres, although primary care professionals play a vital role in identifying the patients who need investigation.

The UK now has a programme for screening all newborns for cystic fibrosis using the Guthrie blood spot test. The initial screen is for raised concentrations of immunoreactive trypsinogen. Positive samples will be tested for common *CFTR* gene mutations followed by a second screen for immunoreactive trypsinogen, if required.

Management

Most patients in the UK and Europe receive care coordinated by a tertiary cystic fibrosis centre, which improves outcomes. However, patients benefit greatly from links with and access to local care, in many cases having formalised 'shared care' with local clinics.

Primary care teams can provide valuable help with surveillance and early treatment of infection; dietary and nutritional support; and social and psychological support for patients and families. Primary care also provides continuity during the difficult transition from paediatric to adult care; an informative patient's perspective of the issues encountered during this period has recently been published.

B. Malignant lung conditions

1. Lung cancer

The current guidance on the management of lung cancer is given in the NICE document CG24.

The **NICE CG24 guideline** suggests some urgent criteria for lung cancer. These are as follows:

◆ An urgent chest X-ray should be offered to patients presenting with haemoptysis, or any of the following if unexplained or present for more than 3 weeks:

- cough
- chest/shoulder pain
- dyspnoea
- weight loss
- chest signs
- hoarseness
- finger clubbing
- signs suggesting metastases (for example, in brain, bone, liver or skin)
- cervical/supraclavicular lymphadenopathy

◆ An urgent referral should be offered to lung cancer MDT (usually the chest physician) while waiting for chest X-ray results if any of the following are present:

- persistent haemoptysis in a smoker or ex-smoker older than 40 years
- signs of superior vena cava obstruction (swelling of the face and/or neck with fixed elevation of jugular venous pressure – consider emergency referral)
- stridor (consider emergency referral)

It is well known that the incidence of adenocarcinoma is rising in comparison to the other types of non-small cell lung cancer. Indeed, adenocarcinoma is now the most common type of lung cancer in the USA. In the UK, however, squamous cell cancer remains the most common subtype.

Whilst many chemicals have been implicated in the development of lung cancer, passive smoking is the most likely cause. Up to 15% of lung cancers in patients who do not smoke are thought to be caused by passive smoking.

Risk factors
Smoking

✦ increases risk of lung Ca by a factor of 10

Other factors

✦ asbestos – increases risk of lung Ca by a factor of five

✦ arsenic

✦ radon

✦ nickel

✦ chromate

✦ aromatic hydrocarbon

✦ cryptogenic fibrosing alveolitis

Factors that are NOT related

✦ coal dust

Note that smoking and asbestos are thought to be synergistic positive risk factors.

Please note carefully the contraindications to lung cancer surgery, including SVC obstruction, FEV <1.5, malignant pleural effusion and vocal cord paralysis.

Surgery is not suitable for a patient diagnosed with small cell lung cancer. The reason for this is that small cell cancer is usually metastatic at the time of presentation. Surgery and radiotherapy are only used for de-bulking, but a good response to chemotherapy can persist for a period of about 4 months.

Operability of lung cancers

Inoperable non-small cell carcinomas are stages IIIb or IV (distant metastasis).
Stage IIIb is either:

✦ N3 (metastasis to contralateral mediastinal lymph nodes, contralateral hilar lymph nodes, ipsilateral supraclavicular lymph nodes) or

✦ T4 (tumour of any size invading mediastinum or involving heart, great vessels, trachea, oesophagus, vertebral body, carina, or presence of malignant pleural effusion)

Further lung function tests are needed (for example, transfer factor, exercise testing) if post-bronchodilator FEV1 <1.5 litres for lobectomy and FEV1 <2 litres for pneumonectomy. Patients with limited chest wall invasion and no evidence of distant metastases are considered potentially curable (stage IIIA).

2. Bronchoalveolar carcinoma

Bronchoalveolar carcinoma is a distinct subtype of adenocarcinoma with a classic manifestation as an interstitial lung disease on chest radiograph.

Bronchoalveolar carcinoma arises from type II pneumocytes and grows along alveolar septa.

This subtype may manifest as a solitary peripheral nodule, multifocal disease, or a rapidly progressing pneumonic form. A characteristic finding in persons with advanced disease is voluminous watery sputum.

3. Superior vena cava obstruction (SVCO)

[This is discussed in Chapter 5.]

C. The impact of systemic disease on the respiratory system

1. Vasculitis

Vasculitis refers to a heterogeneous group of disorders that are characterised by inflammatory destruction of blood vessels. Both arteries and veins are affected. Lymphangitis is sometimes considered a type of vasculitis. Solitary inflammation of veins (phlebitis) or arteries (arteritis), although both occur in vasculitis, on their own are separate entities. Vasculitis affects both arteries and veins. Vasculitis is primarily due to leucocyte migration and resultant damage.

Classification

There are many ways to classify vasculitis. It can be classified by the underlying cause.

Vasculitides can also be classified by the type or size of the blood vessels that they predominantly affect. Apart from the arteritis/phlebitis distinction mentioned above, vasculitis is often classified by the calibre of the vessel affected. However, it should be noted that there can be some variation in the size of the vessels affected.

Causes

Some disorders have vasculitis as their main feature, including:

◆ Kawasaki disease

◆ Behçet's disease

- polyarteritis nodosa
- Wegener's granulomatosis
- cryoglobulinaemia
- Takayasu's arteritis
- Churg-Strauss syndrome
- giant cell arteritis (temporal arteritis)
- Henoch-Schönlein purpura

There are many conditions that have vasculitis as an accompanying or atypical symptom, including:
1. rheumatic diseases, such as rheumatoid arthritis and systemic lupus erythematosus
2. cancer, such as lymphomas
3. infections, such as hepatitis C
4. exposure to chemicals and drugs, such as amphetamines or cocaine

Symptoms
Possible symptoms included in the respiratory system: e.g. nose bleeds, bloody cough, lung infiltrates.

Diagnosis
Laboratory tests of blood or body fluids are performed for patients with active vasculitis. Their results will generally show signs of inflammation in the body, such as increased ESR elevated CRP, anaemia, increased white blood cell count and eosinophilia.

Other possible findings are elevated anti-neutrophil cytoplasmic antibody (ANCA) levels and haematuria. Other organ functional tests may be abnormal. Specific abnormalities depend on the degree of various organs' involvement.

The definite diagnosis of vasculitis is, nonetheless, established after a biopsy of involved organ or tissue, such as lung. The biopsy elucidates the pattern of blood vessel inflammation. An alternative to biopsy can be an angiogram (X-ray test of the blood vessels). It can demonstrate characteristic patterns of inflammation in affected blood vessels.

Treatment
Treatments are generally directed toward stopping the inflammation and suppressing the immune system.

Typically, cortisone-related medications, such as prednisone, are used. Additionally, other immune suppression drugs, such as cyclophosphamide and others, are considered.

Additionally, affected organs (such as the heart or lungs) may require specific medical treatment intended to improve their function during the active phase of the disease.

2. Myasthenia gravis and respiratory complications

Patients with increasingly troublesome symptoms of myasthenia gravis (severe myasthenia gravis) can suffer from potentially fatal respiratory complications including profound respiratory muscle weakness. Acute respiratory failure can occur and prompt the initiation of mechanical ventilation.

Once the precipitating factor(s) of the crisis has been reversed, weaning from ventilatory assistance is begun only if the patient has recovered sufficiently and treatment goals have been realised.

Myasthenic crisis refers to a rapid deterioration in neuromuscular function with respiratory compromise precipitated by ventilatory muscle insufficiency, weakness of upper airway musculature or some combination of these two processes. Crisis may be triggered by multiple factors.

3. HIV/AIDS

Pneumocystis carinii pneumonia

Whilst the organism *Pneumocystis carinii* is now referred to as *Pneumocystis jirovecii*, the term *Pneumocystis carinii* pneumonia (PCP) is still in common use.

- *Pneumocystis jirovecii* is a unicellular eukaryote, generally classified as a fungus but some authorities consider it a protozoa.
- PCP is the most common opportunistic infection in AIDS.
- All patients with a CD4 count <200/mm^3 should receive PCP prophylaxis.

Features

- dyspnoea (often severe)
- dry cough
- fever
- very few chest signs

Extrapulmonary manifestations are rare (1%–2% of cases); may cause:

- hepatosplenomegaly

⬧ lymphadenopathy

⬧ choroid lesions

Investigation

⬧ CXR: typically shows bilateral interstitial pulmonary infiltrates but can present with other X-ray findings, e.g. lobar consolidation. May be normal.

⬧ Exercise-induced desaturation.

⬧ Sputum often fails to show PCP, bronchoalveolar lavage (BAL) is often needed to demonstrate PCP (silver stain).

Management

⬧ co-trimoxazole

⬧ IV pentamidine in severe cases

⬧ steroids if hypoxic (if pO_2 <9.3 kPa then steroids reduce risk of respiratory failure by 50% and death by a third)

D. Specialised respiratory investigations

1. Arterial blood gases

E.g. respiratory alkalosis

Common causes

⬧ anxiety leading to hyperventilation

⬧ salicylate poisoning (usually a mixed respiratory alkalosis and metabolic acidosis)

⬧ CNS disorders: stroke, subarachnoid haemorrhage, encephalitis

⬧ altitude

⬧ pregnancy

⬧ pulmonary embolism

2. Respiratory immunology tests

A radio-allergosorbent test (RAST) determines the amount of IgE that reacts specifically with suspected or known allergens, for example IgE to egg protein. Results are given in grades from 0 (negative) to 6 (strongly positive). It is useful for food allergies, inhaled allergens (e.g. pollen) and wasp/bee venom. Blood tests may be used when skin prick tests are not suitable, for example if there is extensive eczema or if the patient is taking antihistamines.

3. Radiological aspects of respiratory disease

You should ideally revise this with a decent radiological atlas featuring common conditions in respiratory medicine (especially for the MRCP(UK) Part 2 Written). You are unlikely to be presented with radiological images for MRCP(UK) Part 1: please check the current guidelines.

Bilateral hilar lymphadenopathy (BHL)

The most common causes of bilateral hilar lymphadenopathy are:

* sarcoidosis
* tuberculosis
* lymphoma
* other malignancy
* pneumoconiosis, e.g. berylliosis
* fungi, e.g. histoplasmosis, coccidioidomycosis

The staging of the sarcoidosis X-ray is as follows:

    Stage 1 – BHL
    Stage 2 – BHL + infiltrates
    Stage 3 – infiltrates
    Stage 4 – fibrosis

Loefgren's syndrome

Loefgren's syndrome is an acute form of sarcoidosis characterised by bilateral hilar lymphadenopathy (BHL), erythema nodosum, fever and polyarthralgia. It typically occurs in young females and carries an excellent prognosis.

Fibrosis on the chest X-ray

It is important in the exam to be able to differentiate between conditions causing predominately upper or lower zone fibrosis. It should be noted that the more common causes (cryptogenic fibrosing alveolitis, drugs) tend to affect the lower zones.

Fibrosis predominately affecting the upper zones

* extrinsic allergic alveolitis
* coal worker's pneumoconiosis/progressive massive fibrosis
* silicosis
* sarcoidosis
* ankylosing spondylitis (*rare*)
* histiocytosis
* tuberculosis

Fibrosis predominately affecting the *lower* zones

* cryptogenic fibrosing alveolitis
* most connective tissue disorders (except ankylosing spondylitis)
* drug-induced: amiodarone, bleomycin, methotrexate
* asbestosis

After a chest X-ray, a high-resolution CT chest is often diagnostic with good correlation to histological abnormalities. A ground-glass appearance is associated with predominantly cellular appearance on biopsy and more active disease which responds to treatment and has a better prognosis. A reticular pattern is suggestive of destroyed fibrotic lungs.

In cryptogenic fibrosing alveolitis, active inflammation may be suggested by a CT scan. The presence of a predominantly ground-glass appeerence is also an independent predictor of survival.

Drug-induced lung fibrosis

Methotrexate is a recognised cause of pulmonary fibrosis. However, it is sometimes used in the treatment of idiopathic pulmonary fibrosis as a steroid sparing agent.

Pulmonary parenchymal or pleural reactions to chemotherapeutic agents used in the management of patients with malignant diseases are being recognised with increasing frequency. Alkylating agents, asparaginase, bleomycin, methotrexate and procarbazine have all been implicated. Drug-related interstitial pneumonia should also be considered in rheumatoid arthritis patients on methotrexate or newer drugs such as leflunomide.

Causes of a cavitating lesion
Differential diagnosis

+ tuberculosis

+ lung cancer (especially squamous cell)

+ abscess (*Staphyloccus aureus*, *Klebsiella* and *Pseudomonas*)

+ Wegener's granulomatosis

+ pulmonary embolism

+ rheumatoid arthritis

+ aspergillosis, histoplasmosis, coccidioidomycosis

4. Respiratory function tests

Respiratory function tests can be used to determine whether a respiratory disease is obstructive or restrictive. Table 12.4 summarises the main findings in obstructive and restrictive lung diseases.

TABLE 12.4 Obstructive and restrictive lung disesases

Obstructive lung disease	Restrictive lung disease
FEV_1 slightly reduced	**FEV_1 – reduced**
FVC reduced or normal	**FVC – significantly reduced**
$FEV_1\%$ (FEV_1/FVC) – reduced	**$FEV_1\%$ (FEV_1/FVC) – normal or increased**
Asthma	Pulmonary fibrosis
COPD	Asbestosis
Bronchectasis	Sarcoidosis
'Bronchiolitis obliterans'	Acute respiratory distress syndrome
	Infant respiratory distress syndrome
	Kyphoscoliosis
	Neuromuscular disorders

A normal flow volume loop is often described as a 'triangle on top of a semicircle'. Flow volume loops are the most suitable way of assessing compression of the upper airway.

Monitoring progression of COPD

The severity of COPD is categorised using the FEV_1, e.g:

◆ severity FEV_1 (of predicted)

◆ mild 50%–80%

◆ moderate 30%–49%

◆ severe <30%

Measuring peak expiratory flow is of limited value in COPD, as it may underestimate the degree of airflow obstruction.

The following investigations are recommended in patients with suspected COPD:

◆ spirometry to demonstrate airflow obstruction – forced expiratory volume in 1 second (FEV_1) less than 80% of the predicted value and FEV_1/FVC

◆ ratio less than 70%

◆ chest X-ray – hyperinflation, bullae, flat hemidiaphragm

◆ exclusion of lung cancer

◆ full blood count – exclude secondary polycythaemia

E. Specific management problems

1. Smoking cessation

Smoking cessation is critical in the management of many lung conditions, including COPD and lung cancer.

A common scenario is when a smoker has failed to give up smoking, despite nicotine patches. Varenicline (Champix®) is an oral anti-smoking agent with dual action, reducing the craving for cigarettes and also making the smoking of cigarettes less pleasurable. Action on Smoking and Health (ASH) have guidance on its use. It appears to be effective and safe, with the main side effect being nausea. Varenicline appears to be more effective in clinical trials than either bupropion or placebo and is prescribed for 12 weeks in the first instance, with a further 12-week course if craving still persists.

2. Indications for lung transplantation

Lung transplant recipients have a wide variety of underlying disorders.

Lung transplantation in the adult can be categorised into four groups based on aetiology:

◆ non-bronchiectatic obstructive

◆ bronchiectatic

◆ interstitial, and

◆ pulmonary vascular

Non-bronchiectatic obstructive diseases usually are not associated with an infectious process, while bronchiectatic diseases result in an abnormal dilatation and distortion of the bronchi and bronchioles due to recurrent inflammation. Interstitial diseases comprise a group of diffuse inflammatory diseases affecting the lower airways.

Pulmonary vascular diseases typically result in severely increased pulmonary vascular resistance, which leads to hypoxia and right-side heart failure. The majority of lung transplantations are performed for one of four diseases: chronic obstructive pulmonary disease (COPD), idiopathic pulmonary fibrosis (IPF), pulmonary hypertension and cystic fibrosis. Currently, the most common indication is COPD.

3. Guidelines on non-invasive ventilation (NIV)

You should have an understanding of the BTS guidelines on the use of non-invasive ventilation in acute respiratory failure.

Key indicators

◆ COPD with respiratory acidosis pH <7. 30

◆ type II respiratory failure secondary to chest wall deformity, neuromuscular disease or obstructive sleep apnoea

◆ cardiogenic pulmonary oedema unresponsive to CPAP

◆ weaning from tracheal intubation

Recommended initial settings for bi-level pressure support in COPD are as follows:

◆ expiratory positive airway pressure (EPAP): 5 cm H_2O

◈ inspiratory positive airway pressure (IPAP) – RCP advocate 10 cm H_2O whilst BTS suggest 12–15 cm H_2O

◈ back-up rate – 15 breaths/minute

◈ back-up inspiration : expiration ratio – 1 : 3

References

British Thoracic Society Standards of Care Committee, Pulmonary Embolism Guideline Development Group. British Thoracic Society guidelines for the management of suspected acute pulmonary embolism. *Thorax.* 2003; **58**(6): 470–83.

British Thoracic Society, Scottish Intercollegiate Guidelines Network. British guideline on the management of asthma. *Thorax.* 2008; **63**(Suppl. 4): iv1–121.

Davies AC, Alton EW, Bush A. Cystic fibrosis. *BMJ.* 2007; **335**: 1255–9.

Kaye P, O'Sullivan I. BTS asthma guide. *Thorax.* 2001; **56**(8): 666.

MacDuff A, Arnold A, Harvey J; BTS Pleural Disease Guideline Group. Management of spontaneous pneumothorax: British Thoracic Society pleural disease guideline 2010. *Thorax.* 2010; **65**(Suppl. 2): ii18–31.

Maskell NA, Butland RJ; Pleural Diseases Group, Standards of Care Committee, British Thoracic Society. BTS guidelines for the investigation of a unilateral pleural effusion in adults. *Thorax.* 2003; **58** (Suppl. 2): ii8–17.

Chapter 13

Musculoskeletal disorders (and rheumatology)

The Foundation Programme and MRCP(UK) Part 1 syllabus (from the JRCPMTB) specify what is required in terms of competencies, skills and knowledge from junior physicians in core medical training in musculoskeletal disorders/rheumatology. You are advised to consult carefully this syllabus, which emphasises the importance of basic medical sciences as well as a competent level of applied clinical practice.

A. Epidemiology in rheumatology

1. Rheumatoid arthritis

Features

+ peak onset = 30–50 years, although occurs in all age groups
+ F : M ratio = 3 : 1
+ prevalence = 1%
+ some ethnic differences, e.g. high in Native Americans
+ associated with HLA-DR4 (especially Felty's syndrome)

2. Systemic lupus erythematosus

+ much more common in females (F : M = 9 : 1)
+ more common in African–Caribbean and Asian communities
+ onset is usually 20–40 years
+ incidence has risen substantially during the past 50 years (threefold using American College of Rheumatology criteria)

3. Reactive arthritis

- post-sexually transmitted disease reactive arthritis is much more common in men (e.g. 10 : 1)
- the post-dysenteric form is roughly equal in sex incidence

4. Behçet's disease

- more common in the eastern Mediterranean (e.g. Turkey)
- more common in men (complicated gender distribution which varies according to country; overall, Behçet's disease is considered to be more common and more severe in men)
- tends to affect young adults (e.g. 20–40 years old)
- associated with HLA B5 and MICA6 allele
- ca. 30% of patients have a positive family history

B. Common rheumatological diseases

You should be able to answer questions on the symptoms and signs of the rheumatic diseases.

1. Rheumatoid arthritis and associated syndromes

ACR criteria

It would not be unreasonable for the examiners to ask you about the official American College of Rheumatology criteria.

Requires four of the following seven criteria (sensitivity = 92%, specificity = 89%):

- morning stiffness >1 hour (for at least 6 weeks)
- soft-tissue swelling of three or more joints (for at least 6 weeks)
- swelling of PIP, MCP or wrist joints (for at least 6 weeks)
- symmetrical arthritis (for at least 6 weeks)
- subcutaneous nodules
- rheumatoid factor positive
- radiographic evidence of erosions or periarticular osteopenia

Prognostic features

A number of features have been shown to predict a poor prognosis in patients with rheumatoid arthritis, as listed below.

- rheumatoid factor positive
- poor functional status at presentation
- HLA DR4
- X-ray: early erosions (e.g. after <2 years)
- extra articular features e.g. nodules
- insidious onset
- anti-CCP antibodies

In terms of gender there seems to be a split in what the established sources state is associated with a poor prognosis. However, both the American College of Rheumatology and the recent NICE guidelines (which looked at a huge number of prognosis studies) seem to conclude that female gender is associated with a poor prognosis.

 You should attempt to find the Quick Reference Guide for the management of rheumatoid arthritis from NICE (CG79). The full guidelines include the criteria for referral for specialist treatment and the role of disease-modifying and biological drugs.

DMARDS

- Guidance recommends the use of disease-modifying anti-rheumatic drugs (DMARDs) early in the treatment of rheumatoid arthritis, maintaining function and reducing progression of the disease (SIGN Guideline 123, 2011). First-line agents include methotrexate and sulphasalazine, and most subjects receive methotrexate.
- Generally gold is considered more toxic than the former two and hydroxychloroquine is probably less effective.
- Cyclosporin is again rather more toxic than either methotrexate or sulphasalazine, with nephrotoxicity and immunosuppression, and is generally reserved for RhA with systemic features such as vasculitis.
- The tumour necrosis factor alpha (TNFα) antagonists, etanercept and infliximab, are generally reserved for individuals unresponsive to traditional DMARDS.

2. Still's disease in adults

Features

◈ typically affects 16- to 35-year-olds

◈ arthralgia

◈ elevated serum ferritin

◈ rash: salmon pink, maculopapular

◈ pyrexia

◈ lymphadenopathy

◈ rheumatoid factor (RF) and anti-nuclear antibody (ANA) negative

3. Cryoglobulinaemia

Cryoglobulins are immunoglobulins which undergo reversible precipitation at 4°C, dissolve when warmed to 37°. One-third of cases are idiopathic.

Three types

◈ type I (25%): monoclonal

◈ type II (25%): mixed monoclonal and polyclonal – usually with rheumatoid factor (RF)

◈ type III (50%): polyclonal – usually with RF

Type I

◈ monoclonal: IgG or IgM

◈ associations: multiple myeloma, Waldenström's macroglobulinaemia

Type II

◈ mixed monoclonal and polyclonal: usually with RF

◈ associations: hepatitis C, rheumatoid arthritis, Sjögren's, lymphoma

Type III

◈ polyclonal: usually with rheumatoid factor

◈ associations: rheumatoid arthritis, Sjögren's

◈ symptoms (if present in high concentrations):

  ● Raynaud's only seen in type I

  ● cutaneous: vascular purpura, distal ulceration, ulceration

- arthralgia
- renal involvement (diffuse glomerulonephritis)

Targeted investigations

- low complement (especially C4)
- high ESR

Treatment

- immunosuppression
- plasmapheresis

4. Introduction to seronegative spondyloarthritis

Common features

- associated with HLA-B27
- rheumatoid factor negative – hence 'seronegative'
- peripheral arthritis, usually asymmetrical
- sacroilitis
- enthesopathy: e.g. achilles tendonitis, plantar fasciitis
- extra-articular manifestations: uveitis, pulmonary fibrosis (upper zone), amyloidosis, aortic regurgitation

Examples

- ankylosing spondylitis
- psoriatic arthritis
- Reiter's syndrome (including reactive arthritis)
- enteropathic arthritis (associated with inflammatory bowel disease)

5. Ankylosing spondylitis
Features

+ typically a young man who presents with lower back pain and stiffness
+ stiffness is usually worse in morning and improves with activity
+ peripheral arthritis (25%, more common if female)

Other features - the 'A's

+ Apical fibrosis
+ Anterior uveitis
+ Aortic regurgitation
+ Achilles tendonitis
+ AV node block
+ Amyloidosis
+ *And* cauda equina syndrome (!)

Radiology

X-rays are often normal early in disease; later changes include:

+ sacroilitis – subchondral erosions, sclerosis
+ squaring of lumbar vertebrae
+ 'bamboo spine' (*late and uncommon*)

Chest X-ray: apical fibrosis

Spirometry may show a restrictive defect due to a combination of pulmonary fibrosis, kyphosis and ankylosis of the costovertebral joints.

6. Psoriatic arthropathy

Psoriatic arthropathy correlates poorly with cutaneous psoriasis and often precedes the development of skin lesions. Around 10% of patients with skin lesions develop an arthropathy, with males and females being equally affected.

Types

+ rheumatoid-like polyarthritis (30%–40%, most common type)
+ asymmetrical oligoarthritis: typically affects hands and feet (20%–30%)
+ sacroilitis
+ DIP joint disease (10%)

◈ arthritis mutilans (severe deformity of fingers/hand, 'telescoping fingers')

In about 20% of patients there is a chronic, progressive and deforming arthropathy with an asymmetrical pattern, including distal interphalangeal joint involvement.

Management
◈ treat as rheumatoid arthritis
◈ has better prognosis

7. Reactive arthritis
Reactive arthritis is one of the HLA-B27 associated seronegative spondyloarthropathies. It encompasses Reiter's syndrome, a term which described a classic triad of urethritis, conjunctivitis and arthritis following a dysenteric illness during the Second World War. Later studies identified patients who developed symptoms following a sexually transmitted infection (post-STI, now sometimes referred to as sexually acquired reactive arthritis, SARA).

Organisms often responsible for post-dysenteric form
◈ *Shigella flexneri*
◈ *Salmonella typhimurium*
◈ *Salmonella enteritidis*
◈ *Yersinia enterocolitica*
◈ *Campylobacter*

[The organism often responsible for post-STI form is *Chlamydia trachomatis*.]

8. Behçet's syndrome

Behçet's syndrome is a complex multisystem disorder associated with presumed autoimmune mediated inflammation of the arteries and veins. The precise aetiology has yet to be elucidated however. The classic triad of symptoms is oral ulcers, genital ulcers and anterior uveitis.

Features

+ *classically*: (1) oral ulcers (2) genital ulcers (3) anterior uveitis
+ thrombophlebitis
+ arthritis
+ neurological involvement (e.g. aseptic meningitis)
+ gastro-intestinal symptoms: abdominal pain, diarrhoea, colitis
+ erythema nodosum, DVT

Diagnosis

+ no definitive test
+ diagnosis based on clinical findings
+ positive pathergy test is suggestive (puncture site following needle prick becomes inflamed with small pustule forming)

C. Vasculitis

1. Polyarteritis nodosa

Polyarteritis nodosa (PAN) is a vasculitis affecting medium-sized arteries with necrotising inflammation leading to aneurysm formation. PAN is more common in middle-aged men and is associated with hepatitis B infection.

Features

+ fever, malaise, arthralgia
+ hypertension
+ mononeuritis multiplex, sensorimotor polyneuropathy
+ haematuria, renal failure
+ testicular pain
+ abdominal pain (e.g. from mesenteric ischaemia)

◆ perinuclear-antineutrophil cytoplasmic antibodies (ANCA) are found in around 20% of patients with 'classic' PAN

2. Wegener's granulomatosis

Wegener's granulomatosis is an autoimmune condition associated with a necrotising granulomatous vasculitis, affecting both the upper and lower respiratory tract as well as the kidneys.

Features

◆ upper respiratory tract: epistaxis, sinusitis, nasal crusting

◆ lower respiratory tract: dyspnoea, haemoptysis

◆ glomerulonephritis ('pauci-immune', 80% of patients)

◆ saddle-shape nose deformity

◆ also: vasculitic rash, eye involvement (e.g. proptosis), cranial nerve lesions

Investigations

◆ cANCA positive in >90%, pANCA positive in 25%

◆ chest X-ray: wide variety of presentations, including cavitating lesions

◆ renal biopsy: crescenteric glomerulonephritis

Management

◆ steroids

◆ cyclophosphamide (90% response)

◆ plasma exchange

◆ median survival = 8–9 years

3. Churg-Strauss syndrome

Churg-Strauss syndrome is an ANCA-associated small–medium vessel vasculitis.

Features

✦ asthma

✦ blood eosinophilia (e.g. >10%)

✦ paranasal sinusitis

✦ mononeuritis multiplex

✦ pANCA positive in 60%

Leukotriene receptor antagonists may precipitate the disease.

4. Osteoarthritis

Management

The NICE guidelines emphasise the holistic nature of care for patients with osteoarthritis. The NICE guidelines argue that treatment and care should take into account patients' individual needs and preferences. Good communication is essential, supported by evidence-based information, to allow patients to reach informed decisions about their care.

NICE published guidelines on the management of osteoarthritis (OA) in 2008:

✦ All patients should be offered help with weight loss, given advice about local muscle strengthening exercises and general aerobic fitness.

✦ Paracetamol and topical NSAIDs are first-line analgesics. Topical NSAIDs are indicated only for OA of the knee or hand.

✦ Second-line treatment is oral NSAIDs/COX-2 inhibitors, opioids, capsaicin cream and intra-articular corticosteroids. A proton pump inhibitor should be co-prescribed with either drug. These drugs should be avoided if the patient takes aspirin.

✦ Possibly, topical capsaicin for hand or knee osteoarthritis.

✦ Non-pharmacological treatment options include supports and braces, TENS and shock-absorbing insoles or shoes, application of cold to the pain, manipulation and stretching.

✦ If conservative methods fail, then refer for consideration of joint replacement.

The principal goal of systemic therapy is to provide the most effective pain relief with the least associated toxicity. Paracetamol is the initial therapy recommended for the treatment of OA of the hip and knee. Studies have shown that the short-term and long-term efficacy of paracetamol is comparable with that of ibuprofen and naproxen in people with knee osteoarthritis.

Specific COX-2 inhibitors such as celecoxib have clinical benefit similar to that of traditional non-steroidal anti-inflammatory drugs (NSAIDs), but less gastro-intestinal (GI) toxicity, although issues remain regarding their cardiovascular risk. They may be used in patients with GI intolerance of traditional NSAIDs.

Glucosamine

This is a normal constituent of glycosaminoglycans in cartilage and synovial fluid.

A systematic review of several double-blind RCTs of glucosamine in knee osteoarthritis reported significant short-term symptomatic benefits, including significantly reduced joint space narrowing and improved pain scores, however more recent studies have been mixed.

Glucosamine is **not** recommended in the 2008 NICE Guidelines, however.

D. Crystal arthritis (gout, pyrophosphate arthritis)

1. Gout

Gout is a form of microcrystal synovitis caused by the deposition of monosodium urate monohydrate in the synovium. It is caused by chronic hyperuricaemia (uric acid >0.45 mmol/L).

Causes of decreased excretion of uric acid

- drugs: diuretics
- chronic kidney disease
- lead toxicity

Causes of increased production of uric acid

- myeloproliferative/lymphoproliferative disorder
- cytotoxic drugs
- severe psoriasis

Lesch-Nyhan syndrome

◆ hypoxanthine-guanine phosphoribosyl transferase deficiency

◆ inheritance = X-linked recessive

◆ features: gout, renal failure, learning difficulties, head banging

Drug causes

◆ thiazides, furosemide

◆ alcohol

◆ cytotoxic agents

◆ pyrazinamide

Diagnosis

Synovial fluid analysis can confirm the diagnosis by identifying needle-shaped, strongly negatively birefringent urate crystals that are free in the fluid or engulfed by phagocytes.

An elevated serum urate level supports the diagnosis of gout but is neither specific nor sensitive. At least 30% of patients have normal serum urate at the time of an acute attack.

Management

Gout is a form of microcrystal synovitis caused by the deposition of monosodium urate monohydrate in the synovium. It is caused by chronic hyperuricaemia (uric acid >450 μmol/L).

Acute management

◆ NSAIDs

◆ intra-articular steroid injection

◆ colchicine has a slower onset of action; the main side-effect is diarrhoea

◆ if the patient is already taking allopurinol it should be continued

◆ allopurinol prophylaxis (see indications below) – allopurinol should not be started until 2 weeks after an acute attack has settled

◆ initial dose of 100 mg od, with the dose titrated every few weeks to aim for a serum uric acid of <300 μmol/L

◆ NSAIDs or colchicine cover should be used when starting allopurinol

Indications for allopurinol

◆ recurrent attacks – the British Society for Rheumatology recommend 'In uncomplicated gout uric acid lowering drug therapy should be started if a second attack or further attacks occur within 1 year'

◆ tophi

◆ renal disease

◆ uric acid renal stones

◆ prophylaxis if on cytotoxics or diuretics

Lifestyle modifications

◆ reduce alcohol intake and avoid during an acute attack

◆ lose weight if obese

◆ avoid food high in purines, e.g. liver, kidneys, seafood, oily fish (mackerel, sardines) and yeast products

2. Pseudogout

Pseudogout is a form of microcrystal synovitis caused by the deposition of calcium pyrophosphate dihydrate in the synovium.

Features

◆ knee, wrist and shoulders most commonly affected

◆ X-ray: chondrocalcinosis

Risk factors

◆ hyperparathyroidism

◆ hypothyroidism

◆ haemochromatosis

◆ acromegaly

◆ low magnesium, low phosphate

◆ Wilson's disease

Management

◆ aspiration of joint fluid, to exclude septic arthritis and show weakly positively birefringent brick-shaped crystals

◆ NSAIDs or intra-articular, intra-muscular or oral steroids as for gout

3. Discoid lupus erythematous

Discoid lupus erythematous is a benign disorder generally seen in younger females. It very rarely progresses to systemic lupus erythematosus (in less than 5% of cases). Discoid lupus erythematous is characterised by follicular keratin plugs and is thought to be autoimmune in aetiology.

Features

◆ erythematous, raised rash, sometimes scaly

◆ may be photosensitive

◆ more common on face, neck, ears and scalp

◆ lesions heal with atrophy, scarring (may cause scarring alopecia), and pigmentation

Management

◆ topical steroid cream

◆ oral antimalarials may be used second-line, e.g. hydroxychloroquine

◆ avoid sun exposure

4. Sjögren's syndrome

Sjögren's syndrome is an autoimmune disorder affecting exocrine glands resulting in dry mucosal surfaces. It may be primary (PSS) or secondary to rheumatoid arthritis or other connective tissue disorders, where it usually develops around 10 years after the initial onset. Sjögren's syndrome is much more common in females (ratio 9 : 1). There is a marked increased risk of lymphoid malignancy (40- to 60-fold).

Features

◆ dry eyes (keratoconjunctivitis sicca)

◆ dry mouth

◆ vaginal dryness

◆ arthralgia

◆ Raynaud's, myalgia

◆ sensory polyneuropathy

◆ renal tubular acidosis (usually subclinical)

Investigation

- rheumatoid factor (RF) positive in nearly 100% of patients
- ANA positive in 70%
- anti-Ro (SSA) antibodies in 70% of patients with PSS
- anti-La (SSB) antibodies in 30% of patients with PSS
- Schirmer's test: filter paper near conjunctival sac to measure tear formation
- histology: focal lymphocytic infiltration
- also: hypergammaglobulinaemia, low C4

Management

- artificial saliva and tears
- pilocarpine may stimulate saliva production

5. Systemic sclerosis

Systemic sclerosis is a condition of unknown aetiology characterised by hardened, sclerotic skin and other connective tissues. It is four times more common in females.

Three main patterns of disease
Limited cutaneous systemic sclerosis

- Raynaud's may be first sign
- scleroderma affects face and distal limbs predominately
- associated with anti-centromere antibodies
- a subtype of limited systemic sclerosis is CREST syndrome: Calcinosis, Raynaud's phenomenon, oEsophageal dysmotility, Sclerodactyly, Telangiectasia

Diffuse cutaneous systemic sclerosis

- scleroderma affects trunk and proximal limbs predominately
- associated with anti-scl-70 antibodies
- hypertension, lung fibrosis and renal involvement seen
- poor prognosis

Scleroderma (without internal organ involvement)

- tightening and fibrosis of skin

◆ may be manifest as plaques (*morphoea*) or linear

Antibodies

◆ ANA positive in 90%

◆ RF positive in 30%

◆ anti-scl-70 antibodies associated with diffuse cutaneous systemic sclerosis

◆ anti-centromere antibodies associated with limited cutaneous systemic sclerosis

---

BOX 13.1   A note on 'scleroderma renal crisis'

A major complication is the development of **scleroderma renal crisis**. This is characterised by the abrupt onset of severe hypertension, usually with retinopathy, together with rapid deterioration of renal function and heart failure. It develops in 8%–15% of patients with diffuse systemic sclerosis especially associated with rapid progression of diffuse skin disease. It usually presents early, within 3 years of diagnosis. The pathogenic mechanisms leading to renal damage are not known.

The clinical presentation is typically with the symptoms of malignant hypertension, i.e. headaches, blurred vision, fits and/or heart failure.

Renal function is impaired and usually rapidly deteriorates. The hypertension is almost always severe with a diastolic BP over 100 mmHg in 90% of patients. There is hypertensive retinopathy in about 85% of patients with exudates and haemorrhages, and if severe, papilloedema.

Scleroderma renal crisis is a medical emergency. The hypertension should be treated with an ACE inhibitor. The aim is to reduce the blood pressure gradually as an abrupt fall can lead to cerebral ischaemia or infarctions (as in any accelerated hypertension). Calcium channel blockers may be added to ACE inhibitors.

Deterioration in renal function can be rapid, with gross pulmonary oedema, therefore patients with scleroderma renal crisis should be managed in hospitals with facilities for dialysis.

---

6. Dermatomyositis

Overview

+ inflammatory disorder causing symmetrical, proximal muscle weakness and characteristic skin lesions

+ may be idiopathic or associated with connective tissue disorders or underlying paraneoplastic/underlying malignancy (found in 20%–25% – more if patient older)

+ polymyositis is a variant of the disease where skin manifestations are not prominent

Skin features

+ photosensitive

+ macular rash over back and shoulder

+ *'heliotrope'* rash over cheek

+ Gottron's papules – roughened red papules over extensor surfaces of fingers

+ nail fold capillary dilatation

Other features

+ proximal muscle weakness +/− tenderness

+ Raynaud's

+ respiratory muscle weakness

+ interstitial lung disease: e.g. fibrosing alveolitis or organising pneumonia

+ dysphagia, dysphonia

Investigations and management

+ elevated creatine kinase

+ EMG

+ muscle biopsy

+ anti-Jo-1 antibodies are not commonly seen in dermatomyositis – they are more common in polymyositis, where they are seen in a pattern of disease associated with lung involvement, Raynaud's and fever

+ ANA positive in 60%

Management

+ prednisolone

7. Polymyalgia rheumatica

◆ overlaps with temporal arteritis

◆ histology shows vasculitis with giant cells, characteristically 'skips' certain sections of affected artery whilst damaging others

◆ muscle bed arteries affected most in polymyalgia rheumatica

Features

◆ typically patient >60 years old

◆ usually rapid onset (e.g. <1 month)

◆ aching, morning stiffness in proximal limb muscles (not weakness)

◆ also mild polyarthralgia, lethargy, depression, low-grade fever, anorexia, night sweats

Investigations

◆ ESR >40 mm/hour

◆ note CK and EMG normal

◆ reduced CD8+ T cells

Treatment

◆ prednisolone, e.g. 15 mg/od – dramatic response (can be a medical emergency in temporal arteritis, where this condition can cause blindness)

8. Osteoporosis

Risk factors

◆ family history

◆ female sex

◆ increasing age

◆ deficient diet

◆ sedentary lifestyle

◆ smoking

◆ premature menopause

◆ low body weight

◆ Asian and Oriental ethnicity

Diseases which predispose to osteoporosis

◈ endocrine: glucocorticoid excess (e.g. Cushing's, steroid therapy), hyperthyroidism, hypogonadism (e.g. Turner's, testosterone deficiency), growth hormone deficiency, hyperparathyroidism, diabetes mellitus

◈ multiple myeloma, lymphoma

◈ GI problems: malabsorption (e.g. coeliac disease), gastrectomy, liver disease

◈ rheumatoid arthritis

◈ long-term heparin therapy

◈ chronic renal failure

◈ osteogenesis imperfecta, homocystinuria

Secondary prevention

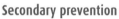

NICE guidelines were updated in 2008 on the secondary prevention of osteoporotic fractures in postmenopausal women.

Management

◈ Treatment is indicated following osteoporotic fragility fractures in postmenopausal women who are confirmed to have osteoporosis (a T-score of −2.5 SD or below). In women aged 75 years or older, a DEXA scan may not be required 'if the responsible clinician considers it to be clinically inappropriate or unfeasible'.

◈ Vitamin D and calcium supplementation should be offered to all women unless the clinician is confident they have adequate calcium intake and are vitamin D replete.

◈ Alendronate is first-line.

◈ Around 25% of patients cannot tolerate alendronate, usually due to upper gastrointestinal problems. These patients should be offered risedronate or etidronate (see treatment criteria below).

◈ Strontium ranelate and raloxifene are recommended if patients cannot tolerate bisphosphonates (see treatment criteria below).

Unfortunately, a number of complicated treatment cut-off tables have been produced in the latest guidelines for patients who do not tolerate alendronate.

Risk factors (for use in the tables below)

◈ parental history of hip fracture

◆ alcohol intake of four or more units

◆ rheumatoid arthritis

TABLE 13.1 T-scores (SD) at (or below) which risedronate or etidronate is recommended when alendronate cannot be taken

Age (years)	No risk factors	1 risk factor	2 risk factors
50–54	Not indicated	–3.0	–2.5
55–59	–3.0	–3.0	–2.5
60–64	–3.0	–3.0	–2.5
65–69	–3.0	–2.5	–2.5
70 or older	–2.5	–2.5	–2.5

TABLE 13.2 T-scores (SD) at (or below) which strontium ranelate or raloxifene is recommended when alendronate and either risedronate or etidronate cannot be taken

Age (years)	No risk factors	1 risk factor	2 risk factors
50–54	Not indicated	–3.5	–3.5
55–59	–4.0	–3.5	–3.5
60–64	–4.0	–3.5	–3.5
65–69	–4.0	–3.5	–3.0
70–74	–3.0	–3.0	–2.5
75 or older	–3.0	–2.5	–2.5

Additional notes on treatment
Bisphosphonates

◆ Alendronate, risedronate and etidronate are all licensed for the prevention and treatment of post-menopausal and glucocorticoid-induced osteoporosis.

◆ All three have been shown to reduce the risk of both vertebral and non-vertebral fractures although alendronate and risedronate may be superior to etidronate in preventing hip fractures.

◆ Ibandronate is a once-monthly oral bisphosphonate.

Vitamin D and calcium

◆ poor evidence base to suggest reduced fracture rates in the general population at risk of osteoporotic fractures – may reduce rates in frail, housebound patients

- raloxifene – this is a selective oestrogen receptor modulator (SERM)
- has been shown to prevent bone loss and to reduce the risk of vertebral fractures, but has not yet been shown to reduce the risk of non-vertebral fractures
- has been shown to increase bone density in the spine and proximal femur
- may worsen menopausal symptoms
- increased risk of thromboembolic events
- may decrease risk of breast cancer

Strontium ranelate

- *'dual action bone agent'* – increases deposition of new bone by osteoblasts and reduces the resorption of bone by osteoclasts
- strong evidence base, may be second-line treatment in near future
- increased risk of thromboembolic events

Teriparatide

- recombinant form of parathyroid hormone
- very effective at increasing bone mineral density but role in the management of osteoporosis yet to be clearly defined

Hormone replacement therapy

This has been shown to reduce the incidence of vertebral fracture and non-vertebral fractures due to concerns about increased rates of cardiovascular disease and breast cancer. It is no longer recommended for primary or secondary prevention of osteoporosis unless the woman is suffering from vasomotor symptoms.

Other measures

- hip protectors
  - some evidence to suggest significantly reduce hip fractures in nursing home patients
  - compliance is a problem
  - falls risk assessment
    - no evidence to suggest reduced fracture rates
    - however, some evidence that they do, however, reduce rate of falls and should be considered in management of high-risk patients

9. Paget's disease of bone

Paget's disease of bone is a disease of increased but uncontrolled bone turnover. It is thought to be primarily a disorder of osteoclasts, with excessive osteoclastic resorption followed by increased osteoblastic activity. Paget's disease is common (UK prevalence 5%) but symptomatic in only one in 20 patients.

Predisposing factors

- increasing age
- male sex
- northern latitude
- family history

Clinical features

NB only 5% of patients are symptomatic

- bone pain (e.g. pelvis, lumbar spine, femur)
- classical, untreated features: bowing of tibia, bossing of skull
- raised alkaline phosphatase (ALP) – calcium and phosphate are typically normal
- skull X-ray: thickened vault, *osteoporosis circumscripta*

Indications for treatment

- include bone pain, skull or long-bone deformity, fracture, periarticular Paget's
- bisphosphonate (either oral risedronate or IV zoledronate)
- calcitonin is less commonly used now

Complications

- deafness (cranial nerve entrapment)
- bone sarcoma (1% if affected for >10 years)
- fractures
- skull thickening
- high-output cardiac failure

10. Chronic fatigue syndrome

The diagnosis and management of chronic fatigue syndrome, or myalgic encephalitis, has recently been reviewed by NICE (2007).

The main features which need to be present to confirm a diagnosis are fatigue that:

+ is new in onset, persistent or recurrent and unexplained by other conditions
+ is characterised by post-exertional malaise
+ results in a substantial reduction in activity level

Associated symptoms include:

+ hypersomnia or insomnia
+ muscle or joint pain without inflammation and
+ painful lymph nodes without lymphadenopathy
+ headaches
+ cognitive dysfunction

'Red flag' symptoms which suggest another diagnosis include:

+ significant weight loss
+ inflammatory arthropathy or connective tissue disease
+ localising or focal neurological signs

11. Systemic lupus erythematosus (SLE)

Systemic lupus erythematosus (SLE) is a multi-system autoimmune connective tissue disorder with various clinical presentations.

Clinical presentation

The widely recognised presentation of a young woman with inflammatory arthritis and a butterfly facial rash is uncommon.

Non-specific symptoms of fatigue, malaise, oral ulcers, arthralgia, photosensitive skin rashes, lymphadenopathy, pleuritic chest pains, headache, paraesthesiae, symptoms of dry eyes and mouth, Raynaud's phenomenon and mild hair loss are more likely presentations.

It is not surprising, therefore, that there is often considerable delay before the diagnosis is considered in patients with low-grade disease.

Patients may present acutely with major organ dysfunction that can affect virtually any organ, and diagnosis hinges on careful and thorough clinical evaluation and recognition of multi-system involvement. Renal involvement (lupus nephritis) presents insidiously, and if it is not detected early, the risk of progression to renal impairment is high.

Diagnosis

The key to early diagnosis is clinical evaluation, which should include a complete systems review and examination and investigations guided by the extent of organ involvement. In primary care, a diagnosis of lupus or a related disorder is often apparent after clinical assessment, and the following:
1. urinalysis for blood and protein
2. basic investigations such as full blood count (often showing anaemia or cytopaenia), renal and liver function, ESR and CRP

(Note also that a high erythrocyte sedimentation rate (ESR) with a normal C-reactive protein (CRP) concentration are characteristic.)

A search for autoantibodies to nuclear antigens (antinuclear and antiDNA antibodies) and rheumatoid factor are the usual starting points while considering referral to specialist care. Antiphospholipid antibodies (anticardiolipin antibodies and the lupus anticoagulant) should be considered in women with previous morbidity in pregnancy or thrombotic events. In secondary care, more extensive testing is usually considered, including detailed assessment of organ dysfunction and further autoantibody testing, including complement levels and antibodies to the extractable nuclear antigens (ENA), such as Ro (SS-A), La (SS-B), ribonucleoprotein (RNP) and Sm.

Principles of management

Most stable patients can be managed jointly between primary and secondary care. Primary care can contribute to monitoring patients with regular urinalysis, measurement of blood pressure, and renal, lipid and glucose profiles, especially in patients on corticosteroids. Blood monitoring of immunosuppressive agents can also be undertaken jointly with shared care protocols. Early identification of disease flares is important, and secondary care facilities should be rapidly accessible for these patients.

Cutaneous lupus

Patients with isolated cutaneous lupus, including discoid lupus, are unlikely to progress to systemic disease and often respond to topical therapies. Weak topical steroid preparations in combination with hydroxychloroquine are often useful.

More recently, topical preparations of tacrolimus and pimecrolimus have shown benefit in small open case series.

Though non-steroidal anti-inflammatory agents (NSAIDs) are widely prescribed for lupus patients with arthralgia, simple analgesics should be used. In particular the COX-2 selective agents are contraindicated because of the potential cardiovascular risks, and even conventional NSAIDs are not without gastrointestinal, renal and cardiovascular risks. Hydroxychloroquine remains the mainstay for patients with mild SLE, especially for those with arthralgia, skin rashes, alopecia, and oral or genital ulceration. It should be considered in all patients as it is well tolerated and is disease modifying as well as having other useful properties including a weak antithrombotic action.

Lupus nephritis
[*See* Chapter 11.]

Neuropsychiatry
Neuropsychiatric manifestations attributable to antiphospholipid syndrome include strokes, seizures, movement disorders, transverse myelopathy, demyelination syndromes, transient ischaemic attacks, cognitive dysfunction, visual loss and headaches including migraine. The treatment of CNS lupus varies according to the particular clinical syndrome – for example, organic brain syndromes and psychosis are managed by multidisciplinary teams with corticosteroids, immunosuppression and antipsychotic medication.

E. Immunological tests in rheumatology
1. Investigations in rheumatological diseases
You should have knowledge of the investigations relevant to the diagnosis and assessment of rheumatic diseases.

Systemic lupus erythematosus
+ 99% are ANA-positive
+ 20% are rheumatoid factor-positive
+ anti-dsDNA: highly specific (>99%), but less sensitive (70%)
+ anti-Smith (anti-Sm): **most specific** (>99%), sensitivity (30%)

Monitoring active disease

+ ESR: during active disease the CRP is characteristically normal – a raised CRP may indicate underlying infection.

+ Complement levels (C3, C4) are low during active disease (formation of complexes leads to consumption of complement).

+ Anti-dsDNA titres can be used for disease monitoring (but note not present in all patients).

Neonatal lupus

The development of neonatal lupus is most closely linked to the presence of anti-Ro/SSA or anti-La/SSB antibodies, which cross the placenta and produce symptoms of neonatal lupus. These include the typical rash and degrees of heart block in the infant. It is rare, occurring in only 2% of mothers with anti-Ro/SSA or anti-La/SSB antibodies.

Immunological tests

For the exam, remember: cANCA, Wegener's granulomatosis, pANCA, Churg-Strauss syndrome + others.

cANCA

+ most common target serine proteinase 3 (PR3)

+ some correlation between cANCA levels and disease activity

+ Wegener's granulomatosis, positive in >90%

+ microscopic polyangiitis, positive in 40%

pANCA

+ most common target is myeloperoxidase (MPO)

+ cannot use level of pANCA to monitor disease activity

+ associated with immune crescentic glomerulonephritis (positive in ca. 80% of patients)

+ microscopic polyangiitis, positive in 50%–75%

+ Churg-Strauss syndrome, positive in 60%

+ Wegener's granulomatosis, positive in 25%

Other causes of positive ANCA (usually pANCA)

◆ inflammatory bowel disease (UC > Crohn's)

◆ connective tissue disorders: RA, SLE, Sjögren's

◆ autoimmune hepatitis

Extractable nuclear antigens

Specific nuclear antigens usually associated with being ANA positive.
   Examples:

◆ *anti*-Ro: Sjögren's syndrome, SLE, congenital heart block

◆ *anti*-La: Sjögren's syndrome

◆ *anti*-Jo-1: polymyositis

◆ *anti*-scl-70: diffuse cutaneous systemic sclerosis

◆ *anti*-centromere: limited cutaneous systemic sclerosis

(*Anti*-Ro antibody is associated with congenital complete heart block (CHB) accounting for the vast majority of cases of CHB.)

F. Rheumatological emergencies

1. Septic arthritis

◆ most common organism overall is *Staphylococcus aureus*

◆ in young adults who are sexually active *Neisseria gonorrhoeae* should also be considered

Investigation of choice for an acute, red, hot joint

The most relevant investigation with anyone with a red, swollen and painful joint would be joint aspiration, sending off for cultures and analysis for crystals. Differential diagnoses include gout (where serum urate may fall during acute attack), pseudogout and infection. All diagnoses would be adequately addressed by joint aspiration.

Management

◆ Synovial fluid should be obtained before starting treatment.

◆ Intravenous antibiotics which cover Gram-positive cocci are indicated. The BNF currently recommends flucloxacillin and fusidic acid together, or clindamycin if penicillin allergic.

◆ Antibiotic treatment is normally given for several weeks (BNF states 6–12 weeks).

◆ Needle aspiration should be used to decompress the joint.

◆ Surgical drainage may be needed if frequent needle aspiration is required.

2. Temporal arteritis

[*See* Chapter 8.]

3. Lower back pain

Please refer to the NICE quick reference guideline 88 on lower back pain.

Specialists now agree that there are in fact a number of warning signs, known as 'red flags', which may indicate that your back pain is actually caused by a more serious condition.

These include:

◆ a high temperature (fever) of 38°C (100.4°F) or above

◆ unexplained weight loss

◆ inflammation or swelling of the back

◆ constant back pain that does not ease after lying down or resting

◆ pain that travels to the chest, or pain that is high up in the back

◆ pain down the legs and below the knees

◆ a recent trauma or injury to the back

◆ loss of bladder control

◆ inability to pass urine

◆ loss of bowel control

◆ numbness around the genitals, buttocks or back passage areas

4. Osteomyelitis

Osteomyelitis is an acute or chronic inflammatory process of the bone and its structures secondary to infection with pyogenic organisms. Adult – *S. aureus* and occasionally *Enterobacter* or *Streptococcus* species. Direct osteomyelitis could be, for example, general (typically *S. aureus*, *Enterobacter* species and *Pseudomonas* species), due to a puncture wound through a shoe (*S. aureus* and *Pseudomonas* species) or sickle cell disease (*S. aureus* and *Salmonellae* species).

Pathology

Osteomyelitis may be localised or it may spread through the periosteum, cortex, marrow and cancellous tissue. The bacterial pathogen varies on the basis of the patient's age and the mechanism of infection. The two primary categories of acute osteomyelitis: haematogenous osteomyelitis and direct or contiguous inoculation osteomyelitis.

History

Haematogenous osteomyelitis usually presents with a slow insidious progression of symptoms. Direct osteomyelitis generally is more localised, with prominent signs and symptoms.

General symptoms of osteomyelitis include the following:

- haematogenous long-bone osteomyelitis (an abrupt onset of high fever, fatigue, irritability, malaise, restriction of movement, local oedema, erythema and tenderness)
- haematogenous vertebral osteomyelitis (insidious onset, history of an acute bacteremic episode, may be associated with contiguous vascular insufficiency, local oedema, erythema and tenderness, failure of a young child to sit up normally)
- chronic osteomyelitis (a non-healing ulcer, sinus tract drainage, chronic fatigue, malaise)

Examination findings

Findings at physical examination may include:

- fever
- oedema
- warmth
- fluctuance
- tenderness to palpation

◈ reduction in the use of the extremity

◈ failure of a young child to sit up normally

◈ sinus tract damage

Management

Osteomyelitis rarely requires emergent stabilisation or resuscitation. The primary challenge for an acute physician is to consider the appropriate diagnosis in the face of subtle signs or symptoms.

Treatment for osteomyelitis predominantly involves the following:

◈ initiation of intravenous antibiotics that penetrate bone and joint cavities

◈ referral of the patient to an orthopaedist or general surgeon

◈ possible medical infectious disease consultation

Physicians are recommended to select the appropriate antibiotics using direct culture results in samples from the infected site, whenever possible.

References

D'Cruz DP. Systemic lupus erythematosus [clinical review]. *BMJ.* 2006; **332**: 890–4.

National Institute for Health and Clinical Excellence. Chronic Fatigue Syndrome/ Myalgenic Cephalitis. NICE guideline 53. London: NIHCE; 2007. http://guidance. nice.org.uk/CG53

National Institute for Health and Clinical Excellence. Low Back Pain: Early Management of Persistent Non-specific Low Back Pain. NICE guideline 88. London: NIHCE; 2009. http://guidance.nice.org.uk/CG88

National Institute for Health and Clinical Excellence. Osteoarthritis. NICE guideline 59. London: NIHCE; 2008. http://guidance.nice.org.uk/CG59

Scottish Intercollegiate Guidelines Network (SIGN). Management of early rheumatoid arthritis: guideline number 123. Edinburgh: SIGN; February 2011. Available at www. sign.ac.uk/pdf/sign123.pdf (accessed 17 September 2011).

Index

Entries in **bold** refer to tables and figures.